THE PHARMACY TECHNICIAN

Third Edition

MARVIN M. STOOGENKE, B.S., R.Ph.

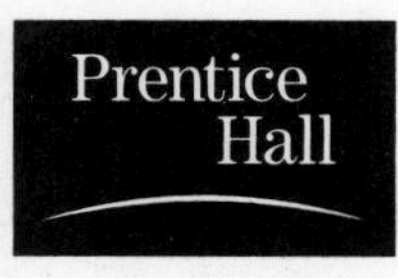

Upper Saddle River, New Jersey 07458

Library of Congress Cataloging-in-Publication Data

Stoogenke, Marvin M.
The pharmacy technician / Marvin M. Stoogenke.—3rd ed.
p.; cm.
Includes index.
ISBN 0-13-060629-4 (alk. paper)
1. Pharmacy technicians. 2. Pharmacy. I. Title.
[DNLM: 1. Pharmacy. 2. Pharmacists' Aides. QV 704 S882p 2001]
RS122.95 .S76 2001
615'.1—dc21 2001037478

Notice:

This textbook is specifically designed to present important aspects of traditional pharmacy practice required by the reader in order to perform typical pharmacy activities. The author and publisher have made a conscientious effort to assure the accuracy, completeness, and compatibility with the standards generally accepted for the information present at the time of publication. Nevertheless, as drug information becomes available as a result of research and experience, changes in the use of drugs and pharmacy practice become necessary. The reader is advised that the author and publisher cannot be responsible for any errors or omissions arising from new information or interpretations.

Publisher: Julie Levin Alexander
Acquisitions Editor: Mark Cohen
Assistant Editor: Melissa Kerian
Director of Production and Manufacturing: Bruce Johnson
Managing Production Editor: Patrick Walsh
Manufacturing Buyer: Pat Brown
Production Liason: Mary Treacy
Marketing Manager: David Hough
Production Information Manager: Rachele Triano
Creative Director: Cheryl Asherman
Cover Designer: Maria Guglielmo Walsh
Compositor: BookMasters, Inc.
Printer/Binder: Banta Harrisonburg

Pearson Education LTD.
Pearson Education Australia PTY, Limited
Pearson Education Singapore, Pte. Ltd.
Pearson Education North Asia Ltd.
Pearson Education Canada, Ltd.
Pearson Educación de Mexico, S.A. de C.V.
Pearson Education—Japan
Pearson Education Malaysia, Pte. Ltd.
Pearson Education, Upper Saddle River, New Jersey

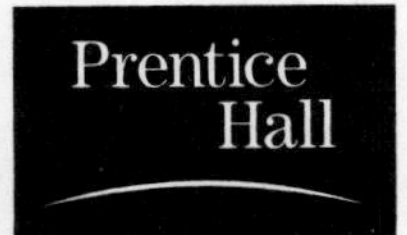

10 9 8 7 6 5 4 3
ISBN 0-13-060629-4

To Judy, my wife and confidante, who continuously holds a light to show me the way. Your inspiration, persistence, tenacity, and support are the greatest part of my motivation. Your practical approaches give reason and purpose to my undertakings.

To my sons, Scott, Jason, and Saul, who are my most gratifying works of art. Your intellectual curiosity and views of life provide me with the energy and balance I need to accomplish my pursuits. Your diverse natures prove that many different roads lead to love.

To my first grandchild, Leah Frances Stoogenke. Her birth at the time of this revision makes the book even more special. Creativity keeps the world dynamic.

Contents

Preface vii

Introduction ix

Unit 1 DISTRIBUTIVE PHARMACY 1

Chapter 1 The Drug Order 3
The Script 4
The Physician's Order 10
Common Pharmaceutical Notations 12

Chapter 2 The Drug Monographs 38
The Status of Pharmacy Practice 38
The Role of Pharmacy Technicians 38
Reviewing Drug Monographs 40
Signs, Symptoms, and Side Effects 45

Chapter 3 Terminology 56
Word Development: Usage and Components 56

Chapter 4 Pharmacy Calculations 81
Decimals 82
Percentage 86
Ratio and Proportion 92
Systems of Measure 94
The Apothecaries' System 96
The Metric System 97

Chapter 5 The Distributive Process 112
The Drug Delivery Process 113
Distribution Begins 115
Safe Medication Practices 120
Handling the Unexpected 122
Patient Monitoring 122
Information Knowledge Is Key 123

Chapter 6 Special Pharmacy Skills 125
Compounding 125
General Compounding Procedures 126
Intravenous Compounding 127
The IV Pharmacy Environment 147
"Computilization" 149
Reference Sources 151
Communication 153
Law 156

Unit 2 DRUGS 165

Chapter 7 Basics of Human Functioning and Pharmacokinetics 167
An Overview of Human Anatomy and Physiology 167

An Overview of Anatomical Systems 169
Pharmacokinetic Basics 192
Chapter 8 Common Disease States and Drug Associations 206
The Condition–Format Explanation 207
Drug–Format Explanation 208
Chapter 9 Drug Classes and Representative Drugs 227
Analgesic 228
Antidiarrheal 229
Antihistamine 229
Anti-Infective 230
Antineoplastic 232
Antiulcer 233
Cardiovascular 234
Diuretic 235
Hormone 236
Laxative 237
Psychotherapeutic 237
Hypotensive 239
Anti-Inflammatory 240
Antigout 240
Muscle Relaxant 240
Bronchodilator 241
Supplement 242
Anticonvulsant 242
Antiarthritic 243
Ophthalmic 244
Hypoglycemic 245
Antinauseant/Antiemetic 245
Blood Modifier 246
Antispasmodic 247
Antiparkinson 247
Antitissue 248
Otic 248
Dermatologic 249
Vaginal 250
Antiobesity 251
Commonly Used Pharmacotherapies 251
Chapter 10 Over-the-Counter Drugs 347

Unit 3 PHARMACY ENVIRONMENTS 353
General Overview 354
Retail Pharmacy 355
Hospital Pharmacy 357

Unit 4 PHARMACY TECHNICIAN COACH 359

Glossary 431

Appendix A The National Pharmacy Technician Certification Examination 435

Appendix B The Professional Pharmacy Technician 436

Appendix C Practice Prescriptions 437

Appendix D Practice Hospital Orders 457

Index 473

Preface

The demand for pharmacy technicians—and the number of positions—continues to grow. The demands on pharmacy technicians are increasing. With these demands, however, come many opportunities. These include specialization (intravenous preparations and compounding), mentoring, and ancillary activities (professional associations, drug ordering, and the Internet). Placement for competent pharmacy technicians has risen. Especially with the advent of the national certification examination, the impact of pharmacy technology on the marketplace has impressed pharmacy administrators in the community and institutional pharmacy environments. As the field of pharmacy technology grows, so do the opportunities. As you enter this career, you will become a vital part of this dynamic and fascinating world of the health professional.

In keeping with the dynamic movement of pharmacy practice, this revision of this textbook reflects additional needs dictated by changes in pharmacy. This textbook is dedicated to the professional development of students interested in this field. The scope of this text and its companion text, *Pharmacy Technician Review and Test Preparation*, further the commitment to providing a sound basis for technical skills and competence in providing the pharmacy services associated with pharmacy practice.

This text and its companion text fulfill the need to prepare for successful completion of national certification for pharmacy technicians. The format is user-friendly. Instead of the many chapters found in the original text, this format focuses on the distributive function of pharmacy practice, the drugs, and the pharmacy settings. Many new drugs have been added and some drugs have been deleted to keep pace and reflect the dynamic activity in pharmacy. In keeping with the movement to self-manage health care, a chapter on over-the-counter drugs has been added to prepare the pharmacy technician for a role in assisting individuals with non-prescription medication needs. *The Pharmacy Technician COACH*, the most recent addition to this textbook, introduces the reader to real excerpts of physician orders and the challenges associated with them.

Each area of study in the text supports and satisfies the needs of the *Code of Ethics for Pharmacy Technicians, the Scope of Pharmacy Practice Project*, and the *Practice Standards of ASHP* (American Society of Health-System Pharmacists). In addition, the scope of this text includes a basic knowledge to successfully complete the National Pharmacy Technician Certification Examination administered by the Pharmacy Technician Certification Board.

Acknowledgments

I want to thank Mary E. Stassi, RNC, Health Occupations Coordinator at St. Charles County Community College for her review of the manuscript for *The Pharmacy Technician.*

Introduction

Acquisition of this text is an indication of your interest in being a pharmacy technician, and of your desire to competently perform those activities associated with pharmacy technology. This text offers you the opportunity to pursue a career as a pharmacy technician by providing you with the knowledge necessary to enter the field of pharmacy technology.

Pharmacy technology deals with the practical, everyday medication needs of the patient. The changes in pharmacy practice and the role of the pharmacist require an enhanced commitment by the pharmacy technician to perform pharmacy practices safely and efficiently.

The pharmacy technician has the charge to handle the traditional distributive pharmacy practice as the requirements for pharmacists to perform clinical pharmacy functions increase. As a result of this professional movement, the role of the pharmacy technician mandates a battery of basic pharmacy skills, as well as the knowledge to perform pharmacy procedures effectively. These procedures ultimately encompass the preparation and distribution of drugs. This text discusses the components of these procedures that comprise the traditional elements of pharmacy delivery. Each skill area has been elaborated upon to provide a basic understanding of pharmacy knowledge, which can be applied in every ambulatory and institutional pharmacy setting.

As you study each unit, you will develop the foundation to practice the skills for each aspect of pharmacy. The units and their respective sections introduce the role of the pharmacy technician, pharmacy terminology, and important abbreviations. They discuss drug monographs, prescription screening, and review hospital Physician's Orders for medication. The necessary components of the prescription are examined, with particular emphasis on common errors made by prescribers. In addition to this sampling of the text material, the content deals with the requirements necessary to dispense the medication properly, including proper labeling, additional information labels for specific situations, and appropriate containers for special drugs.

Weights and measures are traditional rudiments of pharmacy. The text discusses calculating dosages, weights and measures, and conversions. Knowledge of measures must be explicit in order to perform accurately the conversions required for compounding or calculating quantities of drugs for the patient as indicated by the physician. The text reviews ratio and proportion, which is the relationship of quantities of drugs, expressed as a part of the total medication preparation. You will learn to solve problems and convert from one type of measure to another. The calculations discussion is designed to give you the needed tools and methodology that will ultimately make you comfortable with and competent in their use.

Metrology, which is the term used in pharmacy for measures, calculations, and conversions as an aggregate study, is followed by discussions dealing with drugs and pharmacy environments. The aim of the drug discussion is to provide you with an enumeration of drug groups, their intended uses, common representative drugs, and an introduction to common side effects and interactions. One objective of this text is to present solid pharmaceutical knowledge in a very basic manner, which is evidenced, for example, by the pharmacokinetics primer section. The material on pharmacy settings enlightens you to the similarities and differences to expect within each type of practice.

When you have completed your study of the basic needs to practice pharmacy, you will be ready to apply and embellish this knowledge. Each unit is structured to make the learning process friendly and is designed to guide you through an array of information that will be enhanced by your actual on-the-job activities.

Your particular accomplishment as a pharmacy technician, however, depends on your personal commitment to pharmacy and its practice. Use this text as a guide, let it serve you well, and let it help transform your ability into capability.

The publisher and I encourage you to always be inquisitive, enhance your knowledge, and put what you know into practice. Good luck with your career as a pharmacy technician.

UNIT 1

Distributive Pharmacy

CHAPTER 1

The Drug Order

OBJECTIVES

When you have completed this chapter, you will be able to:

1. describe the means used by practitioners to communicate medication needs to the pharmacy
2. list the elements that comprise a prescription
3. identify problem areas that are prone to errors
4. list the appropriate content components of a prescription label
5. interpret a prescription containing common abbreviations used in writing drug orders

The activities of the pharmacy technician begin after a patient has been seen by the physician, the physician has made a diagnosis requiring medication to remedy the ailment, a prescription order is written communicating the physician's drug of choice, and the prescription is presented in a pharmacy to be filled. If the illness is not severe enough to require hospitalization, the physician may order a medication that the patient fills at his or her local pharmacy. The nonhospitalized patient is regarded as ambulatory, as opposed to being hospitalized or an inpatient. Severe or complicated illnesses usually require a hospital stay, in which case the physician orders specific services and medications on a hospital form called the *Physician's Order.*

This chapter deals with prescriptions (often referred to as the *script*) written for ambulatory patients and Physician's Orders. These are the two primary methods used to notify the hospital pharmacy or the retail pharmacy what specific medications are needed, the quantities requested, and the directions for their use. The information contained on the orders and scripts represent the result of the physician's diagnosis, which is based on his or her training, experience, and laboratory test results.

The term *physician* or *doctor* in this text refers to any practitioner legally permitted to prescribe drugs. He or she may be a medical doctor, osteopath, dentist, podiatrist, or veterinarian. For brevity, the terms will be used interchangeably.

Realizing the training and expertise that supports the diagnosis made by a physician, the pharmacy technician must carefully exercise his or her knowledge of drugs and dispensing, assuring that no misinterpretation occurs regarding the strength, the amount to be given, or the directions for use by each patient. Figures 1.1 and 1.2 illustrate examples of a blank script and a hospital Physician's Order. The composition of medication orders indicates that a specific battery of knowledge and skills are necessary in order to prepare and dispense the patient's medications properly. You will see that a basic understanding of mathematics, a knowledge of the Latin terms relevant to pharmacy, an ability to work with mathematical conversions, and a knowledge of what should be contained on pharmacy orders are needed to perform your role as a pharmacy technician appropriately.

Practicing pharmacy competently requires that you learn and use the "tools of the trade," and understand the abbreviations and terminology used frequently by medical and medical-support personnel. The patient's well-being is your primary concern. You must never leave any question unanswered by assumption.

NEVER DISPENSE GUESSWORK

1 PAT SMITH, M.D.
2 27 Oak Leaf Lane
Baltimore, MD 12121
3 Phone: 322 -7890 Name________________ 4
Address________________
Age________ 5

7 Rx

8
9
10

[ ] Contents are labeled unless checked May be refilled 0 1 2 3 4 11

Signed________________ M.D. 12

6 Date________ 20__ DEA No.________ 13

FIGURE 1.1 The script.

Keep this phrase in mind, and make it part of your daily practice. Pharmacy should not be just "counting, pouring, licking, and sticking."

THE SCRIPT

The traditional prescription follows a definite pattern, which is intended to assure patient safety and legal compliance. Although the format has changed somewhat over the years, certain information is necessary in order to prepare the medication properly. You may not expect to find the "Rx" superscription, but you certainly will need to know the drug prescribed, its strength, and the directions for using the drug.

MAJOR ELEMENTS

Referring to the model prescription order in Figure 1.1, note the major elements contained on the ideal prescription:

1. Prescriber's name and title (MD, DDS, DMD, DO, etc.)
2. Prescriber's office address
3. Prescriber's phone number
4. Patient's name and address
5. Patient's age
6. Date on which the prescription was written
7. Superscription (The *Rx* is Latin for "Take Thou.")
8. Drug name, strength, and form (technically known as the *inscription* or body of the prescription)

PATIENT:
AGE:
SEX:
RACE:
CHART NO.

MEMORIAL HOSPITAL
BALTIMORE, MARYLAND
PHYSICIAN'S ORDER RECORD

BEAR DOWN ON HARD SURFACE WITH BALL POINT PEN

GENERIC EQUIVALENT IS AUTHORIZED UNLESS CHECKED IN THIS COLUMN

ALLERGY OR SENSITIVITY

TO__________

NONE KNOWN ☐ SIGNED:__________

DIAGNOSIS

COMPLETED OR DISCONTINUED

	DATE	TIME	ORDERS	PHYSICIAN'S SIG.		NAME	DATE	TIME

PHARMACY COPY

FIGURE 1.2 The physician's order.

9. Quantity of the drug to be dispensed (known as the *subscription)*
10. Clearly written and understandable directions (technically called the *signature*). *Note:* Although directions may be written in Latin abbreviations by the prescribers, directions to the patient must be spelled out in English. The directions should contain the amount of medication to be taken, the frequency, and the route of administration. The directions may also contain the reason for the medication (for example, for pain, for infection) if the prescriber so indicates.
11. Refill instructions
12. Prescriber's signature
13. Prescriber's DEA number, which is required for prescriptions containing controlled drug substances. *Note:* DEA refers to the Drug Enforcement Administration, which is a federal agency within the Department of Justice. This arm of the law oversees controlled drug substances traffic. Controlled drugs, controlled substances, or controlled drug substances (CDS) refer to those drugs that possess a high potential for abuse (e.g., diazepam, codeine, chloral hydrate).

Upon receipt of a properly written script (see Figure 1.3), you are able to prepare or "fill" the prescription without guesswork. In addition, a properly written script also enables you to dispense the medication to the patient in a timely manner. In reality, however, the ideal prescription rarely exists. You will find it necessary to examine the script closely, questioning the patient at times and perhaps phoning the doctor for clarification. There are a number of customary things to look for, and questions to ask:

1. Is this a legitimate prescription blank with the practitioner's name, address, and phone number clearly written on the blank?
2. Is the full name of the patient written on the prescription? (Patient's initials should not be acceptable, because this presents a potential for errors.)

PAT SMITH, M.D.
27 Oak Leaf Lane
Baltimore, MD 12121
Phone: 322 -7890

Name Donna Bell
Address 27 Windsor Place
Balto, MD. 12121 Age 26

Rx

ampicillin 250 mg Caps
Disp. #30
Sig: i cap QID for urinary infection

721723
11/28/01

[ ] Contents are labeled unless checked

May be refilled 0 (1) 2 3 4

Signed P. Smith M.D.
Date 11/27 20 01 DEA No. AS1522209

FIGURE 1.3

3. Check the date the prescription was written. This is important because controlled substances should not be filled or refilled (if refills are indicated) more than 6 months after the script is issued to the patient.
4. The patient's address is a legal requirement for prescriptions containing a controlled drug substance. It is a good practice to complete the address on ALL prescriptions. Many potential errors may be avoided in those cases where family common names occur frequently, or specific names are customary for a particular region.
5. Does the drug, the strength, and the form requested by the practitioner appear on the script? Old drugs with new modifications or uses as well as new drugs are constantly entering the market. Make an effort to establish the drug's existence, and if necessary, contact the doctor if you are unclear regarding the medication.
6. Does the quantity seem adequate? For example, you may question the quantity if a practitioner prescribes an antibiotic for an extremely long period of time, or an antitubercular drug for a very short duration. Lean what the customary course of treatment is for the most common ailments.
7. The directions should be written clearly to avoid any misinterpretation by the patient.
8. If no refill instructions are indicated on the prescription, permit *no refills.* The law clearly defines requirements and time frames for refills. Refills that are dispensed to patients should be entered on the back of the script, noting the date, your initials, and the quantity dispensed.
9. The law requires that a practitioner's signature, DEA number, and office address appear on all prescriptions for controlled substances. You should expect a prescriber to sign prescriptions written in his or her office. A telephoned prescription does not require a signature for noncontrolled drug substances. This also holds true for a limited number of controlled drug substances.
10. Although you would expect the physician to prescribe medications that will not trigger an allergic reaction in the sensitive patient, check for any known drug sensitivities with the patient.

A carefully screened prescription order can avoid many unnecessary problems and confusion.

PROBLEM AREAS

Some areas tend to be more prone to error than others. The following discussion highlights some of these areas.

Last Name Only (Patient) A prescription will often be presented with only the last name of the patient. You must be sure that the prescription is being prepared for the person for whom it is intended. Therefore, it may be necessary to verity the prescription with the patient.

Use of an Initial Rather than a Complete First Name (Patient) This situation can be as harmful as the "last name only" circumstance unless a family profile is maintained by the pharmacy. Use of a letter initial can become a problem even on a family profile if more than one member of the family have first names beginning with the same initial. You should not assume who the patient is, but check with the family or doctor's office.

Address The patient's address is especially important when a number of customers share a common name, when the prescription is to be billed, or when an insurance company is the payer. The address also serves as a check to assure that the person for whom the prescription was intended receives the medication.

Age The age of the patient is important where dosages are crucial. Age is also important where dosage forms (liquids, capsules, tablets, ointments, suppositories, etc.) vary for a particular drug. It is not uncommon for a "rushed" practitioner to prescribe capsules or tablets for children who are too young to swallow solid dosage forms.

Date on Which the Prescription Was Written Undated prescriptions present another problem. The consequence of having an undated prescription order is that the original condition for which the prescription was written may be different from some recently self-diagnosed condition for which the patient is now using the original, unfilled prescription. Some pharmacies may require a new prescription, or verbal confirmation from the doctor, in order to continue an old prescription order beyond 6 months.

Legibility There is no doubt that legibility is the greatest offending factor in prescription error. In order to avoid dispensing guesswork, check with the pharmacist (because he or she is legally responsible for any errors committed by technicians), or with the prescribing practitioner. When questioning the prescription, ask the pharmacist or physician what the prescription reads, rather than asking if the illegible writing is a particular drug. Naming the drug or suggesting the directions (directions are also a cause for question) tends to bias the prescribing practitioner, taking away the total objectivity needed to decipher the illegibility.

Lack of a DEA Number The DEA issues a recorded registry number (DEA number) to eligible practitioners to be used when writing prescriptions for controlled drugs or narcotics. The DEA number is not required on prescriptions for drugs other than narcotics or controlled drugs. When you complete a controlled drug substance prescription, make it evident that the prescription contained a controlled substance by stamping or putting a red-colored "C" on the blank. All prescription forms for controlled substances must also contain the patient's full name and complete address, in addition to the DEA number of the doctor.

Clarity of Directions Legibility has already been addressed. The clarity in this case refers to the intent of the directions. How does a practitioner want the patient to take the medication? The most abused direction is "Take as Directed" (often seen on the prescription order as ut. dict., u.d., ud, or as dir.). Although "Take as Directed" is not a satisfactory direction, it is not your position to interpret the doctor's intent, because this is between the patient and the doctor, based on the doctor's examination and diagnosis. If you see a blatant error that may be harmful, you can be sure that this was not the intent of the practitioner. Type the directions as you perceive them to be for the best use of the drug and the greatest benefit to the patient. However, when asked by the patient how to take the drug, or when left with a feeling that the patient is unsure of the directions, simply ask the patient how the doctor told him or her to take the medication. Should there continue to be any uncertainty, you may call the practitioner's office for clarification, or have the patient reaffirm the instructions with his or her doctor.

Another common direction that confuses many people involves taking the drug while awake (during waking hours) or around the clock (for example, "Take one capsule every four hours"). If there is any doubt regarding how the drug should be taken, first check the literature for specific details. If nothing can be concluded from the information provided, you may be required to make the decision. The literature may set a limit on the amount to be taken (for example, "Do not take more than eight capsules in a 24-hour period"). In the absence of limitations or clarity documented in the literature, a rule of thumb to follow is that antibiotics should be taken around the clock (at least during the initial phase of 24 to 48 hours), pain medications (analgesics) may be taken over a 24-hour period if the patient is awake and the pain is severe enough to require the medication. Other drugs, such as antihistamines, tranquilizers, antidepressants, anti-inflammatory drugs, and so on, should be limited to waking hours. This position may be taken when directions specify a number of times a day (for example, "Take one tablet three times a day").

Refill Instructions If no mention is made of refills, it is safe to assume that no refills were intended. Should the patient insist that the practitioner said refills were allowed, you may agree with the patient (depending on the type of drug being ordered—be careful with controlled drug substances), and verify refill instructions with the doctor at a more convenient time.

THE PRESCRIPTION LABEL

Once you are satisfied with the contents of the prescription and are confident that the information provided enables you to fill the prescription without guesswork, you are ready to fill the order and prepare a label identifying the patient and instructing the patient how to take the medication. Ideally, the label should contain specific information, as illustrated in Figure 1.4. Referring to Figure 1.4, review the contents of the label:

1. A prescription serial number (referred to as the Rx number) and the date the prescription order is filled
2. The patient's full name

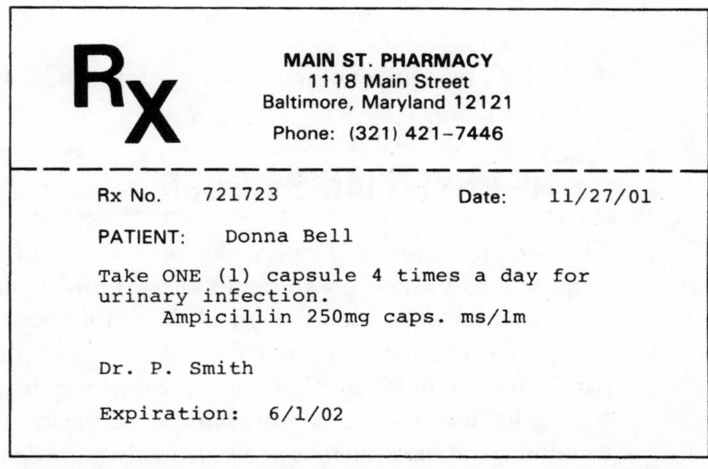

Rx
MAIN ST. PHARMACY
1118 Main Street
Baltimore, Maryland 12121
Phone: (321) 421-7446

Rx No. 721723 Date: 11/27/01

PATIENT: Donna Bell

Take ONE (1) capsule 4 times a day for urinary infection.
Ampicillin 250mg caps. ms/lm

Dr. P. Smith

Expiration: 6/1/02

FIGURE 1.4 The prescription label.

3. Clearly typed instructions for taking the medication. *Note:* The first word of the directions should infer the route of administration. For example:

internal/oral route—"Take"
eye/ear/nose—"Instill" or "Place"
topical lotion/ointment—"Apply"
rectal/vaginal—"Insert"

4. The name of the drug (called *labeling*), unless specifically requested by the practitioner not to label
5. The pharmacist's initials and the initials of the pharmacy technician who prepared the drug for dispensing
6. The practitioner's name
7. The drug's expiration date
8. Additional labels, called "strip" labels (for example, TAKE WITH FOOD OR MILK, DO NOT TAKE WITH ALCOHOL, TAKE ON AN EMPTY STOMACH), may be applied to the bottle containing the medication, informing the patient of a particular way to take the drug that would assure the medication's optimal effect. See Figure 1.5 for additional examples.

FINISH ALL THIS MEDICATION
UNLESS OTHERWISE DIRECTED
BY PRESCRIBER

REFILL ONE TIME

TAKE ON AN EMPTY STOMACH
ONE HOUR BEFORE MEALS OR
TWO HOURS AFTER MEALS

FIGURE 1.5 Strip labels.

9. The number of refills, if any, or no refills, if none

THE PHYSICIAN'S ORDER

The basic principles and care undertaken to examine the ambulatory patient's prescription order also apply to the Physician's Order (illustrated in Figure 1.2) for the hospitalized patient, even though all the script elements discussed do not appear on the Physician's Order. Screening the drug, the strength, the directions for use, and the patient for whom the medication is intended may be more important in the hospital setting, inasmuch as the variety of drugs and the forms for different routes of administration are more numerous and potentially more dangerous than those found in the local retail pharmacy.

MAJOR ELEMENTS

An appropriately written Physician's Order should contain the following elements:

1. Patient's name and hospital number
2. Patient's room or ward location
3. Attending physician
4. Patient's date of birth
5. Allergies or sensitivities to drugs, foods, and so forth
6. Diagnosis
7. Date of admission
8. Patient's condition
9. Services to be performed (i.e., tests, activities, diet, etc.)
10. Medications
11. Strength of each medication
12. Dosage form (tablet, liquid, suppository, injectable, etc.). Dosage form is specified in order to avoid any question regarding the form to be given. For example, nurses prefer to administer drugs in liquid form to patients who have nasogastric tubes, and suppositories or injection are generally used in vomiting patients. Most drugs come prepared in more than one dosage form. Although dosage form is not often written, you can interpret the most appropriate form to use by looking for keynotes such as NGT (nasogastric tube) or age.
13. Directions for the use or frequency of administration for each medication
14. Nurse's or physician's signature and time of entry on the Physician's Order

You should be completely certain of what is wanted, for whom it is ordered, and how it is to be given. Remember, NEVER DISPENSE GUESSWORK.

Most hospitals have a listing of drugs, referred to as a *drug formulary.* The drugs included in the formulary are those medicinal agents that have been reviewed by the hospital's Pharmacy Therapeutics Committee (PT Committee), and have been recommended for inventory based on their therapeutic benefits and economy. Occasionally, only one specific dosage form or strength of a drug will be included in the formulary. Although hospital formularies exist to control costs by limiting the drug inventory, nonformulary drugs may usually be ordered for a particular patient if requested by the prescriber.

Hospital pharmacies usually adopt an automatic stop order policy. The automatic stop order (ASO) may vary for the different categories of drugs for each hospital. For instance, *standing orders* (those medications ordered by the physician that can be presumed to be continued as long as the patient is in the hospital) may specify an automatic stop for narcotics after 72 hours. Therefore, the pharmacy will acknowledge and dispense no more than 72 hours' worth of the drug. A physician would be required to reorder the narcotic after this time. In many hospitals, standing orders are automatically stopped when the patient undergoes surgery or is transferred to another part of the hospital.

The PRN (*Pro Re Nata,* Latin for "as needed") category of drugs refers to the medications that are not used routinely, but only when they are needed. Some examples of this category are nonnarcotic pain medications (e.g., acetaminophen, propoxyphene), sleeping agents (e.g., flurazepam, temazepam), and laxatives. It is your task to learn what the stop order policies are for the specific hospital where you are employed.

COMMON PHARMACEUTICAL NOTATIONS

Hospital staffs generally adopt commonly used abbreviations. Occasionally, however, practitioners may develop their own form of shorthand that is limited to use only in those hospitals in which they are working. Tables 1.1 through 1.4 provide the pharmacy and drug abbreviations commonly used in hospitals, as well as generally accepted medical abbreviations. Concerning those special abbreviations found only within a specific hospital, question their meaning when you have the slightest doubt. Once you determine their meaning, note it in a personal resource file to be used as a reference source when needed.

TABLE 1.1 COMMON ABBREVIATIONS USED IN MEDICAL ORDERS

Abbreviation	Meaning
$\overline{aa}$, aa	of each
a.c.	before meals
ad	to, up to
a.d.	right ear
ad lib.	at pleasure, as desired
a.l.	left ear
A.M.	morning
aq.	water
aq. dest.	distilled water
a.s.	left ear
a.u.	each ear
b.i.d., bd	twice a day
b.m.	bowel movement
b.p.	blood pressure
C	one hundred
$\bar{c}$, c	with
caps.	capsules
comp.	compound
d.	day
dil.	dilute
disp.	dispense
div.	divide
d.t.d.	give of such a dose
el., elix.	elixir
et	and
f., ft.	make, let be made
Gm., g.	gram
gr.	grain
gtt., gtts.	a drop, drops
h.	hour
h.s., hor. som.	at bedtime
IM	intramuscular
IV	intravenously
liq.	liquid, solution
M.	mix
m. dict.	as directed
mixt., mist.	a mixture
no.	number
noc., N, n	night
non. rep.	do not repeat, no refills
O, Oct.	a pint
o.d.	right eye
o.l.	left eye

(continued)

TABLE 1.1 CONTINUED

Abbreviation	Meaning
o.s.	left eye
o.u.	each eye or both eyes
p.c., post. cib.	after meals
P.M.	evening
p.o.	by mouth, orally
p.r.	rectally
p.r.n.	as needed
pulv.	a powder
q	every
qAM	every morning
qd	every day
qh	every hour
q.i.d.	four times a day
q.o.d.	every other day
qPM	every evening
q.s., qs ad	a sufficient quantity, up to
q.v.	as much as you wish
Rx	take, take thou, a recipe, prescription
rep.	let it be repeated
s̄, s	without
s.a.	according to the art (secundum artem)
sat.	saturated
Sig.	label, let it be printed (signa)
sol.	solution
s.q., SQ	subcutaneous
s̄s̄, ss	one half
s.o.s.	if there is a need
stat	at once, immediately
subq	subcutaneously
supp.	suppository
syr.	syrup
tab.	tablet
t.i.d.	three times a day
tr., tinct.	tincture
trit.	triturate
ung.	ointment
ut. dict., u.d., ud	as directed
w.a.	while awake
X	ten

TABLE 1.2 COMMON SYMBOLS USED IN MEDICAL ORDERS

Symbol	Meaning
ʒ	teaspoonful
℥	2 tablespoonsful, 1 fluid ounce, 30 milliliters
℥ss	1 tablespoonful, 15 milliliters
Ⓛ	left
Ⓡ	right
ϕ	none
Δ	change
>	greater than
<	less than
↑	increase
↓	decrease
′	minutes
″	seconds
°	hours
1°	primary
2°	secondary

TABLE 1.3 COMMON DRUG ABBREVIATIONS

Abbreviation	Trade Name	Generic Name	Use
$AgNO_3$	none	silver nitrate	anti-infective
APAP	Tylenol	acetaminophen	analgesic
ASA	Ecotrin	aspirin	analgesic
bicarb	none	bicarbonate (sodium)	antacid/electrolyte
B-1	none	thiamine	vitamin
B-6	none	pyridoxine	vitamin
B-12	none	cyanocobalamin	vitamin
Ca	none	calcium	nutritional supplement
CaCl	none	calcium chloride	electrolyte
$CaCO_3$	Os-Cal	calcium carbonate	nutritional supplement
CT	Chlor-Trimeton	chlorpheniramine	antihistamine
DC	Darvon Compound	propoxyphene, aspirin, caffeine	analgesic
DES	Stilphostrol	diethylstilbesterol	hormone
DHE	D.H.E. 45	dihydroergotamine	vasoconstrictor
dig, digox	Lanoxin	digoxin	cardiac drug
DPH	Benadryl	diphenhydramine	antihistamine
	Dilantin	diphenylhydantoin (generic name changed to phenytoin)	anticonvulsant
DPT	Tri-Immunol	diphtheria, pertussis, and tetanus	vaccine
DSS	Colace	dioctyl sodium sulfosuccinate	laxative
D_5NS	none	5% dextrose in normal saline	intravenous fluid
D_5W	none	5% dextrose in water	intravenous fluid
epi	Adrenalin	epinephrine	bronchodilator/heart stimulant
ETH	none	elixir terpin hydrate	expectorant
ETH c. Cod	none	elixir terpin hydrate with codeine	expectorant/cough suppressant
ETOH	none	ethanol/ethyl alcohol	skin disinfectant
F.A.	Folvite	folic acid	vitamin
$FeSO_4$	Feosol	ferrous sulfate	iron supplement
gent	Garamycin	gentamicin	antibiotic
GG	Robitussin	glyceryl guaiacolate, guaifenesin	expectorant
HC	Cortef	hydrocortisone	steroid
HCTZ	Oretic	hydrochlorothiazide	diuretic
H_2O	none	water	fluid
H_2O_2	none	hydrogen peroxide	antiseptic
INH	INH	Isoniazid	antitubercular
KCI	Kay Ciel	potassium chloride	electrolyte
KI	SSKI	potassium iodide	expectorant
KISS	SSKI	saturated solution of potassium iodide	expectoranty
KPO_4	Neutra-Phos	potassium phosphate	electrolyte
LCD	Zetar	coal tar solution	antipruritic
L-Dopa	Larodopa	levodopa	anti-Parkinson
$LiCO_3$	Eskalith	lithium carbonate	psychotherapeutic drug
LR	none	lactated-Ringers solution	intravenous fluid
mag. cit.	none	magnesium citrate	laxative
mgO	none	magnesium oxide	antacid/laxative
$mgSO_4$	none	magnesium sulfate	anticonvulsant
m.o.	Kondremul	mineral oil	laxative
MOM	none	milk of magnesia	antacid/laxative
MS	none	morphine sulfate	analgesic
MVI	many	multiple vitamins	vitamins
NaCl	none	sodium chloride	electrolyte
$NaHCO_3$, NaBicarb.	none	sodium bicarbonate	antacid/electrolyte
$NaPO_4$	K-Phos	sodium phosphate	electrolyte
NS, NSS	none	normal saline solution	intravenous fluid
PABA	Pabanol	para-aminobenzoic acid	sunscreen
Pb, phenobarb	SK-Phenobarbital	phenobarbital	sedative
PBZ	Pyribenzamine	tripelennamine	antihistamine
PCN	none	penicillin	antibiotic
PCN G	Pfizerpen	penicillin G	antibiotic

(continued)

TABLE 1.3 CONTINUED

Abbreviation	Trade Name	Generic Name	Use
PCN VK	Veetids	penicillin VK	antibiotic
pit	Pitocin	oxytocin	hormone
PPD	Aplisol	purified protein derivative	tuberculin test
PTU	none	propylthiouracil	antithyroid
PZI	none	protamine zinc insulin	blood glucose regulator
RL	none	ringer's lactate	intravenous fluid
sal acid	Keralyt	salicylic acid	keratolytic
SSKI	SSKI	saturated solution of potassium iodide	expectorant
TCN	Sumycin	tetracycline	antibiotic
TNG	Nitrostat	nitroglycerin	antianginal
tobra	Nebcin	tobramycin	antibiotic
TSH	Thytropar	thyroid stimulating hormone	hormone
Vit. C	Cevi-Bid	ascorbic acid	vitamin
Vit. K	Synkavite Mephyton	menadiol phytonadione	vitamin
ZnO	none	zinc oxide	protectant
$ZnSO_4$	Zinc-220	zinc sulfate	nutritional supplement

TABLE 1.4 COMMON HOSPITAL ABBREVIATIONS

Abbreviation	Meaning
ABD	abdomen
abd prep	abdominal preparation
ABG	arterial blood gases
AC lab	anticoagulation laboratory
ACT	activity
ADA	American Dietetic Association
AK	above knee
alk phos	alkaline phosphatase
all	allergy
AMA	against medical advice
amp	ampule
antibio	antibiotics
AP chest	anteroposterior chest X-ray
APhA	American Pharmaceutical Association
ASAP	as soon as possible
ASCVD	arteriosclerotic cardiovascular disease
ASHD	arteriosclerotic heart disease
ASHP	American Society of Health-System Pharmacists
ASO	automatic stop order
BE	barium enema
bili	bilirubin
BK	below knee
BM	bowel movement
BMR	basal metabolic rate
BP	blood pressure
BRP	bathroom privileges
BSA	body surface area
BSS	buffered saline solution
BUN	blood urea nitrogen
C	gallon or the Roman numeral for 100
C&S	culture and sensitivity
C.A.	continuous action
CA	cancer
cap	capsule
cath	catheter
CBC	complete blood count
CBC c. diff	complete blood count with differentials

(continued)

TABLE 1.4 CONTINUED

Abbreviation	Meaning
cc	cubic centimeter
CCU	coronary care unit
CDS	controlled drug substance
Chest AP	*see* AP chest
CHF	congestive heart failure
CICU	coronary intensive care unit
CLD, CL diet	clear liquid diet
cond	condition
cont	continuous
COPD	chronic obstructive pulmonary disease
C section	Cesarean section
CSF	cerebral spinal fluid
CVA	cerebrovascular accident
CXR	chest X-ray
cysto	cystoscopy
D.A.	delayed action
DC, D/C	discontinue or discharge
DEA	Drug Enforcement Administration
decub	decubitus
dig	digoxin
dig level	digoxin blood level
DNI	do not intubate
DNR	do not resuscitate
DR	delivery room
DS	double strength
DSD	dry sterile dressing
Dx	diagnosis
E.C.	enteric coated
ECG or EKG	electrocardiogram
EEG	electroencephalogram
ER	emergency room
FBS	fasting blood sugar
FDA	Food and Drug Administration
Fe	iron
FiO_2	frequency of inspired air
FS	floor stock
FTT	failure to thrive
FUO	fever of unknown origin
Fx	fracture
F(x)	function
GFR	glomerular filtration rate
GI	gastrointestinal
gluc	glucose
Gm., gm., G.	gram
gr.	grain
gtt.	drop(s)
GU	genitourinary
GYN	gynecology
H.A. or HA	headache
HCl	hydrochloride
Hct	hematocrit
HCVD	hypertensive cardiovascular disease
HEENT	head, eye, ear, nose, throat
Hep Lock, H.L.	heparin lock
Hg	mercury
Hgb	hemoglobin
H.O.	house officer
H.P.	high potency
HR	heart rate or hyperalimentation rate
H.T.	hypodermic tablet
HTFN	hold till further notice
Hx	history
Hyperal, HAL	hyperalimentation
I&O	intake and output
ICN	intensive care nursery
ICU	intensive care unit

(continued)

TABLE 1.4 CONTINUED

Abbreviation	Meaning
I.M.	intramuscular
IP	inpatient
IPPB	intermittent positive pressure breathing
IU	international unit
IUD	intrauterine device
IUP	intrauterine pregnancy
I.V.	intravenous
IVF	intravenous fluids
IVP	intravenous pyelogram or intravenous piggyback
IVR	intravenous rate
K^+ level	potassium level
KO	keep open
KVO	keep vein open
L	liter
L.A.	long acting
LAS	label as such
lat	lateral
LDH	lactodehydrogenase
L.E.	lupus erythematosus
LFT	liver function test
LOA	leave of absence
LOC	laxative of choice
LPN	licensed practical nurse
lytes	electrolytes
M&M enema	milk and molasses enema
Mcg., mcg.	microgram
meds	medications
mEq.	millequivalent
Mg., mg.	milligram
MI	myocardial infarction
MIC	minimum inhibitory concentration
ml.	milliliter
MLD	minimum lethal dose
mm.	millimeter
MN	midnight
N, NL	normal
Na^+ level	sodium level
narc	narcotic
N.B.	note well, take notice
NBN	newborn nursery
NC	nasal cannula
NDC	National Drug Code
NF	National Formulary
NGT, NG tube	nasogastric tube
NH	nursing home
NICU	newborn intensive care unit
NKA	no known allergies
NKDA	no known drug allergy
NKMA	no known medication allergy
NPO	nothing by mouth
NS	normal saline
nst	not sent
n/v	nausea and vomiting
O	pint
OB	obstetrics
OD	overdose
oint.	ointment
OJ	orange juice
OOB	out of bed
OP	outpatient
opth.	ophthalmic
OR	operating room
P or p	per, after
P.A.	prolonged action

(continued)

TABLE 1.4 CONTINUED

Abbreviation	Meaning
PA	posteroanterior X-ray, physician's assistant
PBI	protein-bound iodine
PDR	*Physicians' Desk Reference*
Peds	pediatrics
PFT	pulmonary function test
PKU	phenylketonuria
p.o.	by mouth (occasionally "phone order")
Port	portable
post-op	after surgery
PP	post prandial, post partum
PPN	partial or peripheral parenteral nutrition
ppm	parts per million
pr	per rectum
PRBC	packed red blood cells
pre-op	before surgery
pt.	patient
PT	physical therapy, prothrombin time (test for coumadin)
PTT	prothrombin time (test for heparin)
PVB	premature ventricular beat
PVC	premature ventricular contraction
R&M	routine and microscopy
R.A.	released action
RBC	red blood cell
Reg	regular
R.N.	registered nurse
R/O	rule out
ROM	range of motion
RR	recovery room
RTC	return to clinic
RTS	return to stock
S.A.	sustained action or slow-acting
S.C.	sugar coated
sc	subcutaneous
SGOT	serum glutamic oxaloacetic transaminase
SGPT	serum glutamic pyruvic transaminase
s.l.	sublingual
SMA	serial multiple analysis
SOB	shortness of breath
sono	sonogram
S/P	status post, state of a condition
sp. gr.	specific gravity
SQ, sq	subcutaneous
S.R.	sustained release, slow release
STAT	immediately
supp	suppository
T, temp	temperature
T >	temperature greater than
T&A	tonsillectomy and adenoidectomy
tach	tachycardia
TB	tuberculosis
tbsp	tablespoonful
T.D.	timed disintegrating
tele	telemetry
TIA	transient ischemic attack
TLC	tender loving care
TO	transfer orders
TPN	total parenteral nutrition
TPR	temperature, pulse, respiration
T.R.	timed release
trans	transfer
TRH	thyrotropin releasing hormone
TSH	thyroid stimulating hormone
tsp	teaspoonful
T.T.	tablet triturate
TUR	transurethral resection
TV	total volume

(continued)

TABLE 1.4 CONTINUED

Abbreviation	Meaning
TX	treatment
TXC	type and crossmatch
u	unit
U/A, UA	urinalysis
UGI	upper gastrointestinal series
URI	upper respiratory infection
USP	*United States Pharmacopeia*
USPDI	*United States Pharmacopeia Dispensing Information*
UTI	urinary tract infection
VDRL	venereal disease research laboratory
VO	verbal order
VS	vital signs
w.a.	while awake
WBC	white blood cells

EXERCISES

1. What two types of patients are treated by physicians?

2. Never dispense ______________________.

3. When in doubt about directions for taking the prescribed drug, call the ______________________.

4. When in doubt about the name of the patient, check with the ______________.

5. "Take as directed" is an unclear direction and is written on many prescriptions as ______________________, ______________________, or ______________________.

6. The patient should have complete ______________________ of the directions for taking the drug.

7. Physicians communicate their request for medications by using a ______________________ blank for outpatients and a ______________________ for hospitalized patients.

8. Some medications require special instructions that are affixed to the medication container by using a ______________________ label.

9. A properly completed prescription should ideally contain:
   (a) prescriber's name and title
   (b) prescriber's office address
   (c) prescriber's phone number
   (d)
   (e) patient's age
   (f)
   (g) Rx
   (h)
   (i)
   (j)
   (k)

(l) prescriber's signature
(m) DEA number of prescriber

10. Reviewing a Physician's Order specifically for the hospital pharmacy's role in patient care delivery includes screening for the ______________________, ______________________________, route of administration, and directions.

11. A properly completed Physician's Order for a hospital inpatient contains:
(a) patient's name and hospital number
(b) patient's room location
(c) the attending physician's name
(d) patient's date of birth (DOB)
(e)
(f)
(g) date of admission
(h) patient's condition
(i)
(j)
(k)
(l)
(m)
(n) signature of the nurse of physician and the time of entry

12. Most hospitals develop a drug __________________________ or listing that contains medicinal agents reviewed by the hospital's Pharmacy Therapeutics (PT) Committee.

13. Some drugs have a specific duration for which they may be ordered. This is known as an ________________ ________________ ________________, or ASO.

14. Drugs used only when needed are referred to as the ______________category.

15. How do we identify a prescription containing a controlled substance?

16. Review the Physician's Order Records included at the end of this section (Figures 1.6 to 1.15). List each item highlighted by an arrow and explain what it means.

17. Review the prescriptions that follow this section (Figures 1.16 to 1.27). First, identify the missing element(s). Then write the directions for taking the medication in language that is understandable to the patient.

18. What is the USP and what does it mean to pharmacy?

19. What do all the following have in common?
(a) gent
(b) PCN
(c) PCN G
(d) PCN VK
(e) TCN
(f) tobra

PATIENT: AGE: SEX: RACE: CHART NO.	MEMORIAL HOSPITAL BALTIMORE, MARYLAND PHYSICIAN'S ORDER RECORD BEAR DOWN ON HARD SURFACE WITH BALL POINT PEN

GENERIC EQUIVALENT IS AUTHORIZED UNLESS CHECKED IN THIS COLUMN

ALLERGY OR SENSITIVITY TO____ NONE KNOWN ☐ SIGNED:____	DIAGNOSIS		COMPLETED OR DISCONTINUED

DATE	TIME	ORDERS	PHYSICIAN'S SIG.		NAME	DATE	TIME
		Admit to Med C – RM 411					
		Dx: Fever and granulocytopenia metastatic Breast CA					
		Condition – Stable					
		Diet CLD					
		Activity – Bedrest					
		I & O's					
		Meds: amoxicillin 250 mg q 8°					
		Sucralfate 1 Gm AC and q hs					
		Halcion 0.125 mg q hs prn					
		Am Labs EKG (R/O ischemia);					
		CBC c̄ diff.					

PHARMACY COPY

FIGURE 1.6

PATIENT:
AGE:
SEX:
RACE:
CHART NO.

MEMORIAL HOSPITAL
BALTIMORE, MARYLAND
PHYSICIAN'S ORDER RECORD

BEAR DOWN ON HARD SURFACE WITH BALL POINT PEN

GENERIC EQUIVALENT IS AUTHORIZED UNLESS CHECKED IN THIS COLUMN

ALLERGY OR SENSITIVITY TO ______ DIAGNOSIS

NONE KNOWN ☐ SIGNED: ______

COMPLETED OR DISCONTINUED

DATE	TIME	ORDERS	PHYSICIAN'S SIG.		NAME	DATE	TIME
		→ Stat methylprednisolone 250mg bolus					
		→ DPH 50mg IM					
		pt. to go for arteriogram this pm					
		Con't meds:					
		→ MVI i q d					
		→ F.A. i q d					
		→ NPO p̄ MN					

PHARMACY COPY

FIGURE 1.7

PATIENT: AGE: SEX: RACE: CHART NO.	**MEMORIAL HOSPITAL** BALTIMORE, MARYLAND **PHYSICIAN'S ORDER RECORD**
	BEAR DOWN ON HARD SURFACE WITH BALL POINT PEN

GENERIC EQUIVALENT IS AUTHORIZED UNLESS CHECKED IN THIS COLUMN

ALLERGY OR SENSITIVITY TO________ NONE KNOWN ☐ SIGNED:________	DIAGNOSIS		COMPLETED OR DISCONTINUED

DATE	TIME	ORDERS	PHYSICIAN'S SIG.		NAME	DATE	TIME
		Admit to Dr. Smith Med C					
		Dx - CHF					
		Condition - Good					
		Diet: 500mg Na, 1200 cal ADA					
		fluid restrict to 1200 cc/d					
		allergies: ϕ					
		Meds: furosemide 20mg IV BID					
		Dig 0.25 mg on even days					
		TNG Paste - 1" q 6°					
		Isosorbide 2.5mg SL TID					
		Send urine for U/A					
		Send pt. for CXR					
		AM Labs: DIG level					

PHARMACY COPY

FIGURE 1.8

PATIENT:
AGE:
SEX:
RACE:
CHART NO.

MEMORIAL HOSPITAL
BALTIMORE, MARYLAND
PHYSICIAN'S ORDER RECORD

BEAR DOWN ON HARD SURFACE WITH BALL POINT PEN

GENERIC EQUIVALENT IS AUTHORIZED UNLESS CHECKED IN THIS COLUMN

ALLERGY OR SENSITIVITY
TO ______
NONE KNOWN ☐ SIGNED: ______

DIAGNOSIS

COMPLETED OR DISCONTINUED

DATE	TIME	ORDERS	PHYSICIAN'S SIG.		NAME	DATE	TIME
		Dx CVA					
		Activity – with supervision					
		Diet – Soft					
		Meds –					
		ASA 5gr PO QD					
		diltiazem 60mg daily PO					
		MOM 30cc PO q d prn					
		APAP ii q 4° prn					
		flurazepam 15mg hs					
		Maintain H.L.					
		Schedule light PT					

PHARMACY COPY

FIGURE 1.9

PATIENT:
AGE:
SEX:
RACE:
CHART NO.

MEMORIAL HOSPITAL
BALTIMORE, MARYLAND
PHYSICIAN'S ORDER RECORD

BEAR DOWN ON HARD SURFACE WITH BALL POINT PEN

GENERIC EQUIVALENT IS AUTHORIZED UNLESS CHECKED IN THIS COLUMN

ALLERGY OR SENSITIVITY TO → NKDA

NONE KNOWN ☐ SIGNED:

DIAGNOSIS

COMPLETED OR DISCONTINUED

DATE	TIME	ORDERS	PHYSICIAN'S SIG.		NAME	DATE	TIME
		Admit to Med A					
		Condition - Poor					
		→ VS q shift					
		→ D/C Foley cath					
		Regular diet					
		Meds → dig 0.25mg q.o.d					
		→ $FeSO_4$ 325mg q AM p̄ food					
		→ $ZnSO_4$ 220mg q d					
		→ Haloperidol 1mg prn					
		→ triazolam 0.25mg hs prn insomnia					
		→ Δ IV to H.L. in AM					

PHARMACY COPY

FIGURE 1.10

PATIENT:
AGE:
SEX:
RACE:
CHART NO.

MEMORIAL HOSPITAL
BALTIMORE, MARYLAND
PHYSICIAN'S ORDER RECORD

BEAR DOWN ON HARD SURFACE WITH BALL POINT PEN

GENERIC EQUIVALENT IS AUTHORIZED UNLESS CHECKED IN THIS COLUMN

ALLERGY OR SENSITIVITY
TO
NONE KNOWN ☐ SIGNED:

DIAGNOSIS

COMPLETED OR DISCONTINUED

DATE	TIME	ORDERS	PHYSICIAN'S SIG.		NAME	DATE	TIME
		Post-op orders.					
		TO RR					
		Dx - s/p appendectomy					
		Condition - stable					
		NPO I&O's					
		D5 ½NS c̄ 20 KCl @ 125 cc/hr					
		MS 8mg IM or SQ q 3° prn					

PHARMACY COPY

FIGURE 1.11

PATIENT:
AGE:
SEX:
RACE:
CHART NO.

MEMORIAL HOSPITAL
BALTIMORE, MARYLAND
PHYSICIAN'S ORDER RECORD

BEAR DOWN ON HARD SURFACE WITH BALL POINT PEN

GENERIC EQUIVALENT IS AUTHORIZED UNLESS CHECKED IN THIS COLUMN

ALLERGY OR SENSITIVITY
TO
NONE KNOWN ☐ SIGNED:

DIAGNOSIS

COMPLETED OR DISCONTINUED

DATE	TIME	ORDERS	PHYSICIAN'S SIG.	NAME	DATE	TIME
		Admit to Dr. Smith's Service				
		Dx: FUO				
		Diet - LIQ				
		allergies - NKA				
		I & O's.				
		Run IV D5-S KVO				
		Meds - gent 80 mg q 8° IV				
		APAP i-ii q 4 h prn pain				
		D/C CXR for today - reschedule				
		for tomorrow.				
		Do ABG				
		EEG				
		EKG				

PHARMACY COPY

FIGURE 1.12

PATIENT:
AGE:
SEX:
RACE:
CHART NO.

MEMORIAL HOSPITAL
BALTIMORE, MARYLAND
PHYSICIAN'S ORDER RECORD

BEAR DOWN ON HARD SURFACE WITH BALL POINT PEN

GENERIC EQUIVALENT IS AUTHORIZED UNLESS CHECKED IN THIS COLUMN

ALLERGY OR SENSITIVITY
TO____
NONE KNOWN ☐ SIGNED:____

DIAGNOSIS

COMPLETED OR DISCONTINUED

DATE	TIME	ORDERS	PHYSICIAN'S SIG.		NAME	DATE	TIME
		Bolus c̄ 3,000 u heparin IV over 1/2 h.					
		→ PTT @ 8 PM; Call H.O. with results					
		→ Turn off heparin drip in 1 h for 1 h and restart → @ 950 u per h.					
		→ VO Dr Smith					

PHARMACY COPY

FIGURE 1.13

PATIENT:
AGE:
SEX:
RACE:
CHART NO.

MEMORIAL HOSPITAL
BALTIMORE, MARYLAND
PHYSICIAN'S ORDER RECORD

BEAR DOWN ON HARD SURFACE WITH BALL POINT PEN

GENERIC EQUIVALENT IS AUTHORIZED UNLESS CHECKED IN THIS COLUMN

ALLERGY OR SENSITIVITY	DIAGNOSIS		COMPLETED OR DISCONTINUED
TO ______			
NONE KNOWN ☐ SIGNED: ______			

DATE	TIME	ORDERS	PHYSICIAN'S SIG.		NAME	DATE	TIME
		Admit to Floor c̄ telemetry					
		DX – Syncope					
		Condition Fair					
		Allergies – PCN, TCN ⬅					
		Diet: Reg ⬅					
		Activity – OOB c̄ assistance ⬅					
		➡ VS – q shift					
		Meds –					
		➡ procainamide SR 1Gm Q6H					
		➡ DIG 0.125mg Q AM					
		Arrange for Holter monitor ASAP ⬈					

PHARMACY COPY

FIGURE 1.14

PATIENT:
AGE:
SEX:
RACE:
CHART NO.

MEMORIAL HOSPITAL
BALTIMORE, MARYLAND
PHYSICIAN'S ORDER RECORD

BEAR DOWN ON HARD SURFACE WITH BALL POINT PEN

GENERIC EQUIVALENT IS AUTHORIZED UNLESS CHECKED IN THIS COLUMN

ALLERGY OR SENSITIVITY TO ____ NONE KNOWN ☐ SIGNED: ____

DIAGNOSIS

COMPLETED OR DISCONTINUED

DATE	TIME	ORDERS	PHYSICIAN'S SIG.	NAME	DATE	TIME
		admit to Room 815				
		DX: Cholecystitis				
		Condition - Fair				
		VS routine				
		activity OOB as Tolerated				
		IVF: KVO D5 1/2S @125/h				
		FBS				
		Start insulin SQ sliding scale				
		LOC				
		Cefamandole i Gm. IV on call to OR				

PHARMACY COPY

FIGURE 1.15

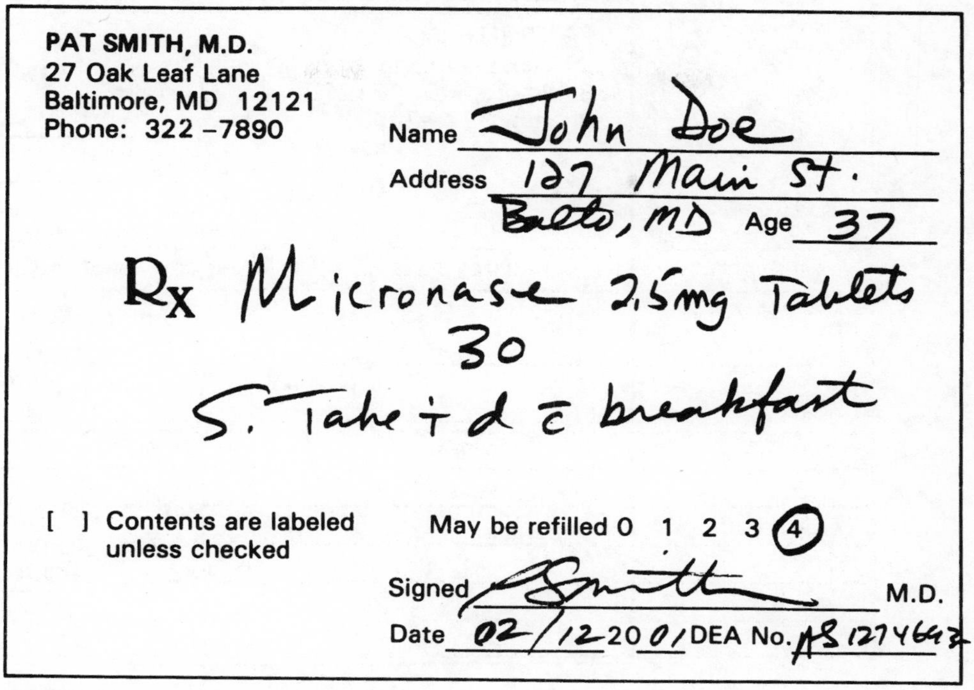

PAT SMITH, M.D.
27 Oak Leaf Lane
Baltimore, MD 12121
Phone: 322 -7890

Name John Doe

Address 127 Main St.
Balto, MD Age 37

Rx Micronase 2.5mg Tablets
30
S. Take i d c̄ breakfast

[ ] Contents are labeled unless checked

May be refilled 0 1 2 3 (4)

Signed P Smith M.D.

Date 02/12 2001 DEA No. AS1274643

FIGURE 1.16

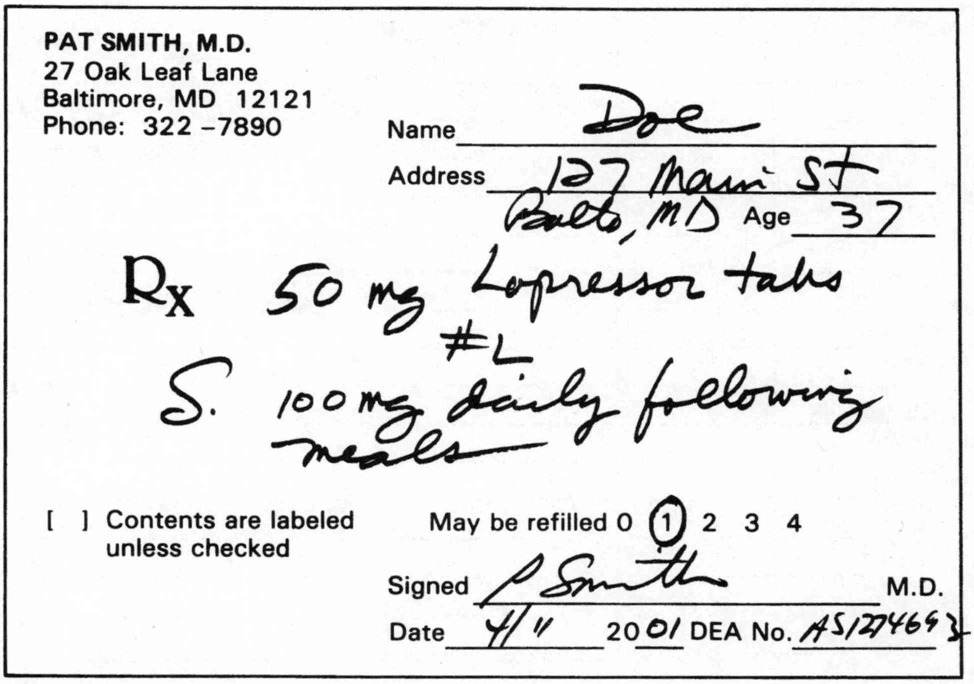

PAT SMITH, M.D.
27 Oak Leaf Lane
Baltimore, MD 12121
Phone: 322 -7890

Name Doe

Address 127 Main St
Balto, MD Age 37

Rx 50 mg Lopressor tabs
#L
S. 100mg daily following meals

[ ] Contents are labeled unless checked

May be refilled 0 (1) 2 3 4

Signed P Smith M.D.

Date 4/11 2001 DEA No. AS1274643

FIGURE 1.17

PAT SMITH, M.D.
27 Oak Leaf Lane
Baltimore, MD 12121
Phone: 322 -7890

Name John Doe
Address
Age 37

Rx Tabs Seldane 60 mg
#60
Dir: i BD during allergy season

[ ] Contents are labeled unless checked

May be refilled 0 1 2 3 4

Signed P Smith M.D.
Date 3 · 2 2001 DEA No. AS 127464

FIGURE 1.18

PAT SMITH, M.D.
27 Oak Leaf Lane
Baltimore, MD 12121
Phone: 322 -7890

Name John Doe
Address 127 Main St
Balto, MD
Age

Rx Ampicillin Susp 125mg/5ml
150 ml
Sig: ℨi q 6 h

[ ] Contents are labeled unless checked

May be refilled 0 1 2 3 4

Signed P Smith M.D.
Date 1/15 2001 DEA No. AS1274693

FIGURE 1.19

PAT SMITH, M.D.
27 Oak Leaf Lane
Baltimore, MD 12121
Phone: 322 -7890

Name John Doe
Address 127 Main St.
Balto, MD Age 37

Rx Theophylline tablets
#50
Sig i q6°

[ ] Contents are labeled unless checked

May be refilled 0 1 2 3 (4)

Signed P Smith M.D.

Date 2·15 20 01 DEA No. 1274693

FIGURE 1.20

PAT SMITH, M.D.
27 Oak Leaf Lane
Baltimore, MD 12121
Phone: 322 -7890

Name John Doe
Address 127 Main St
Balto, MD Age 37

Rx Tabs Conjugated Estrogens 1.25 mg
#30
Sig. i daily

[ ] Contents are labeled unless checked

May be refilled 0 (1) 2 3 4

Signed P Smith M.D.

Date 6/1 / 20 01 DEA No. 1274693

FIGURE 1.21

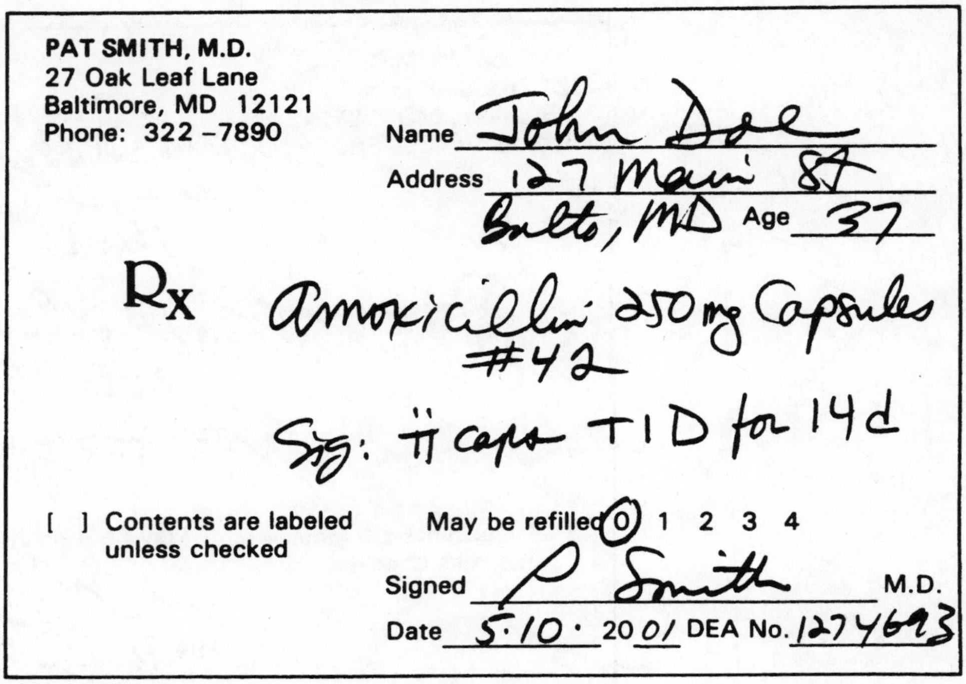

PAT SMITH, M.D.
27 Oak Leaf Lane
Baltimore, MD 12121
Phone: 322 -7890

Name John Doe
Address 127 Main St
Balto, MD Age 37

Rx amoxicillin 250 mg Capsules
#42
Sig: ii caps TID for 14d

[ ] Contents are labeled unless checked

May be refilled (0) 1 2 3 4

Signed P Smith M.D.

Date 5·10· 2001 DEA No. 1274693

FIGURE 1.22

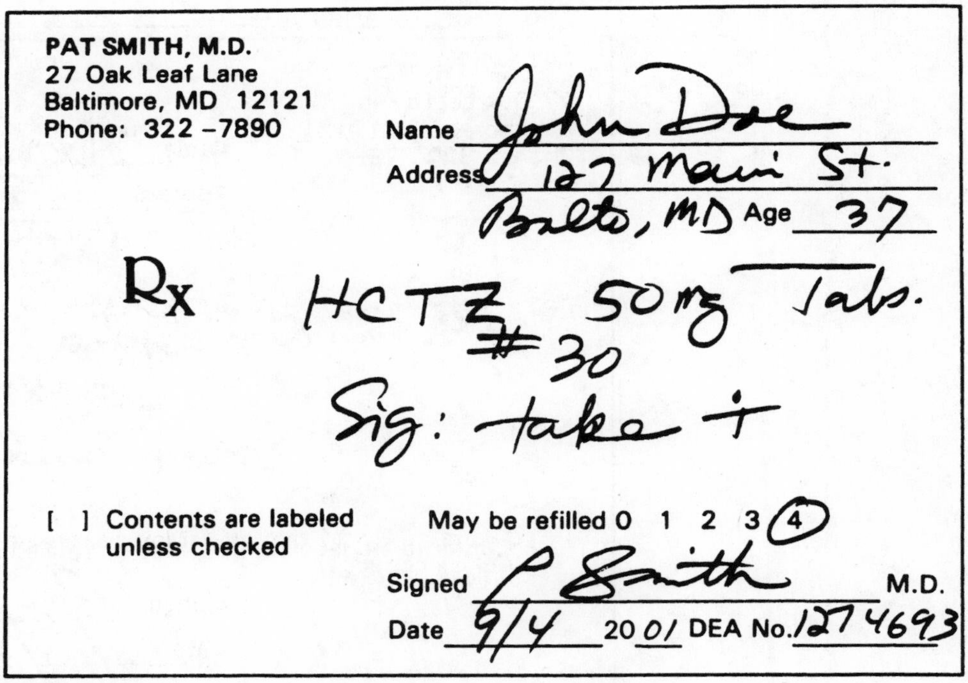

PAT SMITH, M.D.
27 Oak Leaf Lane
Baltimore, MD 12121
Phone: 322 -7890

Name John Doe
Address 127 Main St.
Balto, MD Age 37

Rx HCTZ 50 mg Tabs.
#30
Sig: take i

[ ] Contents are labeled unless checked

May be refilled 0 1 2 3 (4)

Signed P Smith M.D.

Date 9/4 2001 DEA No. 1274693

FIGURE 1.23

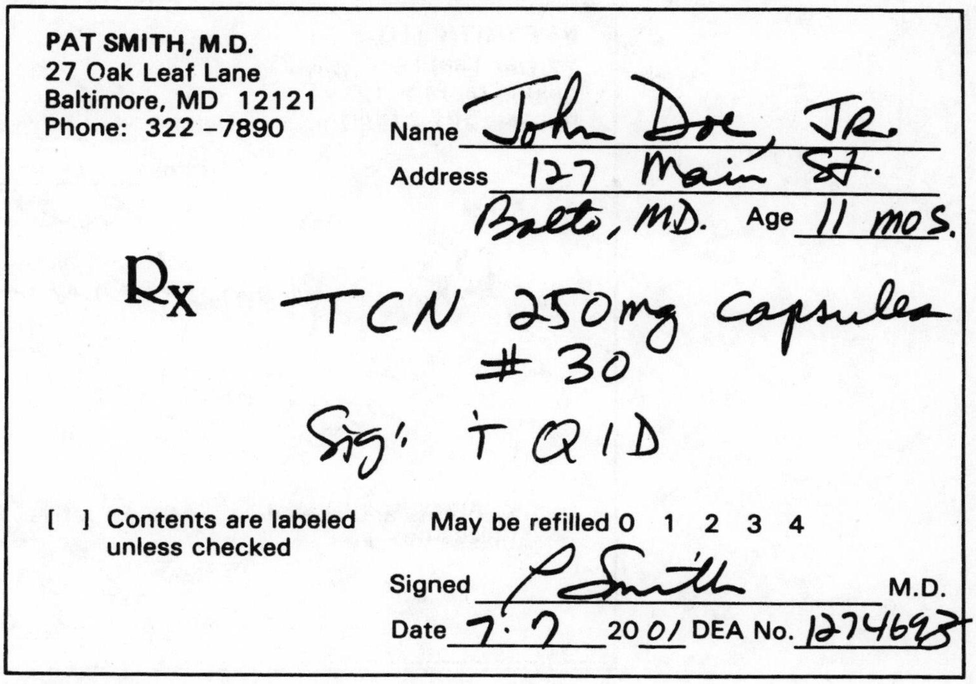

PAT SMITH, M.D.
27 Oak Leaf Lane
Baltimore, MD 12121
Phone: 322 –7890

Name John Doe, JR.
Address 127 Main St.
Balto, MD. Age 11 mos.

Rx TCN 250mg capsules
30
Sig: i QID

[ ] Contents are labeled unless checked

May be refilled 0 1 2 3 4

Signed P Smith M.D.

Date 7·7 20 01 DEA No. 1274693

FIGURE 1.24

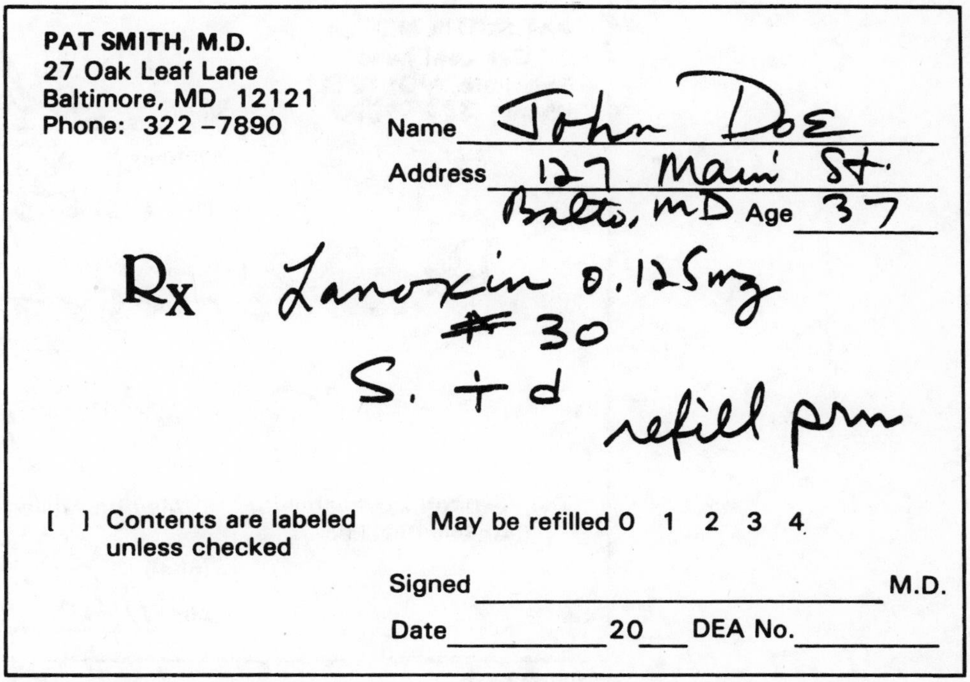

PAT SMITH, M.D.
27 Oak Leaf Lane
Baltimore, MD 12121
Phone: 322 –7890

Name John Doe
Address 127 Main St.
Balto, MD Age 37

Rx Lanoxin 0.125mg
30
S. i d
refill prn

[ ] Contents are labeled unless checked

May be refilled 0 1 2 3 4

Signed ______________ M.D.

Date ________ 20___ DEA No. ________

FIGURE 1.25

PAT SMITH, M.D.
27 Oak Leaf Lane
Baltimore, MD 12121
Phone: 322 -7890

Name John Doe
Address 127 Main St.
Balto, MD Age 37

Rx Phenobarbital 30mg Tabs.
#20
Sig: Take i–ii tablets hs
prn sleep

C

[ ] Contents are labeled unless checked

May be refilled (0) 1 2 3 4

Signed P Smith M.D.
Date 6/12 20 01 DEA No. ______

FIGURE 1.26

PAT SMITH, M.D.
27 Oak Leaf Lane
Baltimore, MD 12121
Phone: 322 -7890

Name John Doe
Address 127 Main St.
Balto, MD Age 37

Rx Lopressor 50mg Tabs.
#30
Sig. Take i qd for HBP

[ ] Contents are labeled unless checked

May be refilled 0 1 2 3 4

Signed P Smith M.D.
Date 11/17 20 01 DEA No. 1234693

FIGURE 1.27

20. Match the following abbreviations with the appropriate definition.

Abbreviations	**Definitions**
1. stat	(a) every other day
2. a.c.	(b) every
3. A.M.	(c) per rectum
4. b.i.d.	(d) after meals
5. disp.	(e) orally
6. elix.	(f) intravenous
7. Gm.	(g) liquid
8. gr.	(h) grams
9. gtts.	(i) grain
10. g.	(j) elixir
11. IM	(k) twice a day
12. liq	(l) before meals
13. h.s.	(m) immediately
14. IV	(n) morning
15. o.d.	(o) dispense
16. p.o.	(p) grams
17. o.s.	(q) drops
18. p.c.	(r) intramuscular
19. o.u.	(s) at bedtime
20. p.r.	(t) right eye
21. p.r.n.	(u) left eye
22. q	(v) both eyes
23. q.i.d.	(w) as needed
24. q.o.d.	(x) four times a day
25. t.i.d.	(y) three times a day
	(z) in vitro

CHAPTER 2

The Drug Monograph

OBJECTIVES

When you have completed this chapter, you will be able to:

1. distinguish between a patient's right of expectation and pharmacy responsibilities
2. list references used in pharmacy practice
3. review a drug monograph with a comprehensive focus on the information
4. list different types of side effects

The scope of this text is to present a basic instructional guide for learning the elements of pharmacy as it pertains to current pharmacy practice and to the pharmacy technician's role changes in the future. Therefore, rather than listing over 100 drugs, their uses, side effects, and interactions, this chapter provides a process for reviewing drugs. The format was designed to accommodate three criteria:

1. The review of drugs should be efficient and effective.
2. The review of drugs should be uniform.
3. The review of drugs should be expandable to provide for new entrants to the marketplace.

Before we get to the drug literature review process, let's look at the status of pharmacy and how the role of the pharmacy technician has developed.

THE STATUS OF PHARMACY PRACTICE

There was a time when pharmacy was an art. The correct compounding process and the final elegance of the product was the state-of-the-art philosophy. Terms such as *secundum artem* (Latin, meaning "according to the art") and *pharmaceutically elegant* evolved during those bygone years.

Pharmacy has substantially changed and is a highly complex scientific field today. Advancements in dispensing hardware (e.g., parenteral and enteral pumps, drug delivery systems, counters, and dispensing systems) and the development of high-powered, potent drugs have created a reduced need for the art and a significantly increased need for knowing and understanding massive amounts of information required to assure the greatest possible safety and effective outcome of drug therapy for patients.

THE ROLE OF PHARMACY TECHNICIANS

Sophisticated advances in technology, changes in social attitudes about health, and concerns over health-care economics have impacted on pharmacy in another way. Pharmacists who traditionally have provided drug dispensing services are now moving into new facets of pharmacy (e.g., computer technology, high-risk drug monitoring, financial management, and specialized pharmacy such as outpatient parenteral chemotherapy and parenteral nutrition). The traditional pharmacy workload (filling drug orders and dispensing) is increasingly handled by pharmacy support staff. This is known as the distributive pharmacy practice and will be discussed later in this unit (Chapter 5). The pharmacy technician's expanding role will require more extensive expertise in the areas of drug dosages, side effects, predictable reactions, and other drug-related issues.

The pharmacy technician is often the final link in the continuity of care between the patient and the illness, and the patient and the drug. The pharmacy technician supplies the drugs and the information, and, as the protector of a patient's health, must make every effort to assure that the patient's rights of expectation are met.

Patient's Rights of Expectation

The patient has the right to expect:

- Protection from unwanted discomfort resulting from drug therapy
- Information regarding side effects, drug reactions, and other drug-related limiting characteristics
- Preparedness for both the expected and unexpected occurrences due to drug therapy
- Vigilant effort to ensure reasonable safety in drug therapy
- Professional service and pharmacy expertise with each drug dispensed
- Complete, comprehendible, and current information on each drug dispensed
- Maintenance of confidentiality

The patient has responsibilities also. These obligations, however, should be expected only after the pharmacy technician has met his or her obligations and presented the patient with appropriate instructions. At times, it may be necessary to remind patients of some of these responsibilities in order to assure the greatest safety and best outcome for the chosen drug therapy.

Patient's Responsibilities

The patient is responsible for:

- Providing complete and accurate information
- Complying with given directions
- Communicating unfavorable signs and symptoms after drug therapy has begun
- Asking questions when instructions are not understood completely

CHANGING ROLES FOR PHARMACY TECHNICIANS

The pharmacy technician's role as a dispenser of medications is destined to grow. Although it is unlikely that any pharmacy technician will be able to learn and retain all the facts about each drug, it is important that he or she provides the correct drug information in compliance with the patient's right of expectation. The purpose of this chapter is to present a tool that will aid you in selecting facts that are pertinent to patients.

NEW ROLES REQUIRE NEW COMPETENCIES

How does the pharmacy technician begin to learn the many facts about each drug? The keys to learning and remembering information are categorizing drug groups, aggregating consistent facts, and making some generalizations. Not all drugs are absolute and fall neatly into a class, category, or set of data. However, the pharmacy technician must screen for potential side effects, interactions, and other potentially limiting outcomes before the patient takes that first dose. The pharmacy technician must make the patient aware of potentially dangerous side effects. The patient must be urged to notify the physician when those signs or symptoms actually occur.

CONFIDENCE BUILDS ON COMPETENCE

First, you must perform an academic exercise that will sharpen your curiosity and desire for probing. Learn to ask WHY? WHERE? and WHAT? After a while, you will become increasingly curious as the knowledge you acquire becomes filled with interest and surprises. As the information expands and the focused process for reviewing data permits you to retain large amounts of noteworthy information, your desire to probe further will sharpen.

Next, you must have an available source of authoritative references. These references include drug compendia, drug monographs, a medical dictionary, and a manual of illness and therapy.

References

- *Physicians' Desk Reference* (PDR)
- *American Hospital Formulary Service Drug Information*
- *AMA Drug Evaluations*
- Compendium of drug therapy
- Dorland, Gould, or Taber medical dictionary
- *The Merck Manual of Diagnosis and Therapy*

(*Note:* These are only a few of the many available references.)

REVIEWING DRUG MONOGRAPHS

Finally, you need the instrument that will help you sort through thousands of pages of data and extract what is necessary for your needs: the drug monograph. Drug monographs have variable formats. Knowing what to review will save you enormous amounts of time. All manufacturer monographs provide the following information about each drug:

- Description
- Action
- Indications
- Contraindications
- Usage in pregnancy
- Adverse reactions
- Dosages (and administration)
- Packaging availability

Additional areas of information are available for drugs when the information is applicable. For instance, many applicable drug monographs may address the following areas:

- Microbiology
- Warnings

- Precautions
- Laboratory interference
- Drug abuse and dependency
- Overdosage
- Pharmacology (and toxicology)
- Drug interactions

THE TOOL

The volume of information available for any drug is massive. It would be nice to learn and retain all the data that exist for each drug. However, the information you need to know about each drug in order to perform your job properly (i.e., select the correct drug, guard patients against unnecessary harm and discomfort, and guide patients in taking drugs appropriately) can be reduced to a realistic workable knowledge of drugs. Whenever possible, try to review as much data about a drug as you can. Practically, however, time may not permit you to indulge in an intensive reading of the material. Therefore, you must focus your reading on the facts pertinent to your needs. The following format is a tool to extract important information. Consistency is also very important in your attempt to retain as much information as possible.

Drug Review Format

1. Generic drug name
2. Representative drug trade name(s)
3. Other identification
4. Primary drug class
5. Intended indications for use
6. Other indications for use
7. Dosage limits
8. Potential drug and/or food interactions
9. Potential unwanted drug effects
10. Potential drug effect on existing disorders
11. Potential drug interference on laboratory tests
12. Noteworthy facts

1. Generic Drug Name The generic name of the drug is the non-proprietary name. There is no legal protection that a manufacturer can obtain for a generic drug product. The implication is that any manufacturer can produce a generic product as long as there are no patented brand name drugs for a generic drug with a patent still in effect.

2. Representative Drug Trade Name(s) Trade names are also referred to as brand names. Manufacturers select these special drug names in order to protect their product under the United States patent laws, which enable the patent holder to be the sole source producer of the drug for the 17-year period during which a patent is in effect. For example, Inderal is the brand name for the generic drug propranolol. In addition, the generic drugs penicillin and phenoxymethyl penicillin have many brand names: Veetids, Pentids, Pen Vee K, Wycillin, V-Cillin K, and many more. (*Note:* Patent holders can license other manufacturers to produce a drug. Once a patent on a drug expires, any company can produce the drug under a new brand name and promote it, using that brand name). Companies can produce the drug under its generic name also.

3. Other Identification Some drugs are given acronyms or "nick-names." Many abbreviated names may be used universally, while others are used in a specific locale, hospital, or geographic section. For example, hydrochlorothiazide may also be written as HCTZ, Chlor-trimeton as CT, tetracycline as TCN, digoxin as dig, and nitroglycerin as TNG or NTG.

4. Primary Drug Class Some drugs may possess more than one clinical use. However, the drug will be categorized under a primary drug class. This class depends on the manufacturer's primary intended use and Food and Drug Administration (FDA) approval. Drugs are commonly found to have therapeutic use for multiple disorders. A prime example is propranolol. This drug was originally marketed as a beta-adrenergic blocking cardiovascular agent indicated for angina. Subsequently, propranolol was found to be effective in the treatment of migraine headaches. The drug is still primarily a cardiovascular agent, but its use for migraine headaches is widely accepted.

5. Intended Indications for Use The disorders for which a drug is to be used are identified only after many years of research and clinical trials on patients. The drug producer submits a new drug application (NDA) to the FDA with an enormous amount of information to support the use and safety of the drug. Upon FDA approval and an assigned national drug code (NDC), the manufacturer is able to market the drug for a particular indication.

6. Other Indications for Use As you saw in item four, Primary Drug Class, subsequent uses are often found for drugs. Consider the few examples in Table 2.1.

7. Dosage Limits The amount of a drug for each dose prescribed by the practitioner and taken by the patient represents the findings of many tests performed by drug producers, research institutions, universities and individual practicing physicians. This dose is referred to as the *usual dose.* Often, dosages are variable to meet the needs of patients without harmful or annoying side effects. Dosage limits indicate the highest dose that can produce a desired therapeutic outcome without adverse effects. Dosage limits documented by drug manufacturers also refer to uncompromised patients (i.e., patients without kidney, liver, or other disorders). Compromised patients require

TABLE 2.1 MULTIPLE USES OF DRUGS

Generic Drug	Intended Indication	Other Indications
acebutolol	hypertension	cardiac arrhythmias
atenolol	hypertension	angina
captopril	hypertension	heart failure (edema)
chlorthalidone	hypertension	edema
clorazepate	anxiety	epileptic seizures alcohol withdrawal
diazepam	anxiety	skeletal muscle spasms alcohol withdrawal
doxepin	depression	peptic ulcer
furosemide	edema	hypertension
nadolol	angina	hypertension
phenytoin	seizures	cardiac arrhythmias

changes in dosages to compensate for their inability to metabolize a drug as in the uncompromised patient. These special drug requirements are addressed in the literature.

8. Potential Drug and/or Food Interactions Generally, drug therapy and drug response are fairly unpredictable. Little has been documented in the area of food/drug interactions. The classic food/drug interaction case occurs in a class of drugs known as monoamine oxidase (MAO) inhibitors. MAO inhibitors are used primarily for the management of patients with depression. Hypertensive crisis has occurred in patients taking MAO inhibitors and ingesting foods in which aging or protein breakdown has been used to increase flavor. These foods include a variety of cheeses, sour cream, wine, beer, chicken liver, and more.

There has been considerable documentation regarding drug/drug interactions. These interactions are measured on their clinical significance (i.e., what percent of the population taking the drug has experienced the interaction?). The documented impact of drug interactions on patients is an important benchmark, because many interactions may not be readily observable or measurably harmful for a majority of patients.

9. Potential Unwanted Drug Effects You may be more familiar with this area referred to as drug side effects, adverse reactions, or untoward reactions. The word *unwanted* is stressed here because some side effects of drugs are desirable. For example, antihistamines are known for their sedative effect. Some companies have marketed sleeping compounds with an antihistamine as the active component.

Review the list at the end of this chapter for an understanding of the myriad of potentially unwanted drug effects. The list includes nearly every side effect that may occur from a drug therapy. These side effects were selected because they are observable by the patient and are, therefore, reportable. Changes in the quantity or quality of blood components have no value without a blood test. These changes are unobservable. However, unusual bruising is observable and may have significant meaning to the patient, physician, pharmacist, and the pharmacy technician.

10. Potential Drug Effect on Existing Disorders You will not find many pharmacists reviewing prescribed drugs for their effect on existing disorders. The relationship between drugs and disorders is significant and should not be overlooked. The consumption of drugs known to affect an existing disorder may either mask the condition, thereby hiding the relevant signs requiring action, or exacerbate (worsen the condition of) the disorder. For example, ulcerative colitis may be worsened by the use of antibiotics such as amoxicillin, ampicillin, penicillin, and cefaclor, or by the use of nonsteroidal anti-inflammatory drugs such as ibuprofen and indomethacin.

11. Potential Drug Interference on Lab Tests Drugs can have a marked effect on the results of blood, urine, and fecal laboratory tests. You should be aware of commonly performed tests, the range of normal measurement, and the drugs that can interfere with the test results.

Many of the following tests are performed routinely on patients:

Blood clotting tests
Complete blood count
Electrolyte tests
Erythrocyte sedimentation rates
Glucose tests
Heart enzyme tests
Kidney function tests
Lipid tests
Liver function tests

Occult blood tests
Routine urinalysis
Thyroid function tests
Uric acid test

12. Noteworthy Facts Up to this point, you have followed a strict information-collecting format that permits little flexibility: Review drug literature and check off the appropriate side effect, disorder, or laboratory test. However, you should also jot down those bits of information often overlooked and never communicated to the patient. For instance:

1. A patient receiving drug therapy to treat hypertension should be reminded to comply with a low-salt diet requirement.
2. Patients being treated for genital herpes (apparent by the use of the antiviral drug, acyclovir) should be reminded that a threat exists of transmitting the virus while the lesions are visible.
3. The effects of allopurinol therapy for gout may first be noticeable between 2 and 6 weeks.
4. Superinfection is always a threat with prolonged use of antibiotic drug therapy.
5. Lactose is an inert ingredient in many preparations but should be noted for lactose-intolerant patients.

These are just a few examples of noteworthy facts. As you proceed to review drugs and build your own reference on drugs, consider what patients have said to you regarding specific drugs. Jot this information down. Remember that all the idiosyncracies of a drug/person response are not contained in the literature, and nothing surpasses firsthand information based on actual experiences.

Review Table 2.2 that lists 25 popularly prescribed drugs. (This list was prepared to guide you with your first selection of drugs to review.)

TABLE 2.2

Generic Name	Trade Name
1. ranitidine	Zantac
2. fluoxetine	Prozac
3. conjugated estrogens	Premarin
4. glyburide	Micronase, Diabeta
5. nifedipine	Procardia
6. omeprazole	Prilosec
7. lovastatin	Mevacor
8. sertraline	Zoloft
9. enalapril	Vasotec
10. diltiazem	Cardizem
11. amoxicillin	Amoxil
12. digoxin	Lanoxin
13. albuterol	Proventil, Ventolin
14. cefaclor	Ceclor
15. warfarin sodium	Coumadin
16. ciprofloxacin	Cipro
17. nambutone	Relafen
18. medroxyprogesterone	Provera
19. captopril	Capoten
20. acetaminophen/codeine	Tylenol w/ codeine
21. clarithromycin	Biaxin
22. propoxyphen-N/APAP	Darvocet-N
23. phenytoin	Dilantin
24. loratadine	Claritin
25. paclitaxel	Taxol

It is much easier to study and remember facts about drugs when you follow a consistent plan. Try to establish "rules of similarity" for drug classes. For example, drugs absorbed from the intestine such as long-acting or sustained-release aspirin, all nonsteroidal anti-inflammatory agents, and beta-lactam antibiotics (e.g., penicillins) should be monitored closely in patient with ulcerative colitis. Study drugs individually within the same drug group. For instance, study each drug in the antibiotic class or cardiac grouping. This method will highlight the similarities shared by each drug within the group.

SIGNS, SYMPTOMS, AND SIDE EFFECTS

WHAT SIGNS AND SYMPTOMS TELL US

Many drug manufacturers perform studies to identify side effects that may occur while using a specific drug. Studies showing the incidence of side effects have not been abundant for many drugs. The subjectivity of many side effects such as drowsiness, cramps, thirst, and tingling presents a shortcoming in determining which side effects are truly significant. Even quantitative studies using blood, urine, and stool samples subjected to laboratory testing result in variable ranges of measurements.

Your role is instrumental because you are the last level of drug monitoring before the patient consumes the drug. You can be of substantive value to many patients by informing them of the high incidence of observable side effects of some drugs. Patients made aware of observable side effects are able to take timely action, which may result in discomfort-free and harm-free therapy.

WHEN A SIDE EFFECT IS SIGNIFICANT

There are few distinct guidelines, if any, to determine when a side effect is due to drug therapy or some other cause. Perhaps a general rule to adopt would be to answer the following questions: How much? How long? How unbearable?

"How much" refers to the quantity of the side effect. This situation can be illustrated nicely by using the common side effect of a rash. There are many types of rashes. The quantity or area affected will vary according to many patients. Quantity will depend on the area covered, the amount of itching or burning, the degree of redness, and other attributes of the rash. Other side effects may be quantified by the number of occurrences (e.g., three sharp shooting pains over a 4-hour period).

"How long" depends on the duration of the side effect. Some patients may not notice a side effect for a period of time. If, however, the degree of side effect makes the patient take more notice, 24 to 36 hours should be ample allowable time to determine if the side effect is lessening. You can see how the quantity and duration may relate to each other.

Finally, a patient will certainly be aware of "how unbearable" or intense a side effect may be. A side effect may cover a large body area, occur often, or last for a period of time, but not be unbearable. For instance, a patient may be covered by a rash on a large area of his or her body and not experience any discomfort. The intensity supersedes "how much" and "how long," resulting in a phone call to the pharmacist or practitioner. Intensity is extremely important, as may be illustrated by severe rashes caused by gold-containing compounds used for arthritis. A physician may weigh the discomfort of the side effect against the benefit of the drug therapy in an effort to determine whether or not to continue with the drug.

You will often be asked questions concerning drug side effects. The most you can do is review the drug monograph for side effects. Then determine from the patient "how much," "how long," "how unbearable," before giving advice to the patient. Check with the pharmacist for concurrence.

GROUPINGS OF SIDE EFFECTS CAN BE SIGNIFICANT

Side effects alone may have little meaning. Groupings of side effects occurring during a period while a patient is on drug therapy may represent an entirely different story. The following groupings of side effects have been prepared to flag situations that require timely intervention. These combinations of signs and symptoms may be suggestive of severe unobservable events.

Symptoms Occurring During Drug Therapy Requiring Immediate Notification of Physician

General Symptoms

joint pain
muscle pain
fever
chills
unusual bleeding
easy bruising
sore throat
sore mouth
discolored tongue
dark urine
wheezing
unusual/uncontrollable fatigue
muscle weakness
chest pain
severe abdominal pain
heart palpitations (pounding)
excessive vomiting
excessive diarrhea
hallucinations
depression
yellowing skin

Specific Combinations of Symptoms

Superinfection (fungal overgrowth)

black tongue
hairy tongue
sore tongue
sore mouth
glossitis

Serum Sickness

chills
fever
arthralgia
edema
pruritus (itching)
fatigue
rash

Excessive Potassium Loss

excessive thirst
tiredness
restlessness
muscle pains/cramps
nausea/vomiting
increased or rapid heart rate/pulse

Jaundice

yellowing skin
yellowing eyeballs

Blood Component Changes

(*Note:* Any combination of the following symptoms may represent a variety of blood changes or disorders such as agranulocytosis, leukopenia, beta-hemolytic anemia, or thrombocytopenia.)

headache	bruising
sore throat/sore mouth	unusual bleeding
muscle weakness	fever
fatigue	chills

Adverse Liver Involvement

fever	right upper quadrant pain
malaise	yellowing skin

Ulcerative Colitis

diarrhea
weight loss

Neuropathy

numbness
weakness
incoordination

Fluid and Electrolyte Disturbances

dry mouth	restlessness
thirst	muscle pain/cramps
weakness	muscle fatigue
lethargy	decreased urinary output
drowsiness	irregular heartbeat/pulse

Sympathomimetic Nervous System Disturbances

muscle cramps	nervousness
insomnia	tremor
nausea	headache
weakness	tachycardia
dizziness	palpitations

Anticholinergic Responses

blurred vision	amnesia
dry mouth	fatigue
mydriasis	urinary retention
change in pulse rate	constipation
drowsiness	

Cholinergic Responses

involuntary repetitive muscular movements	abdominal cramps
	bradycardia
nausea	bronchospasm
vomiting	flushing
diarrhea	lacrimation

miosis
excessive salivation
excessive sweating
urinary urgency
belching

Allergic Reaction

urticaria (hives)
pruritus
clammy skin
flushing
acute bronchospasm
shortness of breath
fluid retention with swelling
throat constriction
cyanosis (blue coloring)
wheezing
fainting

This chapter has covered the development of your importance as a pharmacy technician, patients' expectations, tools needed to properly evaluate drugs, and a means to understand the importance of symptoms and their combinations. Most importantly, as a pharmacy technician you provide patients with an extraordinary service. Where pharmacists move on to new specialties, you must fill the gap. It will be your competence that inspires patients' confidence.

EXERCISES

1. What is meant by *secundum artem?*
2. What can patients expect from us as professional pharmacy practitioners?
3. What should we expect from the patient to assure his or her safety and intended therapeutic outcome?
4. As pharmacy technicians how do we achieve safety, positive therapeutic outcome, and patient affordability?
5. Reviewing drugs by ______________________ makes it easier to learn more about a greater number of drugs.
6. Three important questions to ask when reviewing drugs are ______________________, ______________________, and ______________________.
7. List at least one text for each of the following types of references:
   A drug reference:
   A medical dictionary:
   A medical manual of disease:
8. The ideal drug monograph should contain the following information about each drug:
   (a)
   (b)
   (c)
   (d)
   (e)
   (f)
   (g)
   (h)

9. Additional drug monograph information may include:
   (a)
   (b)
   (c)
   (d)
   (e)
   (f)
   (g)
   (h)

10. What does a functional drug review format enable us to do?

11. What are the elements of a complete working format?
   (a)
   (b)
   (c)
   (d)
   (e)
   (f)
   (g)
   (h)
   (i)
   (j)
   (k)
   (l)

12. What is the generic name of a drug?

13. What is the trade name of a drug?

14. What organization determines and approves the primary therapeutic use of a drug?

15. True or False: Drugs may have more than one therapeutic use.

16. What mechanism enables the drug manufacturer to market a drug?

17. Many drugs used for hypertension as the intended primary indication may have therapeutic benefit for other indications.
   List some of these indications.
   (a)
   (b)
   (c)
   (d)

18. The usual dose is a measurement of ______________________________, which produces a desired benefit with minimal annoying side effects or harm to the patient.

19. Dosage limits represent the ______________________________, which produces the desired therapeutic outcome without adverse effects in the uncompromised patient.

20. In addition to potential drug reactions with other drugs, what represents another possible concern for interaction with prescribed drugs?

21. True or False: Drug side effects are always undesirable.

22. True or False: Drug side effects are not always observable.

23. Some side effects may be inconsequential alone, but significant when appearing in groups. Complete the following by filling in the missing words.
SUPERINFECTION
(a) black tongue
(b)
(c) sore tongue
(d)
(e) glossitis
EXCESSIVE ______________________________ LOSS
(a) excessive thirst
(b) tiredness
(c) restlessness
(d) musclepains/cramps
(e) nausea/vomiting
(f) increased or rapid heart rate/pulse

24. What are the signs and symptoms of serum sickness?

25. True or False: Drugs prescribed for specific conditions may also affect another existing disorder.

26. A term used to indicate a worsening condition is ____________________.

27. True or False: Drugs used as a specific therapy for a condition will never affect laboratory test results performed for that specific condition.

28. What is a compromised patient?

29. Name the following test:
BUN
CBC
PT
ESR
U/A
FBS

30. An inert ingredient in many oral drug preparations that should be noted in persons sensitive to it is called ______________________________.

31. What can cause superinfection?

32. Along with drug therapy for hypertension, what should be discussed with the patient?

33. Where are oral long-acting or sustained-release drugs released?

34. What are typical signs of an allergic reaction?

35. What is the key sign for jaundice?

36. Complete the following abbreviated review forms for each drug listed. It will be necessary to use additional reference sources.

DRUG MONOGRAPH
(Abbreviated Review Form)

DRUG GENERIC NAME: enalapril

Trade Name(s):

Drug Class:

Indications for Use:

Action:

Contraindications:

Adverse Drug Reactions (ADR):

Side Effects:

Dosage Limits:

Drug Interactions:

Warnings:

DRUG MONOGRAPH
(Abbreviated Review Form)

DRUG GENERIC NAME: diltiazem

Trade Names:

Drug Class:

Indications for Use:

Action:

Contraindications:

Adverse Drug Reactions (ADR):

Side Effects:

Dosage Limits:

Drug Interactions:

Warnings:

DRUG MONOGRAPH
(Abbreviated Review Form)

DRUG GENERIC NAME: lovastatin

Trade Name(s):

Drug Class:

Indications for Use:

Action:

Contraindications:

Adverse Drug Reactions (ADR):

Side Effects:

Dosage Limits:

Drug Interactions:

Warnings:

DRUG MONOGRAPH
(Abbreviated Review Form)

DRUG GENERIC NAME: sertraline

Trade Name(s):

Drug Class:

Indications for Use:

Action:

Contraindications:

Adverse Drug Reactions (ADR):

Side Effects:

Dosage Limits:

Drug Interactions:

Warnings:

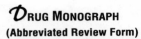

DRUG MONOGRAPH
(Abbreviated Review Form)

DRUG GENERIC NAME: ranitidine

Trade Name(s):

Drug Class:

Indications for Use:

Action:

Contraindications:

Adverse Drug Reactions (ADR):

Side Effects:

Dosage Limits:

Drug Interactions:

Warnings:

DRUG MONOGRAPH
(Abbreviated Review Form)

DRUG GENERIC NAME: fluoxetine

Trade Name(s):

Drug Class:

Indications for Use:

Action:

Contraindications:

Adverse Drug Reactions (ADR):

Side Effects:

Dosage Limits:

Drug Interactions:

Warnings:

DRUG MONOGRAPH
(Abbreviated Review Form)

DRUG GENERIC NAME: nifedipine

Trade Name(s):

Drug Class:

Indications for Use:

Action:

Contraindications:

Adverse Drug Reactions (ADR):

Side Effects:

Dosage Limits:

Drug Interactions:

Warnings:

DRUG MONOGRAPH
(Abbreviated Review Form)

DRUG GENERIC NAME: omeprazole

Trade Name(s):

Drug Class:

Indications for Use:

Action:

Contraindications:

Adverse Drug Reactions (ADR):

Side Effects:

Dosage Limits:

Drug Interactions:

Warnings:

DRUG MONOGRAPH
(Abbreviated Review Form)

DRUG GENERIC NAME: ciprofloxacin

Trade Name(s):

Drug Class:

Indications for Use:

Action:

Contraindications:

Adverse Drug Reactions (ADR):

Side Effects:

Dosage Limits:

Drug Interactions:

Warnings:

DRUG MONOGRAPH
(Abbreviated Review Form)

DRUG GENERIC NAME: glyburide

Trade Name(s):

Drug Class:

Indications for Use:

Action:

Contraindications:

Adverse Drug Reactions (ADR):

Side Effects:

Dosage Limits:

Drug Interactions:

Warnings:

CHAPTER 3

Terminology

OBJECTIVES

When you have completed this chapter, you will be able to:

1. dissect the medical terms in order to decipher the meaning
2. build a vocabulary of medical terms
3. associate word roots with anatomical systems

WORD DEVELOPMENT: USAGE AND COMPONENTS

Language is the foundation of communication. *Jargon* is language that is special to a geographical area, social class, age group, or occupation.

As a pharmacy technician, you should be familiar with where and how a drug works. In order to properly understand the workings of any drug, you must have a basic medical/pharmaceutical vocabulary. You are not expected to know the meaning of every medical term used in anatomy, physiology, or disease condition. Likewise, it is impossible to know every pharmacy term used to express drug activities or sites of action.

Learning some basic principles behind the process of forming medical terms from components will enable you to dissect any word, understand it, and use it appropriately. This chapter addresses word components, their meanings, and word formation.

In medicine, most words follow a general equation for their development:

Prefix + Root + Suffix = Word

(*Note:* You may not always find these three parts in every medical word. In most cases, however, you should find a root and suffix.) The parts of the word are called its components. The prefix usually tells where and how or what. The prefix *sub-,* for example, notes "below" or "less than," as in the word *subcutaneous,* meaning, "beneath the skin." *Tachy-* in *tachycardia* is telling you how the heart is beating or contracting. Tachycardia denotes an increase or acceleration (*tachy-* meaning "rapid or swift") in the heart rate.

The root portion of a medical term tells you what system is being affected. Refer to our previous examples—*subcutaneous* and *tachycardia.* The root portion, *cut-* in subcutaneous, refers to skin, which is part of the integumentary system (this anatomical system includes skin, hair, nails, sweat glands, and sebaceous glands). *Cardi-* in tachycardia is a cardiovascular system root component referring to the heart.

Suffixes may be categorized as diagnostic (e.g., *-itis,* indicating a reddening or inflammation), symptomatic (e.g., *-algia,* expressing a pain symptom), or operative (e.g., *-ectomy,* denoting an excision or "cutting out"). There are many suffixes that may be interpreted differently and cross over these categories. You may question whether a suffix really belongs in a selected category. For the purposes of this text, we merely want to grasp some basic principles involved in word formation. This chapter will enable you to develop an ability to break down most medical and pharmacy terms successfully and understand their appropriate meanings. Experience and exposure to more words through your readings will also help you to develop your own subcategories that you will use to define many words.

You will avoid error and confusion by interpreting medical and pharmaceutical terms from right to left. For example, the word *antibiotic* has a definite prefix, root, and suffix. Reading from right to left, note the following:

suffix: *-(t)ic—t* = one of a number of letters used to connect the components of medical terms; *-ic* means "pertaining to."

root: *bio-* —means "life"

prefix: *anti-* —means "against"

An antibiotic, literally defined, expresses something that is against life or interferes with life. In fact, an antibiotic is an agent that is used to destroy or interfere with the development of harmful organisms (often called pathogenic bacteria).

Let's look at a more complex medical term, which, dissected from left to right, results in a wrong meaning: *osteomalacia.*

Osteomalacia, broken down into its components from left to right, looks like this:

oste—oma—lacia

oste- —denotes "bone"

oma- —refers to tumors

-lacia—this component becomes meaningless

The resulting definition for this word, based on a left-to-right interpretation, erroneously leads you to believe this word refers to a bone tumor.

Correctly broken down from right to left, however, the word becomes:

oste-o-malacia

-malacia—"softening of a part"

o- —a component-combining letter

oste- —denoting "bone"

You now have the true definition of *osteomalacia*—"bone softening."

The components in Tables 3.1 through 3.13 will provide a good foundation upon which to build a solid vocabulary. Always check with any of a number of medical dictionaries for words or components used less often and enter them in your personal reference file.

TABLE 3.1 LETTER COMBINATION SOUNDS AND PLURALIZATION

Letter Combination	Sound	Singular	Plural
ch	k	-a	-ae
cn	n	-ex	-ces
gn	n	-is	-es
ph	f	-on	-a
pn	n	-um	-a
ps	s	-us	-i
rh	r	-itis	-itides

Examples:
chelation sounds like "kelation"
cnemis sounds like "nemis"
gnathion sounds like "nathion"
pharmacy sounds like "farmacy"
pneumonia sounds like "neumonia"
psychogenic sounds like "syckogenic"
rhinitis sounds like "rynitis"

TABLE 3.2 COMMON PREFIXES IN MEDICAL TERMINOLOGY

Prefix	Meaning	Example
a-, an-	lacking	anemia
ab-	away from	abnormal
ad-	above, on top of	adrenal
ambi-	denoting two	ambidexterous
amphi-	around	amphicrania
ana-	up, back again	anabiosis
ante-	just before	antepartum
anti-	oppose, against	antibiotic
apo-	away, separation	apocrine
bi-	two	bilateral
brady-	slow	bradycardia
cata-	down, downward, against	catabolism
contra-	against, opposite	contraceptive
de-	preventing, away from	desensitize
di-	referring to two	dichromatopsia
dia-	through	diaphoresis
dis-	apart, separation	dislocation
dys-	difficult	dyspnea
e-, ec-, ex-, es-	away from, beyond	exophthalmus
ecto-	outside, outer part	ectoretina
erythro-	redness	erythrocyte
extra-	outside, beyond	extrarenal
glyco-	sweetness	glycosuria
hemi-	half	hemigastrectomy
hyper-	excess	hypercalcemia
hypo-	deficiency	hypocalcemia
idio-	individual, distinct	idiopathic
infra-	below	infraorbital
intra-	within	intramuscular
juxta-	of close proximity	juxtacortical
lepto-	thin, narrow, mild, weakness	leptopellic
macro-	large	macroblepharia
meg-, magal-	huge, excessively large	megacolon
mesa-, meso-	middle	mesoderm
meta-	change, transformation	metabolism
micro-	very small	microgastria
olig-	very little	oliguria
omni-	all	omnivorous
pachy-	thickening	pachyostosis
para-	near	paracentesis
per-	puncture, through	percutaneous
peri-	around, enclosed	pericarditis
phaco-	denoting eye lens	phacohymenitis
poly-	excessive	polyuria
post-	after, behind	postclavicular
pre-	before, in front of	prechordal
pro-	before, in front of	prochondral
pseudo-	false	pseudoangina
py-, pyo-	denoting plus	pyorrhea
pyr-, pyreto	fever, heat	pyrogenic
re-	return, back, again	recalcification
retro-	backward	retroflexion
sclero-	hardening, stiffening	scleroderma
semi-	half	semipermeable
skeleto-	denoting the skeleton	skeletization
steno-	constriction, narrowing, shortening	stenocoriasis
sub-	less than, beneath	subcutaneous
super-	above	superalimentation
supra-	above	supranasal
sym-	with, along, beside	symbiosis
syn-	joined together	synanastomosis
tachy-	accelerated	tachycardia
trans-	across, in the process of change	transurethral
tri-	denoting three	triceps
ultra-	beyond, excess	ultraligation
un-	not, reversal	unconsciousness

TABLE 3.3 COMMON ROOTS IN TERMINOLOGY OF THE CARDIOVASCULAR SYSTEM

Root	Meaning	Example
angi-	vessel, vein, artery	angioplasty
cardio-	heart	cardiomegaly
-cardium	heart	pericardium
cor-	heart	percordial
corona-	heart vessels	coronary
-cyte	cell	hematocyte
-emia	blood	hyperemia
hem-, heme-, hemato-	blood	hemapoiesis
lien-	spleen	lienocele
lymphaden-	lymph nodes	lymphadenitis
lymphangi-	lymph vessels	lymphangitis
phlego-	denoting veins	phlebogenous
splen-	spleen	splenectasis
vas-, vaso-	vessel	vasoconstrictor
veni-, veno-	vein	venipuncture

TABLE 3.4 COMMON ROOTS IN TERMINOLOGY OF THE DIGESTIVE SYSTEM

Root	Meaning	Example
arch-	anus	architis
bucca-	cheek	buccoversion
celi-	abdomen	celioma
cheil-	lip	cheilotomy
cholangi-	bile duct	cholangiectasis
cholecyst-	gallbladder	cholecystectomy
choledoch-	bile duct	choledocholithiasis
col-	large intestine	coloptosis
copro-	feces	coprolith
dento-	refers to teeth	dentoid
entero-	small intestine	enteritis
gastro-	stomach	gastritis
gingivo-	gums	gingivitis
gloss-	tongue	glossitis
gnatho-	jaw	gnathodynia
hepato-	liver	hepatitis
labi-	lip	labiomycosis
lapar-	abdominal wall	laparotomy
odont-	tooth	odontalgia
oro-, os-	mouth, opening	osculum
procto-	rectum	proctoscopy
ptyalo-	saliva	ptyalorrhea
recto-	denoting the rectum	rectoclysis
sial-	saliva	sialogogue
staphyl-	palate	staphyloptosis
stoma, stomato-	opening, mouth	stomatalgia
ulo-	gums	uloglossitis
urano-	palate	uranoplasty

TABLE 3.5 COMMON ROOTS IN TERMINOLOGY OF THE GENITO-URINARY SYSTEM

Root	Meaning	Example
colp-	vagina	colporrhagia
cyst-	bladder	cystoscopy
episio-	referring to the vulva	episiotomy
funicul-	small cord	funiculopexy
hyster-	uterus	hysterectomy
metro-	uterus	metrophlebitis
nephr-	kidney	nephrectomy
oophor-	ovary	oophorectomy
orchid-	testicles	orchidopexy
oscheo-	scrotum	oscheocele
pubio-, pubo-	pubic region	pubiotomy
pyel-	part of the kidney	pyelitis
ren-	kidney	renal
salping-	fallopian tubes	salpingostomy
spermo-, spermato-	denotes sperm	spermatocele
trachel-	cervix	trachelectomy
ur-, uro-, urono-	refers to urine and the urinary tract	uroclepsia
vesico-	refers to the urinary bladder	vesicotomy

TABLE 3.6 COMMON ROOTS IN TERMINOLOGY OF THE INTEGUMENTARY SYSTEM

Root	Meaning	Example
cut-	skin	subcutaneous
derma-, dermato-	skin	dermatitis
follic-	secretory sac	folliculoma
histo-	tissue	histoclastic
lipo-	refers to fat tissue	lipoblastoma
mamm-	breast	mammectomy
mast-	breast	mastodynia
onych-	nail	paronychia
pil-, pilo-	hair	pilonidal
sarco-	denotes flesh	sarcoadenoma
thel-	nipple	theleplasty
trich-, tricho-	hair	trichoglossia

TABLE 3.7 COMMON ROOTS IN TERMINOLOGY OF THE MUSCULO-SKELETAL SYSTEM

Root	Meaning	Example
arthr-	joint	arthritis
cheiro-, chiro-	refers to the hand	cheirospasm
chondro-	cartilage	chondrodynia
cranio-	skull	craniopathy
facio-	refers to the face	facioplegia
leiomyo-	smooth muscle	leiomyoma
myelo-	narrow	osteomyelitis
myo-	skeletal muscle	myomalacia
os-	bone	osseous
osteo-	bone	osteoporosis
pod-	refers to the foot	pododynia
rhabdomyo-	striated muscle	rhabdomyanectomy
tendo-, teno-	tendons	tendinoplasty

TABLE 3.8 COMMON ROOTS IN TERMINOLOGY OF THE NERVOUS SYSTEM

Root	Meaning	Example
cephal-	the head	cephalgia
cere-	brain	cerebrosclerosis
encephal-	within the head	encephalitis
meningo-	denotes the membranes covering the brain and spinal cord	meningitis
ment-	mind	dementia
myel-	spinal cord	myelitis
neuro-	nerve	neuralgia
phren-	mind	phrenastenia
psych-	mind	psychosis
rach-	spinal column	rachialgia
spondyl-	vertebrae	spondylopathy

TABLE 3.9 COMMON ROOTS IN TERMINOLOGY OF THE RESPIRATORY SYSTEM

Root	Meaning	Example
broncho-	windpipe	bronchospasm
laryng-	voice box	laryngectomy
naso-	refers to the nose	nasosinusitis
-osmia	smell	hyperosmia
-pnea	act of breathing	dyspnea
pneumo-	lungs	pneumocentesis
pulmo-	lungs	pulmonitis
rhin-	nose	rhinitis
thoraco-	refers to the chest	thoracobronchotomy
trache-, tracheo-	air tube to lungs	tracheaectasis
trachelo-	denotes neck	trachelodynia

TABLE 3.10 COMMON ROOTS IN TERMINOLOGY OF THE SENSE ORGANS

Root	Meaning	Example
audit-	hearing	auditory
auri-	ear	auripuncture
bleph-, blephar-	eyelid	blepharitis
dacryaden-	tear gland	dacryadenitis
dacryo-	tears	dacryagogue
dacryocyst-	tear sac	dacryocystocele
derat-	cornea	keratitis
irid-	iris	iridectomy
myring-	eardrum	myringotomy
oculo-	denoting the eye	oculomotor
ophthalm-	eye	ophthalmology
-opia	vision, sight	diplopia
optico-, opto-	relating to the eye or vision	opticopupillary
ot-	ear	otitis
palpebr-	eyelid	palpebral
phaco-	eye lens	phacoma

TABLE 3.11 DIAGNOSTIC SUFFIXES

Suffix	Meaning	Example
-cele	swelling, growing out	hydrocele
-ectasis	swelling, dilation	cardiectasis
-gram	tracing	electrocardiogram
-graph	record	encephalograph
-iasis	state or condition of, pathologic state	mydriasis
-itis	inflammation, reddening	gastritis
-malacia	softening	osteomalacia
-mania	irrational, madness	megalomania
-oid	denoting resemblance	carcinoid
-oma	denoting a tumor	dermatoma
-osis	denoting a deteriorating condition	osteomiosis
-pathy	a condition	dermatopathy
-phobia	fear	photophobia
-ptosis (pt = "t")	dropping, downward displacement	blepharoptosis
-rrhage, -rrhagia, -rrhagic	bursting forth	hemorrhage
-rrhea	flow	dysmenorrhea
-rrhexis	broken, burst	cardiorrhexis
-sthen, -sthenia	weakness	myasthenia

TABLE 3.12 OPERATIVE SUFFIXES

Suffix	Meaning	Example
-centesis	puncture	thorancentesis
-desis	binding	arthrodesis
-ectomy	excision, cutting out	gastrectomy
-oscopy	looking into	gastroscopy
-ostomy	making an opening	colostomy
-otomy	incision	gastrotomy
-pexy	fixing an organ in place	gastropexy
-plasty	shaping or forming	rhinoplasty
-rrhaphy	suture	gastrorrhaphy

TABLE 3.13 SYMPTOMATIC SUFFIXES

Suffix	Meaning	Example
-aemia, -emia	denoting blood	uremia
-algia	pain	myalgia
-dynia	pain	gastrodynia
-esthesia	denotes sensation	parasthesia
-genia	origin, production	myogenic
-osis	excessive	leukocytosis
-penia	lack	leukocytopenia
-trophy	denotes growth	hypertrophy

EXERCISES

These exercises contain excerpts from medical texts, references, professional journals, and other readings. See Figures 3.1 to 3.12. Review the words highlighted by arrows. Develop their meanings by using the prefix-root-suffix approach. List each word and its component development on the charts provided in this section (Figures 3.13 to 3.17).

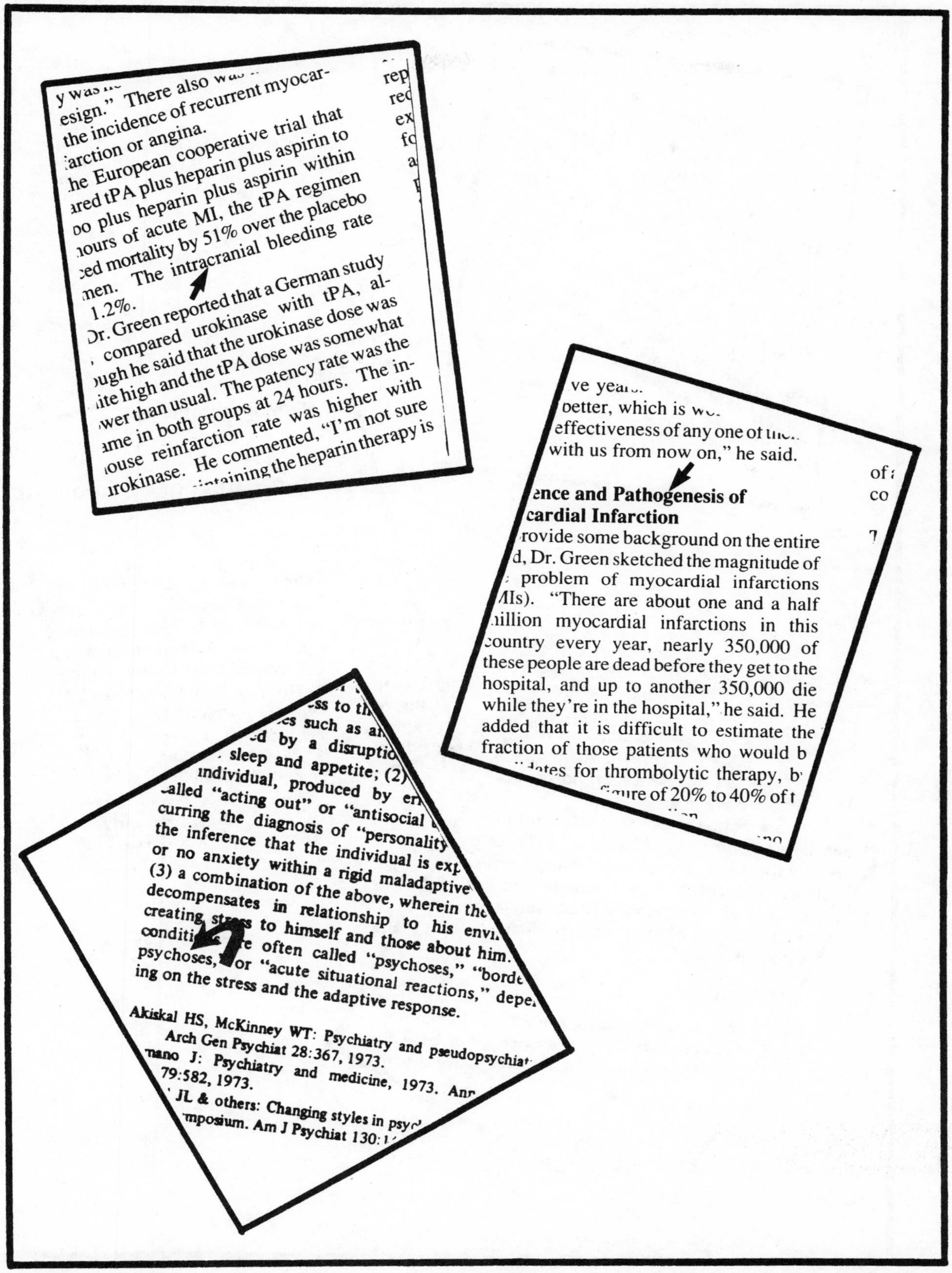

y was ...
esign." There also was ...
the incidence of recurrent myocar-
arction or angina.
he European cooperative trial that
ared tPA plus heparin plus aspirin to
oo plus heparin plus aspirin within
hours of acute MI, the tPA regimen
ced mortality by 51% over the placebo
men. The intracranial bleeding rate
1.2%.
Dr. Green reported that a German study
, compared urokinase with tPA, al-
ough he said that the urokinase dose was
ite high and the tPA dose was somewhat
wer than usual. The patency rate was the
ame in both groups at 24 hours. The in-
ouse reinfarction rate was higher with
urokinase. He commented, "I'm not sure
...ntaining the heparin therapy is

rep
rec
ex
fo
a

ve years.
better, which is w...
effectiveness of any one of the...
with us from now on," he said.

ence and Pathogenesis of
cardial Infarction

rovide some background on the entire
d, Dr. Green sketched the magnitude of
problem of myocardial infarctions
MIs). "There are about one and a half
nillion myocardial infarctions in this
country every year, nearly 350,000 of
these people are dead before they get to the
hospital, and up to another 350,000 die
while they're in the hospital," he said. He
added that it is difficult to estimate the
fraction of those patients who would b
...dates for thrombolytic therapy, b
...figure of 20% to 40% of t

of
co

ss to th
es such as an
d by a disruptio
sleep and appetite; (2)
individual, produced by en
called "acting out" or "antisocial
curring the diagnosis of "personality
the inference that the individual is exp
or no anxiety within a rigid maladaptive
(3) a combination of the above, wherein the
decompensates in relationship to his envi
creating stress to himself and those about him.
conditi... re often called "psychoses," "borde
psychoses," or "acute situational reactions," depe
ing on the stress and the adaptive response.

Akiskal HS, McKinney WT: Psychiatry and pseudopsychia...
Arch Gen Psychiat 28:367, 1973.
...mano J: Psychiatry and medicine, 1973. Ann
79:582, 1973.
... JL & others: Changing styles in psyc...
...mposium. Am J Psychiat 130:1...

FIGURE 3.1

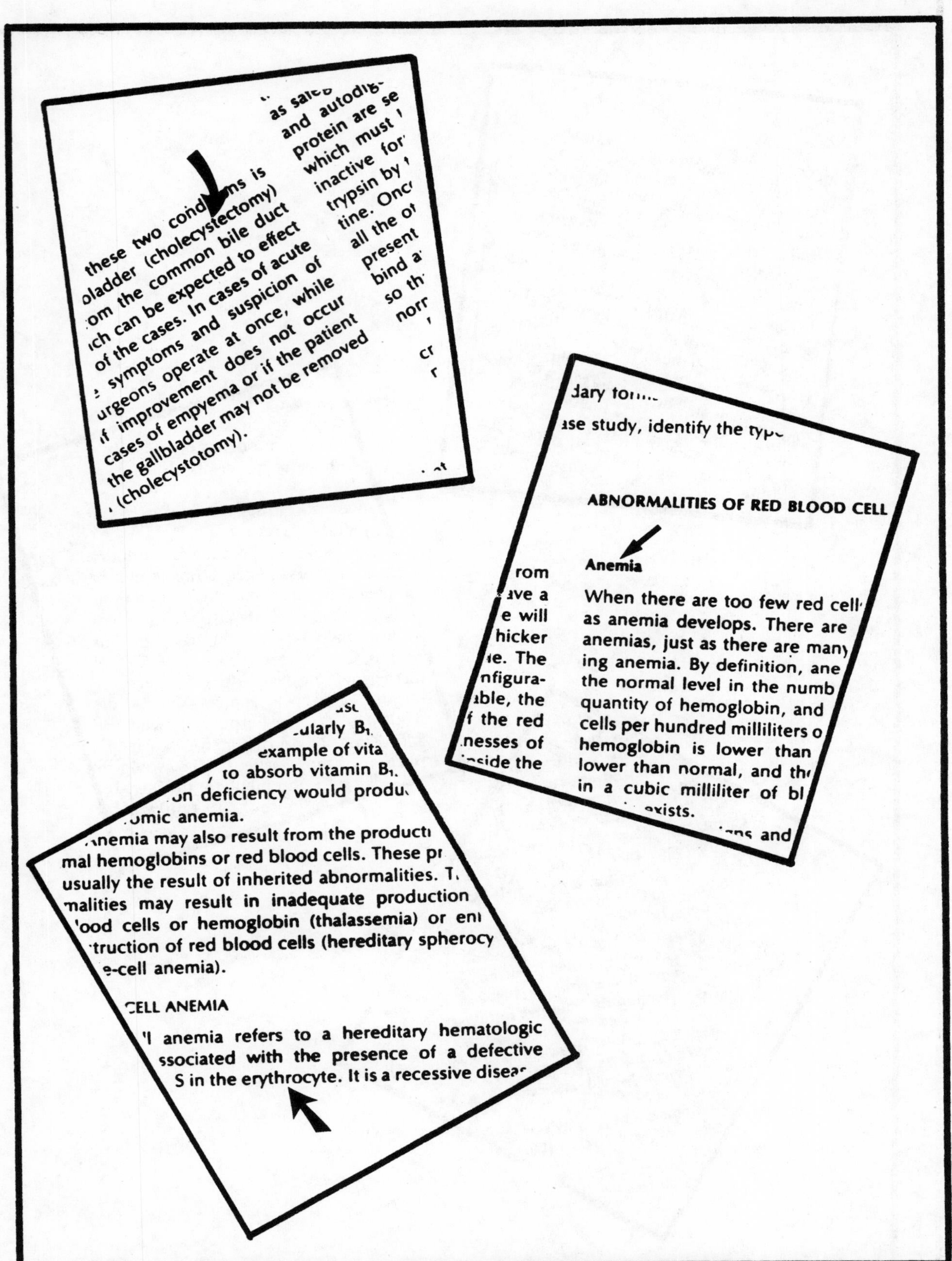
as saleo
and autodig-
protein are se
which must
inactive for
trypsin by
tine. Once
all the ot
present
bind a
so th
norr
these two conditions is
oladder (cholecystectomy)
om the common bile duct
ich can be expected to effect
of the cases. In cases of acute
symptoms and suspicion of
urgeons operate at once, while
f improvement does not occur
cases of empyema or if the patient
the gallbladder may not be removed
(cholecystotomy).
dary form
ase study, identify the type
ABNORMALITIES OF RED BLOOD CELL
Anemia
When there are too few red cell
as anemia develops. There are
anemias, just as there are many
ing anemia. By definition, ane
the normal level in the numb
quantity of hemoglobin, and
cells per hundred milliliters o
hemoglobin is lower than
lower than normal, and th
in a cubic milliliter of bl
exists.
and
rom
ave a
e will
hicker
ie. The
nfigura-
able, the
f the red
nesses of
inside the
ularly B
example of vita
to absorb vitamin B
on deficiency would produ
omic anemia.
Anemia may also result from the producti
mal hemoglobins or red blood cells. These pr
usually the result of inherited abnormalities. T
malities may result in inadequate production
lood cells or hemoglobin (thalassemia) or en
truction of red blood cells (hereditary spherocy
e-cell anemia).
CELL ANEMIA
l anemia refers to a hereditary hematologic
ssociated with the presence of a defective
S in the erythrocyte. It is a recessive disea

FIGURE 3.2

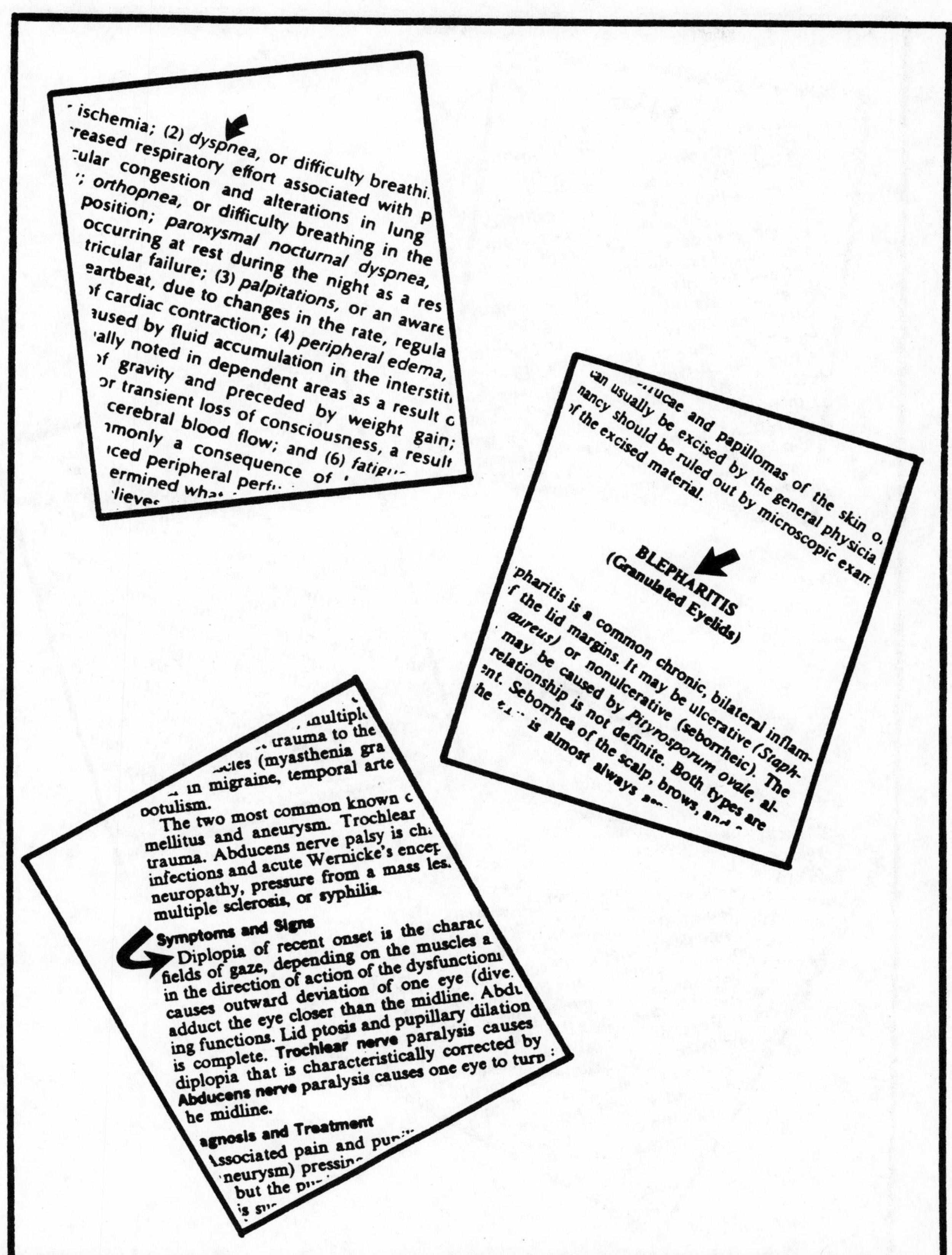

ischemia; (2) *dyspnea*, or difficulty breathi
reased respiratory effort associated with p
ular congestion and alterations in lung
; *orthopnea*, or difficulty breathing in the
position; *paroxysmal nocturnal dyspnea*,
occurring at rest during the night as a res
tricular failure; (3) *palpitations*, or an aware
eartbeat, due to changes in the rate, regula
of cardiac contraction; (4) *peripheral edema*,
aused by fluid accumulation in the interstit
ally noted in dependent areas as a result o
of gravity and preceded by weight gain;
or transient loss of consciousness, a result
cerebral blood flow; and (6) *fatig*
nmonly a consequence of
ced peripheral perf
ermined wha
lieve

rrucae and papillomas of the skin o
can usually be excised by the general physicia
nancy should be ruled out by microscopic exam
of the excised material.

BLEPHARITIS
(Granulated Eyelids)

pharitis is a common chronic, bilateral inflam-
f the lid margins. It may be ulcerative (*Staph-*
aureus) or nonulcerative (seborrheic). The
may be caused by *Pityrosporum ovale*, al-
relationship is not definite. Both types are
ent. Seborrhea of the scalp, brows, and
he e is almost always

multipl
trauma to the
scles (myasthenia gra
in migraine, temporal arte
botulism.

The two most common known c
mellitus and aneurysm. Trochlear
trauma. Abducens nerve palsy is ch
infections and acute Wernicke's encep
neuropathy, pressure from a mass les
multiple sclerosis, or syphilis.

Symptoms and Signs

Diplopia of recent onset is the charac
fields of gaze, depending on the muscles a
in the direction of action of the dysfunction
causes outward deviation of one eye (dive
adduct the eye closer than the midline. Abd
ing functions. Lid ptosis and pupillary dilation
is complete. **Trochlear nerve** paralysis causes
diplopia that is characteristically corrected by
Abducens nerve paralysis causes one eye to turn
he midline.

agnosis and Treatment

Associated pain and pu
neurysm) pressin
but the pu
is su

FIGURE 3.3

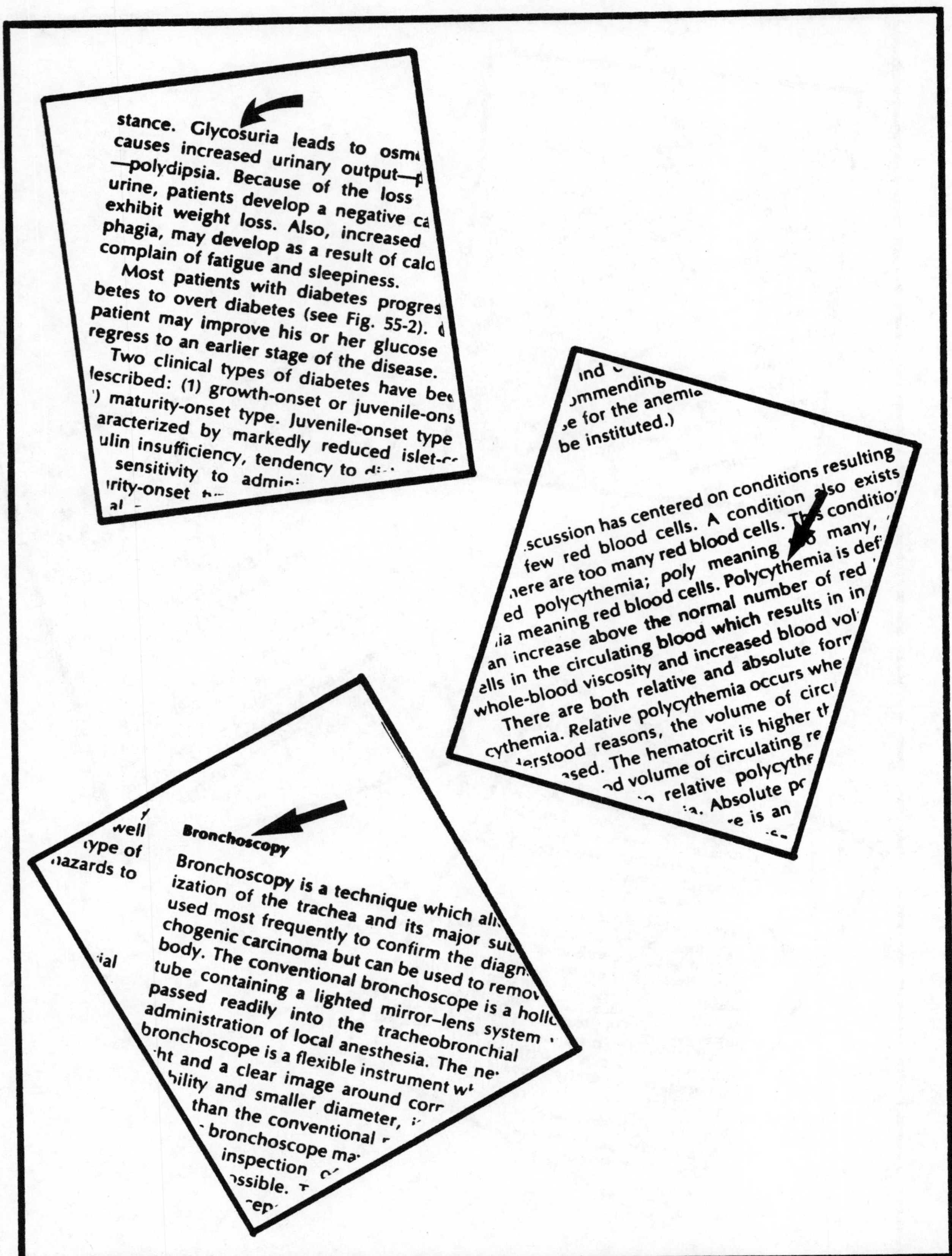

stance. Glycosuria leads to osm
causes increased urinary output—
—polydipsia. Because of the loss
urine, patients develop a negative ca
exhibit weight loss. Also, increased
phagia, may develop as a result of calo
complain of fatigue and sleepiness.
Most patients with diabetes progres
betes to overt diabetes (see Fig. 55-2).
patient may improve his or her glucose
regress to an earlier stage of the disease.
Two clinical types of diabetes have bee
lescribed: (1) growth-onset or juvenile-ons
) maturity-onset type. Juvenile-onset type
aracterized by markedly reduced islet-c
ulin insufficiency, tendency to
sensitivity to admin
rity-onset

ind
ommending
e for the anemia
be instituted.)

scussion has centered on conditions resulting
few red blood cells. A condition also exists
here are too many red blood cells. This conditio
ed polycythemia; *poly* meaning many,
ia meaning red blood cells. Polycythemia is def
an increase above the normal number of red
ells in the circulating blood which results in in
whole-blood viscosity and increased blood vol
There are both relative and absolute form
cythemia. *Relative* polycythemia occurs whe
derstood reasons, the volume of circ
ased. The hematocrit is higher th
d volume of circulating re
relative polycythe
a. Absolute p
e is an

well
type of
hazards to

ial

Bronchoscopy

Bronchoscopy is a technique which al
ization of the trachea and its major su
used most frequently to confirm the diagn
chogenic carcinoma but can be used to remov
body. The conventional bronchoscope is a holl
tube containing a lighted mirror–lens system
passed readily into the tracheobronchial
administration of local anesthesia. The ne
bronchoscope is a flexible instrument w
ht and a clear image around corr
bility and smaller diameter,
than the conventional
bronchoscope ma
inspection o
ssible.

FIGURE 3.4

route of excretion for these meta
lites.[2] Further metabolic disturban
may develop including acute re
failure, cardiac arrhythmias, or sud
death.[3]

Manifestations of acute tumor lysis syndrome

Hyperuricemia

Hyperuricemia (> 8.0 mg/dl)
one of the most common manifes
tions of acute tumor lysis syndrom
This metabolic disturbance may re
from increased production or
creased excretion of uric acid,

potassium
en up into functio
uptake limited only by
ply.[1] This provides the basis
cintigraphic imaging of per-
eas of the heart. Since vessels
ed up to 80% may still meet
l cardiac demands at resting
rate level, imaging offers no
nostic evidence of CAD when
formed under these conditions.[1]
herefore, a state of vasodilation
must be induced, whereby the perfu-
sion gradient between occluded and
nonoccluded vessels increases.[1,2,3] This
may be obtained by stressing the
patient to 90% of his/her maximal
rate. Traditional stress-testing
ertion presents prob-
not be maxi-
to

education
because i
informat
to you
would
terial
this
dep
Co
Ph
W

ate
ce amphc
ity in animals.[15]
munosuppressive agent
steroid with an undetermined b
in the reduction of the febrile reac
and potential for toxicity should
avoided in the compromised host wit
systemic mycosis.

Nephrotoxicity

Impairment of renal function is the
most common and important toxic
effect of therapy with amphotericin B
and is observed in greater than 80
percent of treated patients.[2,16-19] Al-
hough preexisting renal disease does
t appear to predispose patients to
manent renal damage caused b
otericin B, advanced a
e the risk.[19] The
rized by
al

1.
cr
the
days
patien
kidn

FIGURE 3.5

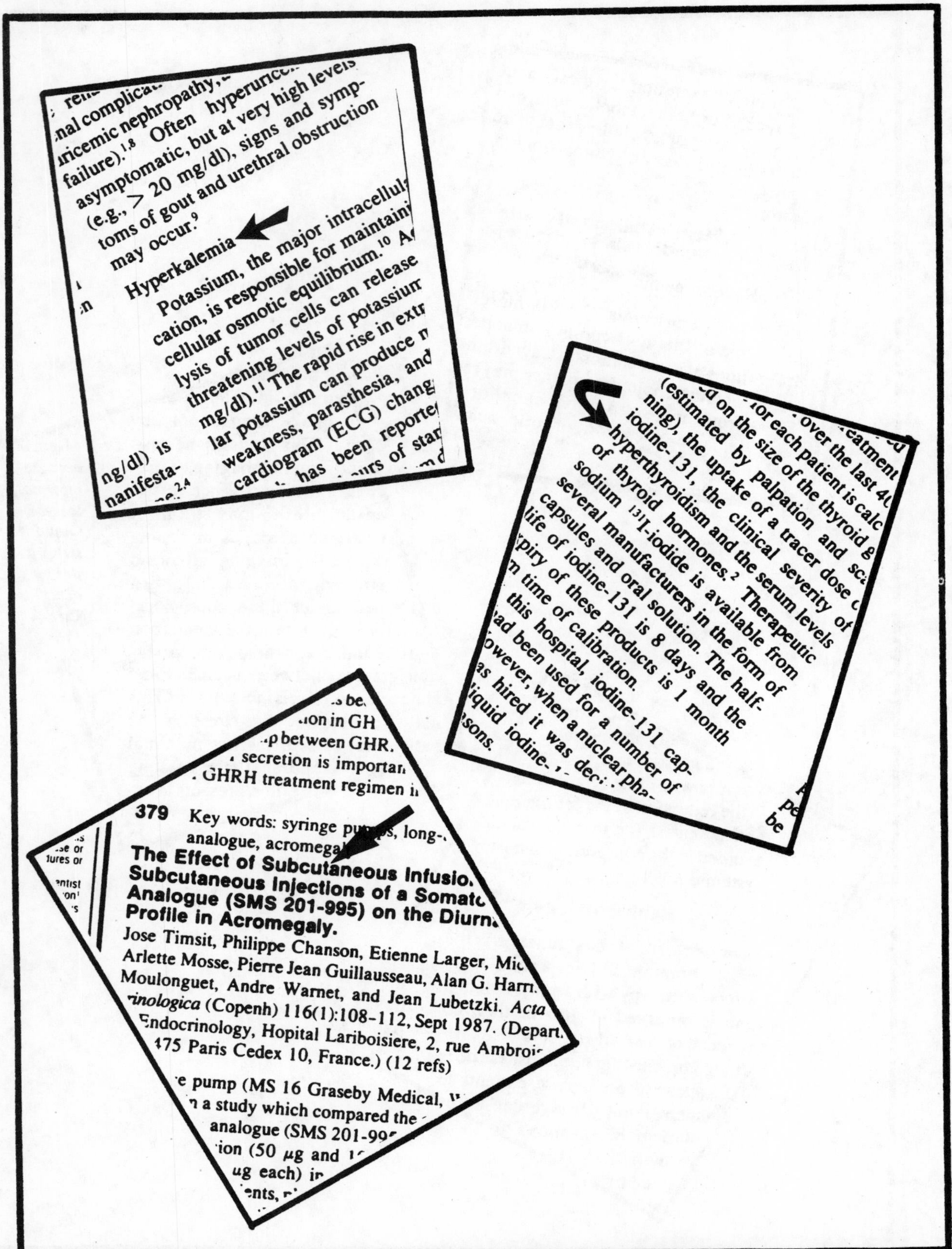

nal complicat
ıricemic nephropathy,
failure).[1,8] Often hyperuricem
asymptomatic, but at very high levels
(e.g., > 20 mg/dl), signs and symptoms of gout and urethral obstruction
may occur.[9]

Hyperkalemia

Potassium, the major intracellul
cation, is responsible for maintain
cellular osmotic equilibrium.[10] A
lysis of tumor cells can release
threatening levels of potassium
mg/dl).[11] The rapid rise in extr
lar potassium can produce m
weakness, parasthesia, and
cardiogram (ECG) chang
has been reporte

ng/dl) is
nanifesta-

eatment
over the last 4
for each patient is calc
d on the size of the thyroid g
(estimated by palpation and sc
ning), the uptake of a tracer dose o
iodine-131, the clinical severity of
hyperthyroidism and the serum levels
of thyroid hormones.[2] Therapeutic
sodium ^{131}I-iodide is available from
several manufacturers in the form of
capsules and oral solution. The half-
life of iodine-131 is 8 days and the
piry of these products is 1 month
n time of calibration.
this hospital, iodine-131 cap-
ad been used for a number of
owever, when a nuclear pha
as hired it was deci
liquid iodine-1
sons.

ion in GH
p between GHR.
secretion is importan
GHRH treatment regimen i

379 Key words: syringe pumps, long-
analogue, acromegal

The Effect of Subcutaneous Infusio
Subcutaneous Injections of a Somato
Analogue (SMS 201-995) on the Diurn
Profile in Acromegaly.

Jose Timsit, Philippe Chanson, Etienne Larger, Mic
Arlette Mosse, Pierre Jean Guillausseau, Alan G. Harr
Moulonguet, Andre Warnet, and Jean Lubetzki. *Acta*
rinologica (Copenh) 116(1):108–112, Sept 1987. (Depart.
Endocrinology, Hopital Lariboisiere, 2, rue Ambroi
175 Paris Cedex 10, France.) (12 refs)

e pump (MS 16 Graseby Medical,
n a study which compared the
analogue (SMS 201-99
ion (50 μg and 1
μg each) in
ents,

FIGURE 3.6

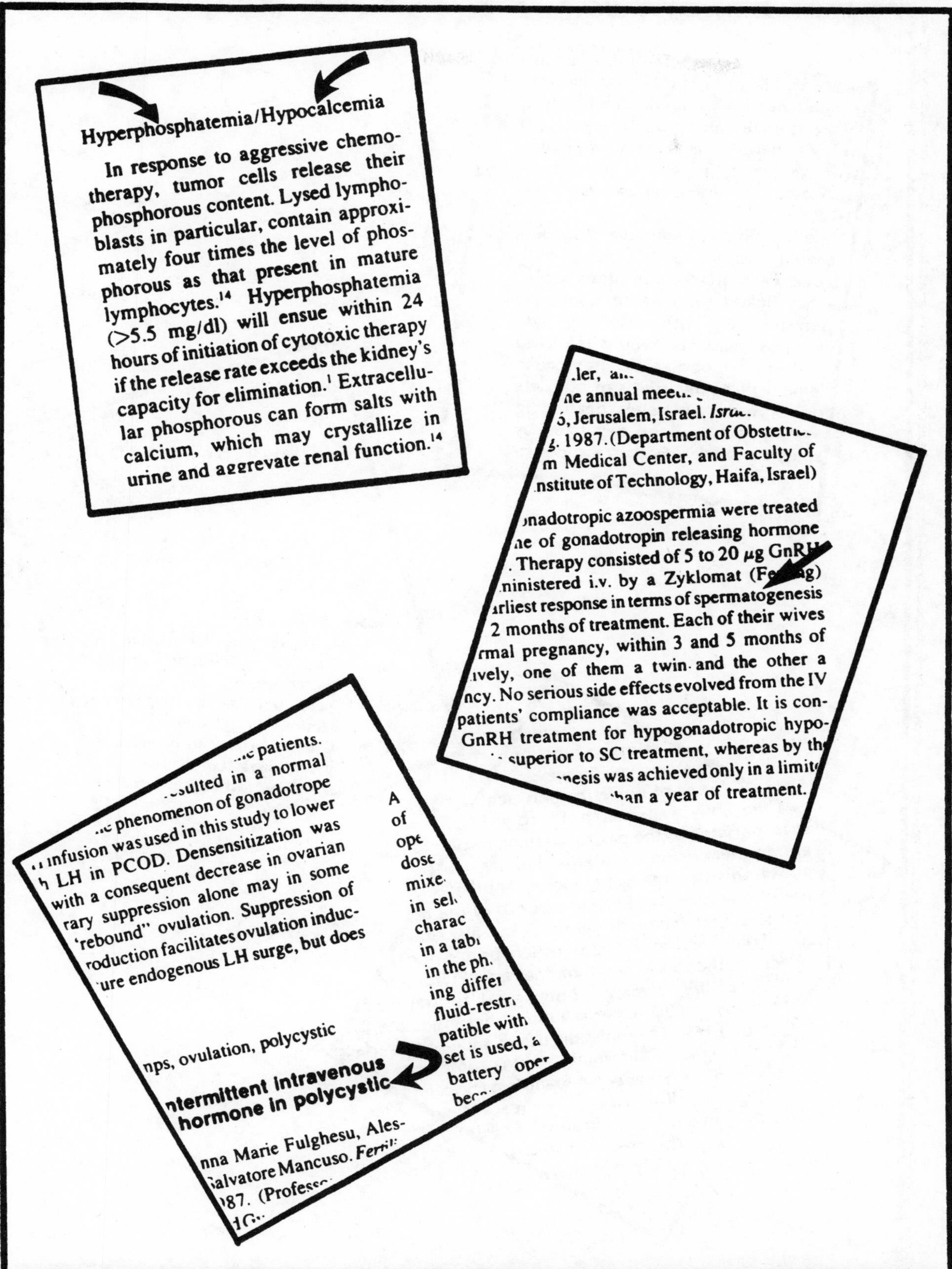

Hyperphosphatemia/Hypocalcemia

In response to aggressive chemotherapy, tumor cells release their phosphorous content. Lysed lymphoblasts in particular, contain approximately four times the level of phosphorous as that present in mature lymphocytes.[14] Hyperphosphatemia (>5.5 mg/dl) will ensue within 24 hours of initiation of cytotoxic therapy if the release rate exceeds the kidney's capacity for elimination.[1] Extracellular phosphorous can form salts with calcium, which may crystallize in urine and aggrevate renal function.[14]

.ler, a...
ne annual mee...
5, Jerusalem, Israel. *Isra...*
g. 1987. (Department of Obstetri...
m Medical Center, and Faculty of
nstitute of Technology, Haifa, Israel)

nadotropic azoospermia were treated
ne of gonadotropin releasing hormone
. Therapy consisted of 5 to 20 μg GnRH
ninistered i.v. by a Zyklomat (Fe...g)
arliest response in terms of spermatogenesis
2 months of treatment. Each of their wives
rmal pregnancy, within 3 and 5 months of
ively, one of them a twin and the other a
ncy. No serious side effects evolved from the IV
patients' compliance was acceptable. It is con-
GnRH treatment for hypogonadotropic hypo-
... superior to SC treatment, whereas by th
...nesis was achieved only in a limit
...han a year of treatment.

...c patients.
...sulted in a normal
...c phenomenon of gonadotrope
... infusion was used in this study to lower
h LH in PCOD. Densensitization was
with a consequent decrease in ovarian
rary suppression alone may in some
'rebound" ovulation. Suppression of
roduction facilitates ovulation induc-
ure endogenous LH surge, but does

nps, ovulation, polycystic

ntermittent intravenous
hormone in polycystic

nna Marie Fulghesu, Ales-
Salvatore Mancuso. *Ferti...*
987. (Profess...
1G...

A
of
ope
dose
mixe
in sel
charac
in a tab
in the ph
ing differ
fluid-restr
patible with
set is used, a
battery oper
bec...

FIGURE 3.7

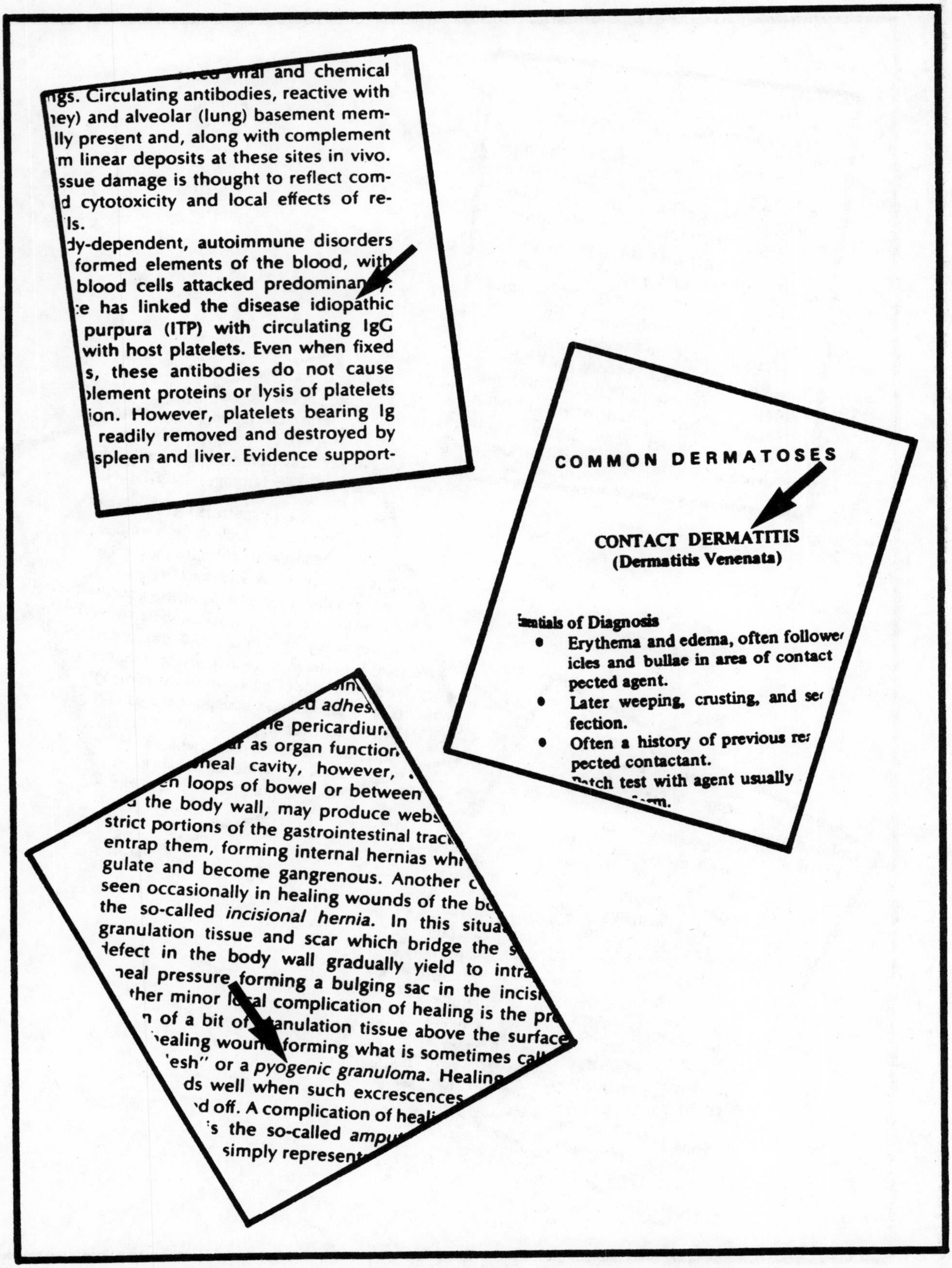

...wed viral and chemical
ngs. Circulating antibodies, reactive with
ney) and alveolar (lung) basement mem-
lly present and, along with complement
m linear deposits at these sites in vivo.
ssue damage is thought to reflect com-
d cytotoxicity and local effects of re-
ls.
dy-dependent, autoimmune disorders
formed elements of the blood, with
blood cells attacked predominantly.
e has linked the disease idiopathic
purpura (ITP) with circulating IgG
with host platelets. Even when fixed
s, these antibodies do not cause
plement proteins or lysis of platelets
ion. However, platelets bearing Ig
readily removed and destroyed by
spleen and liver. Evidence support-

COMMON DERMATOSES

CONTACT DERMATITIS
(Dermatitis Venenata)

...ntials of Diagnosis
- Erythema and edema, often followe... icles and bullae in area of contact ... pected agent.
- Later weeping, crusting, and se... fection.
- Often a history of previous re... pected contactant.
- Patch test with agent usually ...

...ed *adhes*...
...e pericardiu...
...r as organ functio...
...neal cavity, however, ...
...en loops of bowel or between
... the body wall, may produce webs
strict portions of the gastrointestinal trac...
entrap them, forming internal hernias wh...
gulate and become gangrenous. Another c...
seen occasionally in healing wounds of the bo...
the so-called *incisional hernia*. In this situa...
granulation tissue and scar which bridge the ...
defect in the body wall gradually yield to intra...
neal pressure forming a bulging sac in the incis...
ther minor local complication of healing is the pr...
n of a bit of granulation tissue above the surface
healing wound forming what is sometimes cal...
esh" or a *pyogenic granuloma*. Healing
ds well when such excrescences
d off. A complication of heal...
s the so-called *ampu*...
simply represent...

FIGURE 3.8

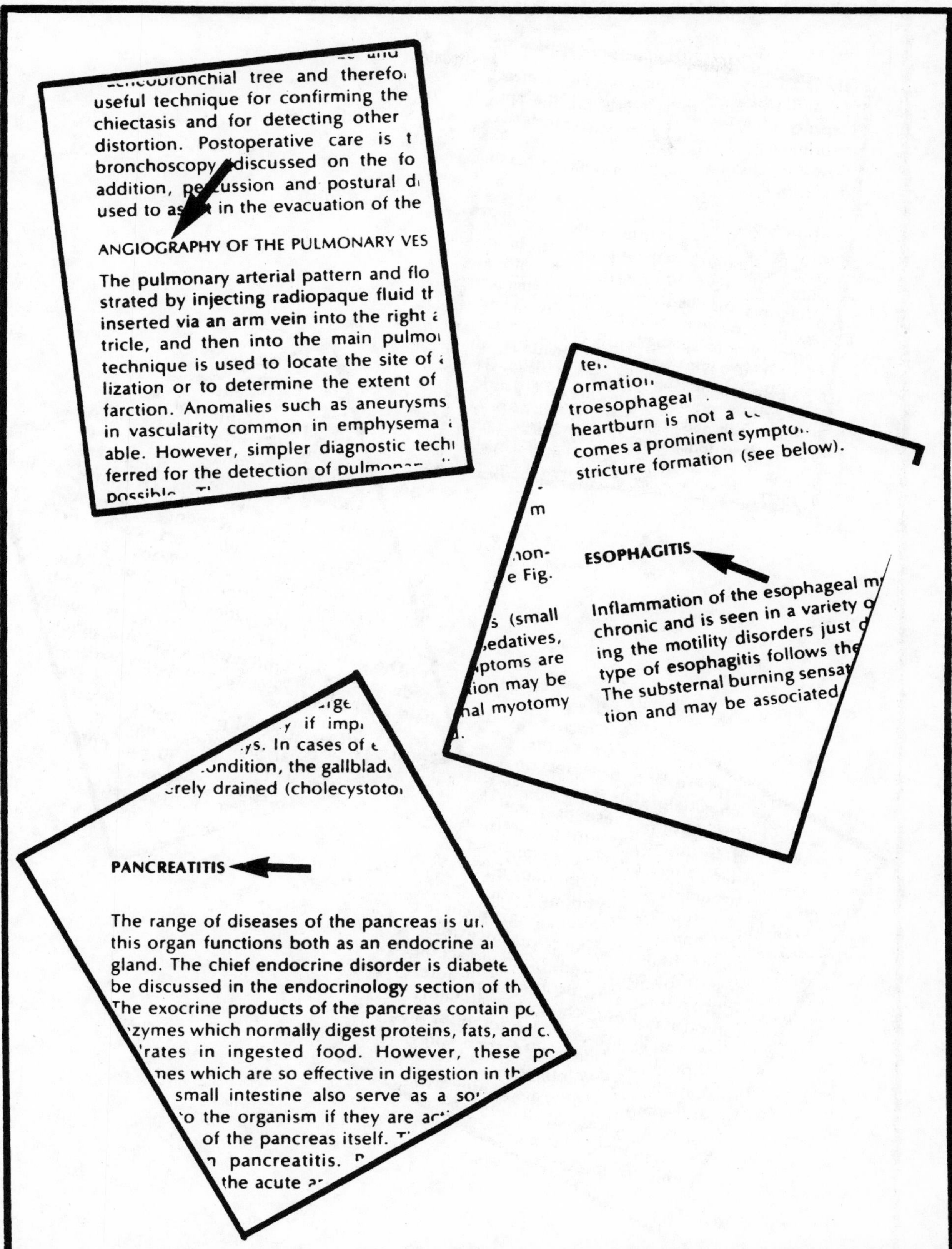

tracheobronchial tree and therefo
useful technique for confirming the
chiectasis and for detecting other
distortion. Postoperative care is t
bronchoscopy discussed on the fo
addition, percussion and postural d
used to assist in the evacuation of the

ANGIOGRAPHY OF THE PULMONARY VES

The pulmonary arterial pattern and flo
strated by injecting radiopaque fluid th
inserted via an arm vein into the right a
tricle, and then into the main pulmo
technique is used to locate the site of a
lization or to determine the extent of
farction. Anomalies such as aneurysms
in vascularity common in emphysema a
able. However, simpler diagnostic techi
ferred for the detection of pulmon
possible.

ormation
troesophageal
heartburn is not a
comes a prominent sympto
stricture formation (see below).

ESOPHAGITIS

Inflammation of the esophageal m
chronic and is seen in a variety o
ing the motility disorders just d
type of esophagitis follows the
The substernal burning sensat
tion and may be associated

ys. In cases of
condition, the gallblad
erely drained (cholecystoto

PANCREATITIS

The range of diseases of the pancreas is ur
this organ functions both as an endocrine a
gland. The chief endocrine disorder is diabete
be discussed in the endocrinology section of th
The exocrine products of the pancreas contain po
zymes which normally digest proteins, fats, and c
rates in ingested food. However, these po
nes which are so effective in digestion in th
small intestine also serve as a so
o the organism if they are ac
of the pancreas itself.
pancreatitis.
the acute a

FIGURE 3.9

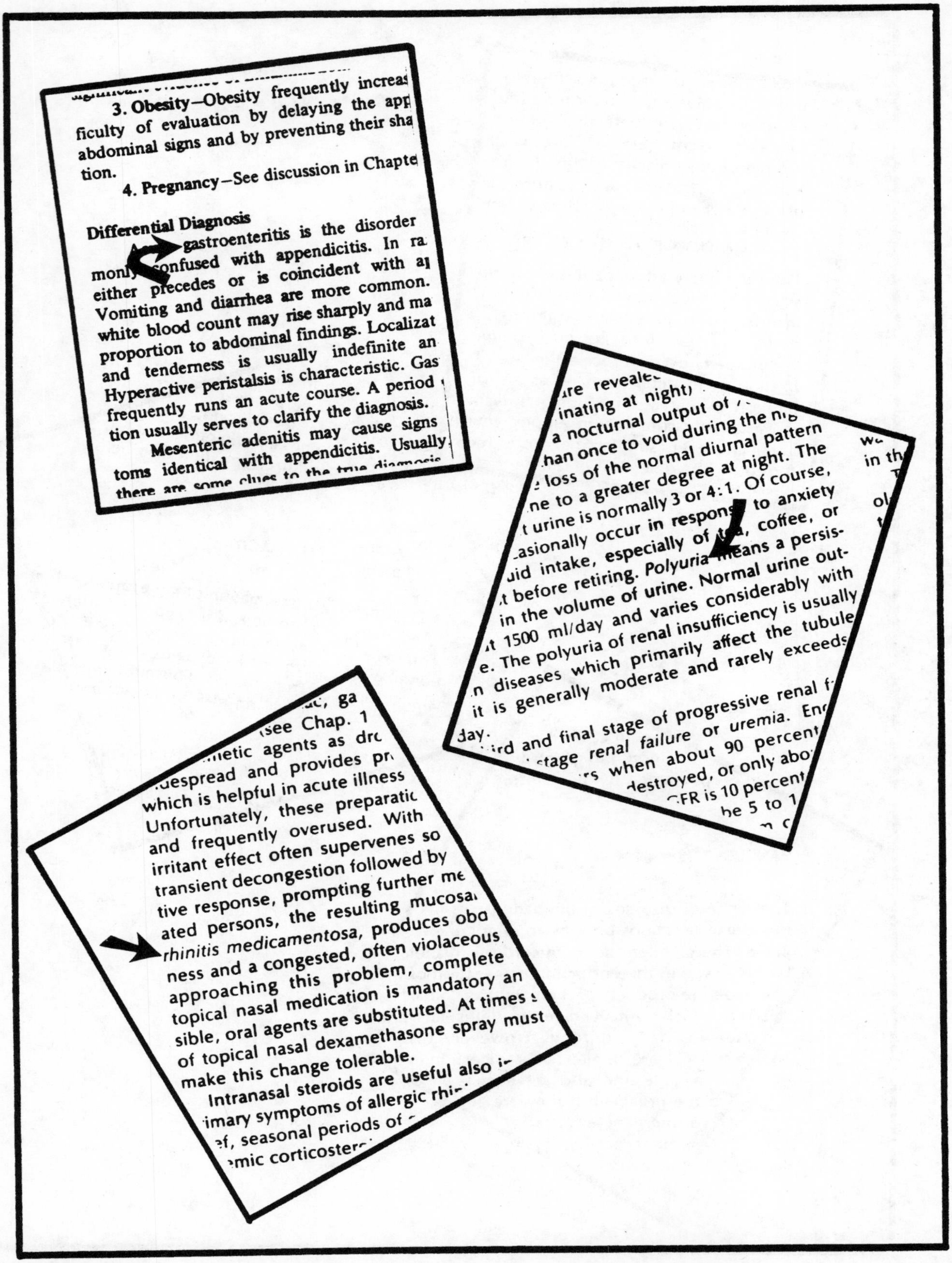

3. **Obesity**—Obesity frequently increas
ficulty of evaluation by delaying the app
abdominal signs and by preventing their sha
tion.
4. **Pregnancy**—See discussion in Chapte

Differential Diagnosis
gastroenteritis is the disorder
monly confused with appendicitis. In ra
either precedes or is coincident with ap
Vomiting and diarrhea are more common.
white blood count may rise sharply and ma
proportion to abdominal findings. Localizat
and tenderness is usually indefinite an
Hyperactive peristalsis is characteristic. Gas
frequently runs an acute course. A period
tion usually serves to clarify the diagnosis.
Mesenteric adenitis may cause signs
toms identical with appendicitis. Usually
there are some clues to the true diagnosis

re reveale
inating at night)
a nocturnal output of
han once to void during the nig
loss of the normal diurnal pattern
ne to a greater degree at night. The
t urine is normally 3 or 4:1. Of course,
asionally occur in response to anxiety
uid intake, especially of tea, coffee, or
t before retiring. *Polyuria* means a persis-
in the volume of urine. Normal urine out-
t 1500 ml/day and varies considerably with
e. The polyuria of renal insufficiency is usually
n diseases which primarily affect the tubule
it is generally moderate and rarely exceeds
day.
ird and final stage of progressive renal f
stage *renal failure* or *uremia*. En
rs when about 90 percent
destroyed, or only abo
GFR is 10 percent
he 5 to 1

ac, ga
(see Chap. 1
metic agents as dr
despread and provides pr
which is helpful in acute illness
Unfortunately, these preparatic
and frequently overused. With
irritant effect often supervenes so
transient decongestion followed by
tive response, prompting further me
ated persons, the resulting mucosa
rhinitis medicamentosa, produces obo
ness and a congested, often violaceous
approaching this problem, complete
topical nasal medication is mandatory an
sible, oral agents are substituted. At times
of topical nasal dexamethasone spray must
make this change tolerable.
Intranasal steroids are useful also i
imary symptoms of allergic rhi
ef, seasonal periods of
emic corticoster

FIGURE 3.10

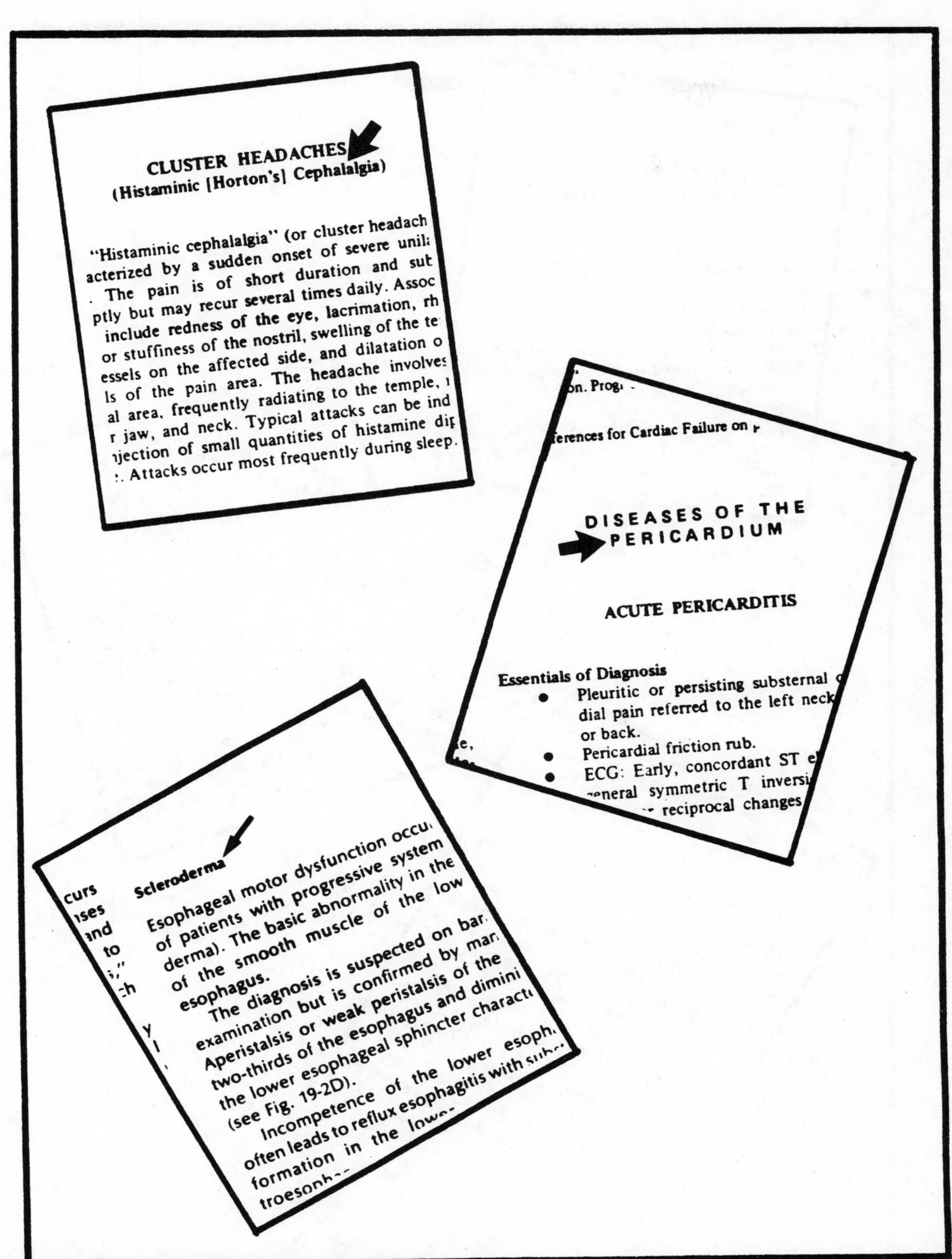

CLUSTER HEADACHES
(Histaminic [Horton's] Cephalalgia)

"Histaminic cephalalgia" (or cluster headach
acterized by a sudden onset of severe unil
. The pain is of short duration and sub
ptly but may recur several times daily. Assoc
include redness of the eye, lacrimation, rh
or stuffiness of the nostril, swelling of the te
essels on the affected side, and dilatation o
ls of the pain area. The headache involves
al area, frequently radiating to the temple,
r jaw, and neck. Typical attacks can be ind
njection of small quantities of histamine dip
:. Attacks occur most frequently during sleep.

n. Prog

ferences for Cardiac Failure on

DISEASES OF THE
PERICARDIUM

ACUTE PERICARDITIS

Essentials of Diagnosis
- Pleuritic or persisting substernal
  dial pain referred to the left neck
  or back.
- Pericardial friction rub.
- ECG: Early, concordant ST e
  general symmetric T inversi
  reciprocal changes

Scleroderma

Esophageal motor dysfunction occu
of patients with progressive system
derma). The basic abnormality in the
of the smooth muscle of the low
esophagus.

The diagnosis is suspected on bar
examination but is confirmed by man
Aperistalsis or weak peristalsis of the
two-thirds of the esophagus and dimini
the lower esophageal sphincter charact
(see Fig. 19-2D).

Incompetence of the lower esoph
often leads to reflux esophagitis with sub
formation in the lowe
troesoph

FIGURE 3.11

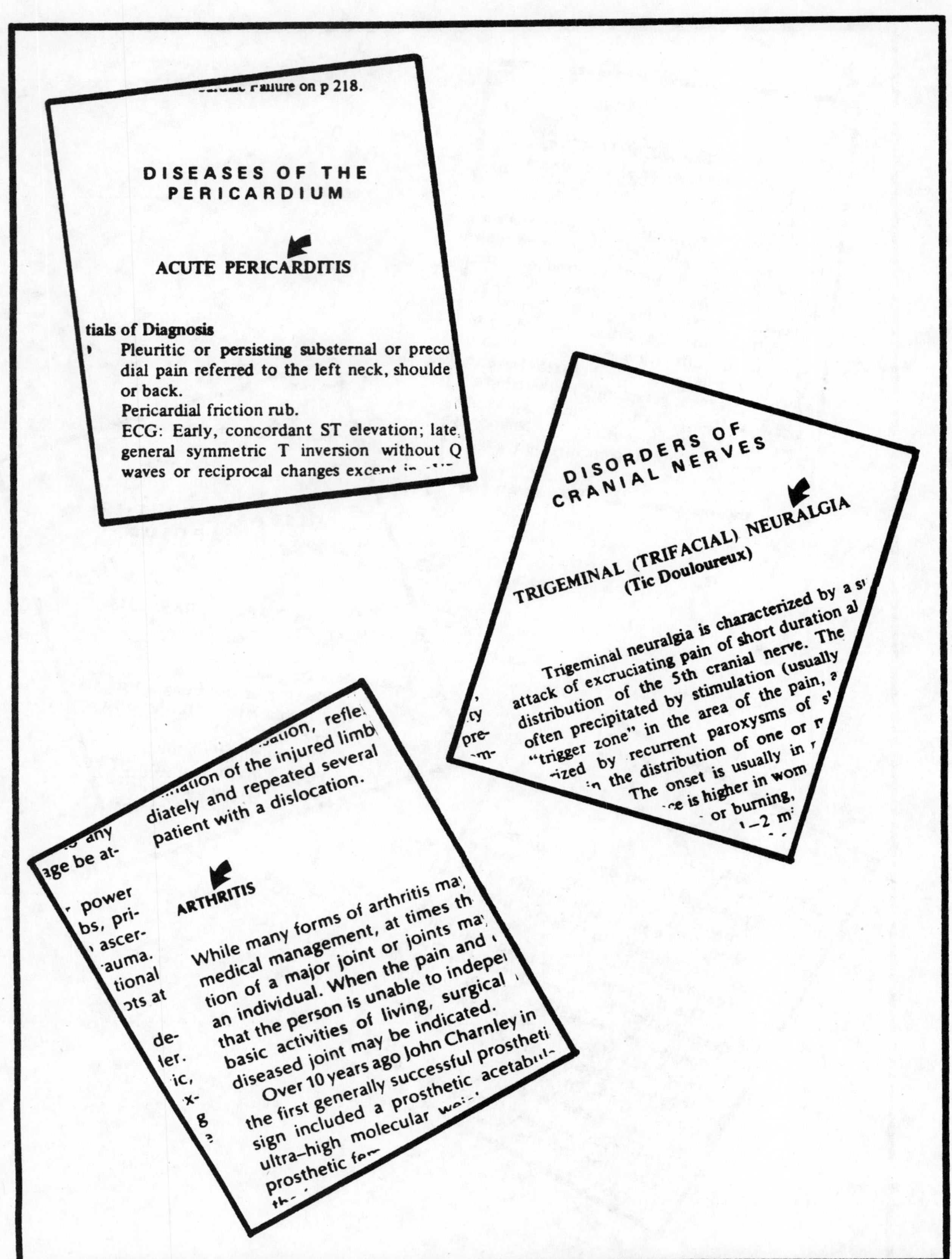

Cardiac Failure on p 218.

DISEASES OF THE PERICARDIUM

ACUTE PERICARDITIS

tials of Diagnosis

- Pleuritic or persisting substernal or preco dial pain referred to the left neck, shoulde or back.
- Pericardial friction rub.
- ECG: Early, concordant ST elevation; late general symmetric T inversion without Q waves or reciprocal changes except in

DISORDERS OF CRANIAL NERVES

TRIGEMINAL (TRIFACIAL) NEURALGIA (Tic Douloureux)

Trigeminal neuralgia is characterized by a s attack of excruciating pain of short duration al distribution of the 5th cranial nerve. The often precipitated by stimulation (usually "trigger zone" in the area of the pain, a rized by recurrent paroxysms of s in the distribution of one or The onset is usually in ce is higher in wom or burning, 1–2 m

mation of the injured limb diately and repeated several patient with a dislocation.

ARTHRITIS

While many forms of arthritis ma medical management, at times th tion of a major joint or joints ma an individual. When the pain and that the person is unable to indepe basic activities of living, surgical diseased joint may be indicated.

Over 10 years ago John Charnley in the first generally successful prostheti sign included a prosthetic acetabu ultra–high molecular wei prosthetic fe

FIGURE 3.12

Word	Prefix	Root	Suffix	Meaning

FIGURE 3.13

ADDITIONAL EXERCISES

The following key terms have been extracted from a variety of journal readings. Using references in addition to your text, explain each term.

1. hemodynamic monitoring
2. meniscectomy
3. thrombophlebitis

Word	Prefix	Root	Suffix	Meaning

FIGURE 3.14

4. gynecomastia
5. venography
6. intrathecal
7. intrahepatic therapy
8. percutaneous
9. extravasation

Word	Prefix	Root	Suffix	Meaning

FIGURE 3.15

10. hemodialysis

11. liposomes

12. monoclonal antibodies

13. antiarrhythmic

14. bradycardia

15. tachycardia

Word	Prefix	Root	Suffix	Meaning

FIGURE 3.16

16. bacteremia
17. sepsis
18. leukopenia
19. in vitro
20. in vivo

Word	Prefix	Root	Suffix	Meaning

FIGURE 3.17

DIAGNOSIS

Define each of the following diagnoses that have been taken from actual physician medical orders.

21. cholecystitis

22. UTI

23. dehydration
24. CVA
25. syncope
26. dysrrhythmia
27. CHF
28. HTN
29. aortic stenosis
30. vertigo
31. rheumatoid arthritis
32. asthma
33. urosepsis
34. pyelonephritis
35. TIA
36. cellulitis
37. hyperglycemia
38. metastatic cancer
39. pneumonia
40. exacerbation of bronchiectasis
41. lymphoma
42. colitis
43. abscess
44. anemia
45. colonic polyp
46. ataxia
47. hydrocephalus
48. malnutrition
49. edema
50. SOB
51. MI
52. angina pectoris
53. bronchospasm
54. bulemia
55. leukoplakia

CHAPTER 4

Pharmacy Calculations

OBJECTIVES

When you have completed this chapter, you will be able to:

1. perform pharmacy calculations
2. crosswalk between decimals and fractions
3. perform decimal operations according to standard rules
4. perform percentage calculations
5. use ratio and proportion to perform pharmacy calculations
6. differentiate between various systems of measurement

Specific skills are needed for every occupation. An individual completing the tasks required by the job should be proficient in those skills if he or she is going to perform the activity properly. Pharmacy technology requires a proficiency in mathematical procedures, concepts, and numbers manipulation. Pharmacy calculations is a title given to a fundamental tool required in pharmacy. The importance of mathematics and calculations cannot be stressed enough.

At one point, the importance of calculations in pharmacy was debatable. Drug companies manufactured drugs in prescribed dosages and forms (liquids, tablets, capsules, suppositories, etc.). The compounding of medications that was required in the past diminished. "Old-time" physicians who prescribed their specially compounded remedies and potions became fewer and fewer.

However, as drugs became more potent and the state of the art of pharmacy progressed, pharmacy calculations ironically became even more critical. Potent drugs required tailored dosage calculations based on body weight, body surface area, age, and laboratory test results. The gap between *therapeutic drug levels* (the level at which research shows a drug to provide an effect that has a positive outcome) and *toxic levels* (levels that can cause harm in an individual) narrowed. The role of calculations as a tool in pharmacy took on renewed emphasis. Specific calculations for antibiotics, newborn intensive care units, intravenous admixtures, and hyperalimentation supported and demanded the need for proficiency in pharmaceutical calculations. It follows, therefore, that you should be thoroughly acquainted with basic arithmetic operations, fundamental mathematical concepts (decimals, percentages, and ratio and proportion), and simple algebraic procedures.

This text presumes that you have a basic knowledge of mathematics and its operations. However, this section is designed to refresh those mathematical skills in areas that specifically involve pharmacy and its computations. Once the review of decimals, percentages, and ratio/proportion is completed, you will see how to apply this knowledge to problems reflecting contemporary pharmacy practice. Many of these problems are derived from actual Physician's Orders and prescriptions.

Consult a basic arithmetic and math text to sharpen those rarely used fundamental skills in math that are especially important to those operations involving pharmacy practice. A basic knowledge in pharmacy calculations will enable you to handle the array of calculations customarily associated with pharmacy.

DECIMALS

Can you complete the following problems?

1. Convert 0.30 to a fraction.
2. Convert $\frac{1}{4}$ to a decimal.
3. Add $0.260 + 1.9 + 4.32 + 2$
4. Multiply 4.9 by 2.3876
5. Divide 11.49 by 3.83
6. Subtract 6.72 from 12.9

Were your answers as follows?

1. $\frac{3}{10}$
2. 0.25
3. 8.48
4. 11.69924
5. 3.0
6. 6.18

If you got these answers, you should have no difficulty with decimals. However, if you were not too successful, this chapter should refresh some decimal operations that perhaps have been forgotten.

A decimal is a way to express fractions ($\frac{1}{4}$, $\frac{1}{2}$, $\frac{30}{72}$, etc.) as whole numbers. It is much easier to work with numbers in a decimal notation than to work with numbers expressed as fractions. Pharmacy drug measurements are often expressed in amounts less than 1. These measurements can be indicated in fractional notation. In many instances they are so noted. For example, you may see bottles of phenobarbital (a sedative drug) expressed in strengths of $\frac{1}{4}$ gr. and $\frac{1}{2}$ gr.; nitroglycerin (a heart medication used for angina) as $\frac{1}{100}$ gr., $\frac{1}{150}$ gr., $\frac{1}{200}$ gr.; thyroid extract (a drug used for an underactive thyroid) as $\frac{1}{4}$ gr., $\frac{1}{2}$ gr., and so on. In order to make the process of calculating amounts for specific compounding orders or special prescription requests, it is much easier to convert fractions to their decimal notations (i.e., $\frac{1}{4} = 0.25$, $\frac{1}{2} = 0.50$, $\frac{3}{8} = 0.375$, etc.). In the decimal form, numbers are treated as whole numbers, with the only difference being the position of the decimal point.

There are a number of rules to follow when working with decimals.

Rule Pay close attention to the position of the decimal point. When adding and subtracting decimal numbers, be sure that the decimal points are lined up. The decimal point must also be lined up in the answer.

The RIGHT Way:	The WRONG Way:
1.2345	1.2345
12.3456	12.3456
1234.56	1234.56
7	7
0.3456	0.3456

Rule In the multiplication of decimals, the sum of the number of figures to the right of the decimal point in the multiplicand and multiplier equals the number of places after the decimal point in the resulting product.

Example:

(multiplicand)	2.57	(two numbers follow the decimal point)
(multiplier)	$\times$ 3.4	(one number follows the decimal point)
(product)	8.738	(three figures follow the decimal point). (This represents the sum of the numbers following the decimal point in the multiplicand and the multiplier)

Rule In the division of decimals, move the decimal point in the divisor to the right until the number becomes a whole number. Keep count of the number of times you moved the decimal point. Move the decimal point the same number of places in the dividend.

Example:

$$\text{divisor}\overline{)\text{dividend}}^{\ \text{quotient}} \text{ or dividend/divisor} = \text{quotient}$$

$$679.684/14.63$$

Moving the decimal point two places to the right changes the decimal-fraction divisor, 14.63, to a *whole* number, 1463. Following the rule, move the decimal point in the dividend two places to the right. The dividend is now changed from 679.684 to 67968.4.

Be sure the decimal point is lined up in the quotient directly above the decimal point in the dividend. Complete the division operation. The answer (the quotient) should read: 46.4.

The final division process leaves you with a remainder of 582. How do you treat this remainder? You can complete the problem in a variety of ways.

1. If the remainder is greater than one-half of the divisor, increase the last digit in the quotient by 1. Note, therefore, that the remainder of 582 is more than one half of the divisor (i.e., 582/1463 = 0.58). (*Note:* $\frac{1}{2} = 0.5$, therefore, 0.58 is greater than $\frac{1}{2}$.) You have an option of making the resulting quotient 46.5. This is referred to as "rounding."

2. Another option is to add zeros after the last digit in the dividend without changing the numerical value of the dividend (67968.4 = 67968.40 = 67968.400, etc.). The number of places you want to carry a number after the decimal point will determine the number of zeros you must add on to the dividend. For instance, if you want to carry the number to three decimal places, you would add two zeros to the dividend, thereby making three places after the decimal point. The division process continues with the following result:

   $$67968.400/1463 = 46.458$$

   Again, after completing the division, you find that you still have a remainder of 346, which is less than one-half of the divisor. You may drop this remainder and leave the quotient at 46.458.

There may be times which warrant "rounding off." In the previous example, you may want to reduce the number of places beyond the decimal to fewer than you have currently chosen. If you want to take your answer to two places beyond the decimal point, your quotient would read 46.46 (i.e., rounding 46.458, the last digit, 8, is greater than 5, which permits you to increase the number to the left of the 8 by one digit, or in this case, the 5 becomes a 6). If you were to take the number to only one place beyond the decimal point, you would follow the same procedure. The quotient, 46.458, becomes 46.46, which when rounded to the ones place beyond the decimal point becomes 46.5 (the last 6 in 46.46 being greater than 5 enables you to increase the 4 after the decimal point to 5, resulting in the final quotient of 46.5).

Note: The magic number of 5 is not magic at all. The decimal (from the French meaning "tenth") system is based on 10, which is also the basis for the metric system. Therefore, the halfway point from 1 to 10 is 5. Any number greater than 5 is obviously more than half. A final note to remember is the rule of rounding when your remainder is 5 or a 5 follows the digit you want to round up or down. If the number to be rounded is an odd number followed by 5, round up the odd number by 1. If the number to be rounded is an even number followed by 5, the even number remains unchanged.

There are times when it is necessary to convert fractions to decimals. This is done simply by dividing the numerator by the denominator. For example, the fraction $\frac{1}{4}$ is converted to a decimal by dividing the numerator (top number) by the denominator (bottom number).

$$4\overline{)1.000}^{\,0.250} \quad 0.250 = \text{decimal fraction } \tfrac{1}{4}$$

It is a good practice to hold a position to the left of a decimal point with a zero if there is no whole number, such as in the preceding example. It is quite easy to leave the number as .250 with no whole number to the left of the decimal. Identifying this position with a zero does not change the value of the number and has the benefit of preventing potential errors caused by inadvertent markings or incorrect placement of the decimal point.

Convert the following fractions to decimal numbers:

$$\tfrac{4}{10},\ \tfrac{11}{52},\ \tfrac{12}{13},\ \tfrac{3}{2},\ 1\tfrac{1}{2}$$

The correct answers are:

$$\tfrac{4}{10} = 0.4$$

$$\tfrac{11}{52} = 0.21$$

$$\tfrac{12}{13} = 0.92$$

$$\tfrac{3}{2} = 1.5$$

$$1\tfrac{1}{2} = 1.5$$

Observe that in the last two answers the procedure for converting the fraction to a decimal remains the same. These numbers are unique in that they are mixed numbers. The number $\frac{3}{2}$ was specifically selected to show that $\frac{3}{2}$ is the same as $1\frac{1}{2}$, which is the same as 1.5, and although a mixed number may appear, simply follow whichever arithmetic process is easier for you.

As a final refresher on decimals, let's discuss the identification of *place values*. Each position following the decimal point to the right is associated with a named place value.

XX.XXXX

whole numbers.part of the whole number

whole numbers = one, two, tens, twenties, etc.

parts of the whole number = tenths, hundredths, thousandths, ten thousandths

1.1 is one and one tenth

1.01 is one and one hundredth

1.001 is one and one thousandth

1.0001 is one and one ten thousandth

The fractional part is named by the last number beyond the decimal point. For example, 1.1 is one and one tenth, 1.11 is one and eleven hundredths (*not* one and eleven tenths.)

A zero as the last digit has no value significance. The number 1.10 is still one and one tenth. However, 1.01 is one and one hundredth.

Try reading this one: 10.1234. You should have read it as ten and one thousand two hundred thirty-four ten thousandths.

PRACTICE PROBLEMS

1. A physician wants 10 capsules of a specially formulated drug. Each capsule is to contain 0.375 Gm. of the active ingredient. How many grams must be weighed out to prepare the physician's prescription?
2. The physician has ordered a patient to take a medication for 3 days. For the first 2 days the patient is to take $1\frac{1}{2}$ Gm. doses 3 times a day. For the last day the patient is to take only one dose that contains half the amount of the drug. How much drug will you need to prepare the order?
3. In problem 2 the prescription permits refills. You find that you have 19.9 Gm. of the drug in the bottle. How many times will you be able to refill this prescription with the amount of drug you have available?
4. How many grams are in the following doses? (Aloud name the numbers.)
   (a) 0.025 Gm.
   (b) 2.74 Gm.
   (c) 10.001 Gm.
   (d) 1.1000 Gm.
   (e) 110.011 Gm.
5. Convert the following numbers to decimals (if a fraction) or to fractions (if a decimal):
   (a) $\frac{1}{10} =$
   (b) 0.125 =
   (c) $\frac{3}{4} =$
   (d) 0.11 =
   (e) $\frac{23}{4} =$

Answers

1. 0.375 Gm. of drug × 10 capsules prescribed = 3.750 Gm. total drug needed for 10 capsules.
   (*Note:* The zero on the end of the decimal has no value. You would weigh out 3.75 Gm. of the drug.)
2. Three days = total.
   For each of the first 2 days:
   1.5 Gm. three times a day = 4.5 Gm. per day.
   For the first 2 days this will add up to 9.0 Gm.
   For the last day:
   One dose of half the amount is equal to 0.75 Gm.
   Total amount of drug needed = 9.75 Gm.
   (9.0 Gm. for the first 2 days + 0.75 Gm. for the last day.)
3. With 19.9 Gm. of drug on hand, you will be able to refill the prescription only one time (19.9 Gm. /9.75 Gm. = 2.04 or enough drug for the original prescription plus one refill).
4. **(a)** 0.025 Gm. = twenty-five thousandths of a gram
   (b) 2.74 Gm. = two and seventy-four hundredths grams
   (c) 10.001 Gm. = ten and one thousandth grams
   (d) 1.1000 Gm. = one and one tenth grams
   (e) 110.011 Gm. = one hundred ten and eleven thousandths grams
5. **(a)** $\frac{1}{10} = 0.1$
   (b) 0.125 = 125/1000, which can be reduced to $\frac{1}{8}$
   (c) $\frac{3}{4} = 0.75$
   (d) $0.11 = \frac{11}{100}$
   (e) $\frac{23}{4} = 5.75$

PERCENTAGE

The next order of review is a mathematical expression that is very important to pharmacy practice. You often see drug products prepared in specific strengths expressed as a percentage. For instance, hydrocortisone ointment, lotions, and sprays come in strengths of 0.5% and 1%; phenylephrine nose drops are available in strengths of $\frac{1}{4}$%, $\frac{1}{2}$%, and 1%. Profits/loss, pricing, and many management applications are also expressed in terms of percentage.

Percentage is a method of expressing fractional parts. In pharmacy the use of percent is very common and useful. The basis of percent is that the *whole* is divided into 100 parts (percent is a Latin derivative meaning "by the hundred"). For instance, you know that one dollar is made of 100 individual pennies or cents. If you measure one cent as a part of the dollar, the result is 1 percent, or 1%. Similarly, if you take 50 cents of this dollar and express it as a percentage of the dollar, the result is 50%.

Logic may lead you to believe that the maximum that can be achieved is 100%, or the "whole thing." But you can exceed 100%. A five-dollar bill, for example, is simply 5 times the one-dollar bill, or 500%.

You may find percentages in excess of 100% when you evaluate profits or customer traffic. Pharmaceutical preparations, however, *do not* exceed a 100% concentration. A saturated solution of potassium iodide (KI) contains 1 gram (Gm.) of KI in each milliliter (ml.) of solution. This solution has a 100% concentration.

The values of percentages can also be less than 1%. It is very common to see drug preparations in concentrations of $\frac{1}{8}$%, $\frac{1}{4}$%, 0.5%, and so on. This should not be confusing as long as you adhere strictly to the basic mathematical operations using percentages.

What should you know to feel comfortable with percentages? There are three elements to percentage:

1. The resulting percent
2. The parts involved
3. The "whole" with which you are dealing

In the application of percentages, you may be asked to find:

1. The *percent,* which is the part divided by the whole,
2. The *part,* which is the percent times the whole, or
3. The *whole,* which is the part divided by the percent.

Although the percent notation is commonly used to describe the parts of the whole or drug product concentration, it is necessary to convert this percent notation to a workable form, the decimal. This is easily accomplished by simply following the rule: *To change a percent to a decimal, move the decimal point two places to the left and drop the percent symbol.* For example, to change 21% to a decimal, move the decimal point two places to the left (21.0% becomes 0.21) and drop the % sign, resulting in a decimal 0.21 ($\frac{21}{100}$ is the fractional form). Observe that this system is based on 100.

The decimal fraction is the usable form for accomplishing the necessary mathematical operations you will encounter. Practice using decimal fractions until you feel comfortable with the operations. These calculations become critical in preparing intravenous formulations, among other pharmacy preparations.

Moving the decimal point two places to the left also works with numbers greater than 100%. Try the number 218%. What decimal would you use in working out a drug compounding problem? If you said 2.18, you are correct. The number 2.18 says:

1. 2.18 is 2.18 times greater than the "whole." If a manager says that the prescriptions in his department have increased by 218%, he is indicating an increase in prescription volume of 2.18 prescriptions for every prescription his department did previously.
2. 2.18 is the same as $2\,\frac{18}{100}$ or $\frac{218}{100}$
3. 2.18 is the decimal notation for 218%

Change the following percents to decimal fractions:

$$5\%,\ \tfrac{1}{2}\%,\ 32\%,\ 176\%,\ 4.87\%$$

Your decimal fractions should be:

$$0.05,\ 0.005,\ 0.32,\ 1.76,\ 0.0487$$

There are three basic types of percentage problems you will encounter. Follow the steps as they appear in each example.

A. *Find Percent:* What percent of 8 is 3?

Given: 8 = the whole, 3 = the part

Find: the percent

Operation: part/whole

$\frac{3}{8} = 0.375$ (decimal fraction)

Convert the decimal fraction to a percent.

$0.375 \times 100 = \%$ (multiplying by 100 is the same as moving the decimal point two places to the right)

Answer: 37.5%

Rule To change a number from a decimal to a percent, move the decimal point two places to the right and add the % symbol.

B. *Find the Part:* What number is 16% of 62?

Given: 16% = the percent, 62 = the whole

Find: the part

Operation: percent × whole

You cannot work with 16%. Therefore, you must convert 16% to a decimal fraction. Your decimal fraction is 0.16. Take $0.16 \times 62 = 9.92$, or 9.92 is the part of 62 that represents 16%.

C. *Find the Whole:* 60 is 4% of what number?

Given: 60 = the part, 4% = the percent

Find: the whole

Operation: part/percent

$$\frac{60}{4\%} = 60/0.04 = 1500.0\text{, or 60 represents } 4\% \text{ of } 1500$$

Did you notice the logic used to solve these examples? Working out word problems is often made easier by listing three major elements:

1. The information given,
2. What you are asked to find, and
3. The operation used to solve the problem.

Therefore, using scratch paper, restate the problem in a way you understand. Write the heading *Given* and list the information given, write the heading *Find* and state what you are seeking, and finally, solve the problem step-by-step with the information you have (including information found elsewhere such as conversions used in weights and measures).

PRACTICE PROBLEMS

1. The owner of the pharmacy has purchased a quantity of vitamins for $108.00. The quantity consists of two cases with 24 bottles of vitamins in each.
   (a) If he sells each bottle for $2.95, what percent profit will the owner be making?

(b) What percent of the bottles must be sold for the owner to break even (i.e., make an amount of money equal to his investment of $108.00)?
(c) What price should each bottle sell for in order to realize a 50% profit on the owner's investment?

The following practice problems use percentages as they apply to pharmaceutical preparations.

2. The hospital in which you are working makes a number of its bulk products in the pharmacy. You are assigned to the pharmacy manufacturing room on the day the Minor Surgery Department needs more of its disinfecting solution. You review the pharmacy's compounding manual and find the following formula for bronchofibroscopic disinfecting solution (minor surgery):

povidone-iodine solution	50%
70% ethyl alcohol	25%
distilled water	25%

Prepare a total volume of 4000 ml. How much of each ingredient will you need?

3. A special order is written by a physician in the radiology department. The order requires the pharmacy to prepare a Hypaque solution in a 3.33% concentration. The pharmacy has bottles already prepared with 8 grams of Hypaque powder in each bottle. How much diluent must be added to the powder to prepare the prescribed preparation?

4. You receive a call from a physician who is concerned about the availability of calcium in a calcium preparation he or she is prescribing for a patient. You review the label on a bottle of calcium glucobionate and determine that there is 9.5% available calcium in 1200 milligrams (mg.) of calcium glucobionate. How many milligrams of calcium do you tell the physician are available?

5. The chief pharmacist has assigned you the special task of identifying the major causes of improperly completed prescriptions. You have identified the following problems as major reasons for improperly completed prescriptions:
(a) no refill instructions
(b) incomplete patient name
(c) missing addresses on prescriptions for controlled drug substances (including narcotics)
(d) out-of-date prescriptions
(e) inappropriate drug strengths
(f) illegible physician signature

After reviewing and tallying the prescriptions for a 5-day period, you have gathered the following information:

Total number of prescriptions received: 637
Total number of prescriptions for controlled drugs and narcotics: 197 (this number is included in the 637 count)
The number of prescriptions with problems contained in the major categories:

(a) no refill instructions: 142
(b) incomplete patient name: 299
(c) missing addresses on controlled prescriptions: 11
(d) out-of-date prescriptions: 7
(e) inappropriate strengths: 14
(f) illegible physician signature: 473

The chief pharmacist wants you to report to him the percent of prescriptions showing each problem. He will then take the necessary actions to correct the problems based on the degree of abuse. The results you present to the chief become very important. What does your report look like? (Note: Many prescriptions contain multiple problems. Therefore, there are 946 problems in 637 prescriptions.)

Answers

1. **(a)** Given: purchase price = \$108.00
quantity = 2 cases with 24 bottles per case
(total of 48 bottles)
selling price = \$2.95
Find: percent profit (the profit is the amount of money made in excess of the purchase price)
Operations: \$2.95 (selling price per bottle) × 48 (number of bottles)

\$141.60 (gross sales)
−\$108.00 (cost of merchandise)
\$33.60 (profit)

\$33.60/\$108.00 = 31.1% profit made by the owner on his investment of \$108.00

(b) Given: \$2.95 = selling price per bottle
\$108.00 = owner's investment in 48 bottles
Find: the number of bottles which must be sold to break even
Operations: \$108.00/\$2.95 = 36.6 or 37 bottles (rounded off)

To answer the question of what percent of the merchandise must be sold to break even, consider the number of bottles sold to break even a percent of the total number of bottles purchased by the owner.

$\frac{37}{48}$ = 0.77, or 77% of the merchandise must be sold before the owner starts to make a profit.

(c) Given: \$108.00 = purchase price of merchandise
48 = number of bottles purchased
Find: the selling price for each bottle of vitamins to result in a 50% profit to the owner.
Operations: 50% of \$108.00 = 0.50 × \$108.00 = \$54.00

\$108.00 owner's investment
\$ 54.00 50% profit
\$162.00 total sales required to give the owner a 50% profit on his investment

Now, to determine the sales price for each bottle of vitamins:

\$162.00/48 = \$3.38 selling price per bottle

In other words, selling all 48 bottles at \$3.38 each will give the owner a 50% profit (\$54.00) on his investment of \$108.00.

2. Given: total volume required is 4000 ml.
% of each ingredient in formula
Find: amount of each ingredient in the final product
Operations: % × whole

providone-iodine solution: 50% × 4000 ml. = 0.50 × 4000 ml. = 2000 ml.

70% ethyl alcohol: $25\% \times 4000$ ml. $= 0.25 \times 4000$ ml. $= 1000$ ml.
distilled water: $25\% \times 4000$ ml. $= 0.25 \times 4000$ ml. $= 1000$ ml.

Note: If you add up the amount of each ingredient in the problem, the result is a total of 4000 ml., the required amount to be prepared.

3. Given: Hypaque powder = 8 grams
required concentration = 3.33%
Find: volume of diluent required to make the preparation
Operations: part/percent

$$8/3.33\% = 8/0.0333 = 240 \text{ milliliters of diluent}$$

In other words, by adding 240 ml. of diluent to the 8 grams of Hypaque, you will have a final solution containing a 3.33% concentration of Hypaque. Check your answer: $\frac{8}{240} = 0.0333$, or 3.33%.

4. Given: 1200 mg. of calcium glucobionate
9.5% available calcium
Find: amount of calcium available in the formulation
Operations: % × whole

$$9.5\% \times 1200 \text{ mg.} = 0.095 \times 1200 = 114 \text{ mg.}$$

You are able to inform the physician that there are 114 mg. of calcium available in every 1200 mg. of calcium glucobionate.

5. Given: 637 total prescriptions
197 controlled drug and narcotic prescriptions

Problem Category	Number of Problems
a	142
b	299
c	11
d	7
e	14
f	473

Find: percent each problem represents of all the prescriptions
Operations: part/whole

(a) $\frac{142}{637} = 0.2229 = 22.29\%$ or 22.3%

(b) $\frac{299}{637} = 0.4693 = 46.93\%$ or 46.9%

(c) The total number of prescriptions in this problem category is only the number of controlled drug and narcotic prescriptions. Therefore, your whole number becomes 197 and you determine the percentage based on these specific prescriptions.

$$\frac{11}{197} = 0.0558 = 5.58\% \text{ or } 5.6\%$$

(d) $\frac{7}{637} = 0.0109 = 1.09\%$ or 1.1%

(e) $\frac{14}{637} = 0.0219 = 2.19\%$ or 2.2%

(f) $\frac{473}{637} = 0.7425 = 74.25\%$ or 74.2%

You have now provided the chief pharmacist with a substantial report. He will be able to establish a corrective plan based on priorities set by these percentages.

RATIO AND PROPORTION

You have completed some very important basic mathematical tool reviews. You should feel comfortable with the concepts behind decimals and percentages and the way to use them properly. You have built the foundation for a commonly used mathematical operation in pharmacy called *ratio and proportion.*

By definition, a *ratio* is an expression of the relative value of one number to another. For example, the number $\frac{1}{2}$ shows the relationship between the numbers 1 and 2. The quantity 1 is half of the quantity 2.

Whole numbers also show a relationship between quantities. Take the number 2. Written as a ratio, "2" is expressed as $\frac{2}{1}$ or 2:1. (*Note:* ratios may be written as fractions, or with a colon, :). The relationship in this instance is that the quantity "2" is twice as great as the quantity "1."

Two equal ratios form a proportion. Therefore, it is necessary to have four numbers to complete a proportion. Practically, a *proportion* may be defined as an extension of a ratio. Take the ratio 1:2 or $\frac{1}{2}$. You know that $\frac{1}{2}$ is equal to $\frac{2}{4}$, $\frac{3}{6}$, $\frac{4}{8}$, and so on. Each of these ratios is equal to any other listed—2:4::4:8, 2:4::3:6, 1:2::12:24. When one ratio is set equal to another, this forms a proportion. For instance, $\frac{2}{4} = \frac{4}{8}$ is a proportion that shows that the relationship of each number in each ratio is the same. In the first ratio, $\frac{2}{4}$, 2 parts are half of the 4 parts. The same is true with the second ratio, in which 4 parts are half of the 8 parts. The ratios are equal even though the numbers are different. This proportion may also be written as 2:4::4:8 (the colon means "is to"; the double colon means "as"). This equation is spoken as "2 is to 4 as 4 is to 8." The numbers 4 and 4 are called the means and the numbers 2 and 8 are referred to as the extremes.

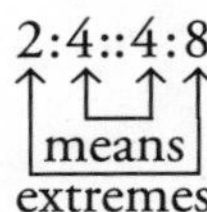

You will see the importance of applying your knowledge of proportions when you prepare different quantities of a drug from a given compounding order. You may need to determine new prices or amounts from given prices and amounts. Other applications are available also.

There are rules that are true for all proportions:

1. The product of the means equals the product of the extremes. Using the example of 2:4::4:8, the product of the means, or $4 \times 4 = 16$, and the product of the extremes, or $2 \times 8 = 16$, are equal.
2. The product of the means divided by one extreme equals the other extreme. The product of the means, or $4 \times 4 = 16$, divided by one of the extremes, 8, equals the other extreme, 2 (that is, $\frac{16}{8} = 2$).
3. The product of the extremes divided by one mean gives the other mean. The test of this rule will be left up to you to verify using our example.

In order to see how these rules apply, consider the following situation. A patron hands you a prescription for 100 tablets of pseudoephedrine 60 mg. (a nasal decongestant). You inform the patron that the prescription will cost her $16.00 for 100 tablets. The patron decides that she would prefer to try some of the medicine before purchasing the entire prescription. She asks for only 25 tablets. What do you charge for the 25 tablets?

You may reason that $16.00 for 100 tablets is equal to $0.16 per tablet ($16.00/100 tablets = the cost per tablet). Therefore, 25 tablets should logically cost $4.00 (25 tablets × $0.16 per tablet).

Using this example to illustrate the use of ratio and proportion may appear extreme for such a simple problem. However, a working skill of proportions will enable you to tackle and solve any problem with any degree of difficulty. Using this method of proportion, you can state the given information:

Given: 100 tablets = $16.00

Find: the charge for 25 tablets

Operations: set up a proportion

tablets/tablets as dollars/dollars
100:25::$16.00:? (? = unknown)

Referring to rule two, the product of the means divided by one extreme equals the other extreme.

25 × 16.00 divided by 100 = $4.00

Hint: Keep similar labels together. In this case you can associate tablets "is to" tablets as dollars "is to" dollars.

The price $4.00 for 25 tablets is the same as $16.00 for 100 tablets. The price for each tablet remains the same, but because the total quantity changed, there was a *proportional* change in the charge to the patron. Also, by keeping like labels together, you knew that solving for the unknown in this case was solving for dollars.

See if the other rules of proportion apply to this example. There are no gray areas in mathematics. Familiarize yourself with ratio and proportion. You will encounter the need for its use in solving pharmacy compounding problems, intravenous mixtures, pricing, and other nonpharmacy needs.

Complete the practice problems before continuing with what follows on weights and measures.

PRACTICE PROBLEMS

1. The nurse in the Newborn Intensive Care Unit (NICU) of the hospital calls the pharmacy with a request to determine how many milliliters of calcium gluconate injection will provide 150 mg. of calcium. The vial of calcium gluconate states 9.3 mg. of calcium is contained in each milliliter. How many milliliters must the nurse administer to the infant patient to provide 150 mg. of calcium?

2. Referring to the first problem, if each calcium gluconate vial contains 10 ml., how many vials will be needed to provide the required amount of drug?

3. Again referring to the first problem, a medical student calls the pharmacy to find out how many milliequivalents (mEq.) of calcium are contained in the 150 mg. of calcium. After checking the appropriate sources (in this instance the label on the vial contains the mEq. content), you determine that 9.3 mg.

of calcium equals 0.465 mEq. How many mEq. of calcium equals 150 mg. of calcium?

4. You are preparing bottles in the intravenous (IV) pharmacy when you receive an order for a change in flow rate (the rate at which the contents of an IV has been determined to flow into the patient) from 40 ml. per hour to 50 ml. per hour. Liter (1000 ml.) bottles are prepared for a 24-hour period. You have already prepared one bottle for the patient. Will the bottle be enough? If not, how many more will be required for the 24-hour period?

5. The owner of the pharmacy in which you are working has just purchased a "deal" on tubes of allergy cream. The deal consists of a gross (12 dozen or 144 individual pieces) of tubes of allergy cream. The owner of the pharmacy normally stocks 12 tubes of the cream and allots a foot and one-half of shelf space for them. The owner does not want to spare more than 24 inches of shelf space for the "deal." He wants you to figure out the number of tubes needed to stock the increased shelf space allotment. Also, if he sells 18 tubes of cream per week, how many weeks will the "deal" last?

Answers

1. 16.1 ml.
2. 1.61 vials. The pharmacy will send two vials of 10 ml.-size calcium gluconate to the NICU. The nurse will withdraw 16.1 ml. of calcium gluconate, which will provide the required 150 mg. of calcium.
3. 7.5 mEq.
4. No. We know that 960 ml. of a 1000 ml. (one liter) bottle is used over a 24-hour period. Proceed to the next step and determine whether increasing the flow rate by 10 ml. per hour requires the preparation of additional bottles. Yes, one more bottle will be necessary although only a portion (200 ml.) will be used.
5. 16 tubes. An additional 4 tubes will be needed. *Hint:* Convert the measure to like labels. You cannot work with feet and inches. Change the labels to either feet or inches. This "deal" will last 8 weeks.

SYSTEMS OF MEASURE

Now that you have completed a review of the fundamental arithmetic operations important to pharmacy, you can proceed with the science of weights and measures known as *metrology* (from the Greek *metrologia,* meaning "theory of ratios"). The essence of pharmacy historically surrounded the accurate measurement of herbs and other medicinal ingredients used in preparing potions, salves, elixirs, and so on. Today, even though most drugs are premade, one of the fundamental activities of pharmacy remains the measurement of drug quantities for compounding medications. A knowledge of weights and measures is needed to properly adjust existing drug dosage strengths when necessary. The science dealing with medication dosages is called *posology* (from the Greek word *posos,* meaning "how much").

A number of measurement systems have been used for pharmacy calculations. These include the apothecaries' system, metric system, Troy weight, avoirdupois, and even household measurements. Each system of measurement has established standards of weight and volume (except for avoirdupois, which measures weight only). However, because pharmacy deals with the measurement of minute quantities, only two systems could adequately be used to measure these small amounts. The systems are the apothecaries' system and the metric system. These two systems became the accepted measurements for drugs.

The metric system is currently the primary measurement used by drug companies and those involved in pharmacy practice. Dr. A. S. Blumgarten, author of *Textbook of Materia Medica and Therapeutics,* wrote, "In this country, the apothecaries' system is still used, but it is gradually being superseded by the metric system. It is simply a question of time when the apothecaries' system will be abandoned entirely." The apothecaries' system is no longer used in pharmacy as an official pharmaceutical system of measurement.

In addition to the metric system, this section will look briefly at the apothecaries' measurement and two other measures seen in pharmacy practice. The avoirdupois (pronounced "avoe-du-pwah") and household measures are occasionally used in compounding and dosage directions on prescriptions, respectively. However, the extent of their value and use is so limited that it is important to remember only a few necessary measurements and their conversions to other systems.

The acceptance of the avoirdupois pound was the result of relations between France and England. The king of England adopted the avoirdupois pound, which is equivalent to 16 ounces. The importance of this 16-ounce avoirdupois pound to pharmacy is only that it should not be confused with the 12-ounce apothecary pound.

Historically, avoirdupois measure was used for bulk weights of raw drug products. Apothecary measure was used for much smaller drug quantities used in the actual compounding of specific medications.

Household measure is used primarily by patients who take medicine at home. Because they are not familiar with grams, milliliters, and fluid measures (such as fluid drams and fluid ounces), it becomes the pharmacist or pharmacy technician's responsibility to assure the person that he or she is taking the correct dosage. Therefore, it is necessary to know the equivalents among the various systems of measurement. The pharmacy technician will then be able to convert the dosage from "pharmacy language" to everyday household language, which readily enables a person to take medication with a teaspoon, tablespoon, or dropper.

Tables 4.1 and 4.2 show the most common equivalents you will encounter.

Points to Remember

1. A standard teaspoonful has been established to contain approximately 5 ml.
2. 60 gtt. (gtt. = drops) = 1 teaspoonful (also written 1 ʒ)
3. 3 teaspoonsful = 1 tablespoonful (also written ℥ ss, ss = $\frac{1}{2}$)
4. 1 teaspoonful = approximately 5 Gm. (Gm. = grams)
5. 1 teaspoonful = approximately 60 gr.

TABLE 4.1 COMMON PHARMACY CONVERSIONS

Household	Apothecaries'	Metric
1 drop	1 minim	0.06 ml.
1 teaspoonful	1 fluid dram	4–5 ml.
1 tablespoonful	4 fluid drams	15 ml.
2 tablespoonsful	1 fluid ounce	30 ml.
1 glassful	8 fluid ounces	240 ml.

TABLE 4.2 COMMON PHARMACY EQUIVALENTS

Avoirdupois
437.5 gr. (gr. = grains) = 1 oz. (oz. = ounce)
7000 gr. = 16 oz. = 1 lb. (lb. = pound)
Apothecary
480 gr. = 1 ℥ (℥ = ounce)
12 ℥ = 5760 gr. = 1 lb.

THE APOTHECARIES' SYSTEM

Although this system of measure for pharmacy has been officially replaced by the metric system, we should at least be familiar with the apothecary standard.

The standard unit of measure for weight (solid substances) in the apothecaries' system is the *grain* (abbreviated gr.). Fluids (liquid volumes) in the apothecaries' system are measured by the unit called the *minim* (abbreviated ♏.). You may see a number of different symbols used in apothecaries' measurement. Table 4.3 summarizes the most commonly encountered symbols and their meanings. Occasionally a physician will write prescriptions using apothecaries' measure.

Table 4.4 summarizes units used in the apothecaries' system.

TABLE 4.3 COMMON PHARMACY SYMBOLS

Symbol	Meaning
♏.	minim
ʒ	dram or drachm (pronounced "dram")
fʒ	fluid dram, fluid drachm
℥	ounce
f℥	fluid ounce
O or pt.	pint
qt.	quart
C or gal.	gallon
gr.	grain
℈	scruple
lb.	pound

TABLE 4.4 COMMON APOTHECARY CONVERSIONS

Capacity (fluid measure usually refers to liquids)		
60 minims	=	1 fluid dram
8 fʒ	=	1 fluid ounce
16 f℥	=	1 pint
2 pints	=	1 quart
4 quarts	=	1 gallon
Weight (solids)		
60 gr.	=	1 dram (ʒ)
480 gr.	=	8 ʒ = 1 ounce (℥)

Note: The ʒ symbol and the ℥ symbol are used in both the dry and liquid apothecaries' measure. The letter f preceding the symbol denotes fluid for the liquid measure (fʒ or f℥).

THE METRIC SYSTEM

The metric system is the official system of measure for pharmacy practice. After the French Revolution, at the end of the eighteenth century, France adopted the metric system of measurement. In 1837, the French made the metric system a law and everybody in France was obliged to use this system. The United States Congress, in 1866, made the metric system legal in this country, even though the system was not commonly used here. Then, in 1890, the United States Pharmacopeia (USP) adopted metric measure. This action by the USP was especially important because the USP is the legally recognized compendium of standards for drugs.

The advantages of the metric system are that it is simple, brief, adaptable, and universal. There are metric measures for length, area, volume, weight, temperature, and even money. Pharmacy, however, is concerned mainly with weights and volumes of drugs.

The metric system is a decimal system that can be divided into any parts that are a multiple of 10 (10, 100, 1,000, etc.). Greek and Latin prefixes are used to show what multiple is used. For instance, *milli-* is a Latin prefix meaning one thousandth ($\frac{1}{1000}$). Joining the prefix *milli-* to the word *liter* (a measure of liquid volume) forms the word *milliliter* (abbreviated ml. or mL.), which means one thousandth of a liter.

The standard unit of metric measure for capacity or volume is the *liter.* The *gram* is the standard unit of metric measure for weight. You have already seen how the Latin prefix *milli-* was used to denote a proportion of the unit measure, the *liter.* The other prefix commonly used is *centi-*. This Latin prefix defines a unit of measure to be one hundredth ($\frac{1}{100}$) of the unit. Finally, an infrequently used Latin prefix is *deci-*, which means one tenth of the unit.

The most commonly used Greek prefix is *kilo-*, which denotes "one thousand times" the unit. You will often see measures in kilograms, which equal 1,000 times the grams (e.g., 2 kilograms = 2,000 grams). Drug manufacturers determine drug dosages using body weight measured in kilograms. For example, a 165-pound person weighs 75 Kg. (Kg. or kg. = kilogram). The kilogram label is often referred to as "kilos." A drug monograph lists the amount of drug to be given based on the patient's weight in kilograms.

At one time I would have disregarded the unit of measure for length—the meter. However, developments have been made in dosage forms that are measured in linear measure. Two examples are a nitroglycerin ointment (abbreviated NTG or TNG ointment) and a nitroglycerin patch. You may encounter prescriptions for NTG ointment with a dosage measured in inches. Nitroglycerin patches are measured in square centimeters (cm.^{2}).

Although a patient may be directed to apply the nitro (jargon for nitroglycerin) ointment in inch measures, a resident doctor in a hospital may exercise his or her newly acquired metric expertise. The nitro patches, however, are actually measured in square centimeter areas—5 cm.^{2} (cm.^{2} = square centimeters), 10 cm.^{2}, 20 cm.^{2}, and so forth.

The following units, once memorized, will enable you to solve nearly all of those rarely occurring problems involving metric linear measure:

2.54 cm. (cm. = centimeter) = 1 inch

1 cm. = 0.01 M. (M. = meter)

1 mm. (mm. = millimeter) = 0.001 M.

meter (m. = meter) = metric unit for linear measure

1 Km. (Km. = kilometer) = 1000 M.

There are two metric measures that predominantly apply to pharmacy. As a pharmacy technician, your primary use of metric measure will be for both the volume or cubic measure (for liquids) and weight measure (for solids) of drugs and medicinal ingredients used in compounding special prescription orders.

In the metric system, the unit of volume or capacity is the liter (abbreviated L. or l.). Large-volume solutions are referred to by their liter size. You may hear a nurse say she needs 20 K in a liter of D5W. What the nurse is saying is that she needs one liter of 5% of dextrose (a sugar) in water (D5W) with 20 milliequivalents of potassium (K) incorporated into the liter.

Liter-size IVs are prepared by major pharmaceutical companies such as Baxter, McGaw, and Abbott Laboratories. Many different fluids are purchased in liter sizes. Such preparations include D5W, normal saline (NS), half-normal saline ($\frac{1}{2}$ NS), and 5% dextrose in normal saline (D5NS), and are among a vast variety of liters available from companies.

Other pharmacy activities involving metric volumetric calculations use fractional parts of the liter. These fractional parts are usually expressed in milliliters (ml.) or cubic centimeters (cc.). *The milliliter and cubic centimeter are equivalent.* In your practice of pharmacy, these designations are interchangeable. You will often see liter or milliliter measure. It is, therefore, very important for you to remember that:

1 liter = 1,000 milliliters

1 milliliter = 0.001 liter

For example, 0.5 L. = 500 ml. or 500 cc.

The metric unit of weight is the *gram* (Gm., gm., or G.). The kilogram (1,000 grams), originally used as the unit of weight, was too large to meet the practical needs of pharmacy. The gram has been standardized as the weight of 1 milliliter of distilled water at 4 degrees Celsius (centigrade). It is important that you remember:

1 gram = 1,000 milligrams

1 milligram = 0.001 gram

The gram and the milligram are the most frequently used designations for weight measure in pharmacy practice. Note that the weight 0.250 Gm. may be read as "point two hundred and fifty grams" or 250 milligrams (1 gram = 1,000 milligrams, 0.250 gm. × 1,000 mg. per gram = 250 mg.).

Occasionally you will encounter a drug measured in micrograms (μg. or mcg.). Remember that:

1 Gm. = 1,000,000 mcg.

1000 mg. = 1,000,000 mcg.

1 mg. = 1,000 mcg.

1 mcg. = 0.001 mg.

Thyroid agents such as levothyroxine and liothyronine are measured in both milligrams and micrograms. You will commonly see levothyroxine labels listing strengths of 25 mcg. (0.025 mg.), 50 mcg. (0.050 mg.), 100 mcg. (0.1 mg.), 125 mcg. (0.125 mg.), and so on, through 300 mcg. (0.3 mg.).

Microgram measure is also used in defining how a drug distributes itself in the body after it is absorbed. The distribution is measured in mcg./ml. (micrograms per milliliter). Traditional pharmacy drug references such as the *Physicians' Desk Reference (PDR), Drug Information Handbook for the Allied Health Profession*, and others contain information about these concentrations. The Minimum Inhibitory Concentration (MIC) of an antibiotic (the least amount of an antibiotic needed to inhibit the growth of a bacteria) is also measured in mcg. per ml.

You will frequently encounter Physicians' Orders and prescriptions for special medications or dosage forms that require a conversion within the same system (e.g., convert 0.350 Gm. to 350 mg.—the quantities are both metric, but for convenience you may find using milligrams preferable) or from one system to another (e.g., convert 170 pounds to 77 kilograms because most drug dosage requirements are determined by body weight in kilograms). The translation of quantities from one system to another or within a system is called a *conversion.* Most physicians are not familiar with the various systems that exist and, therefore, write orders in a way that may appear to be jumbled quantities.

The pharmacy technician can easily adjust the Physician's Order and process it by knowing a few key conversions. We have already discussed the most common conversions within the metric system (liter/milliliters and gram/milligrams/micrograms). There are convenient equivalents that help you go from one system to another. These should be memorized. All pharmacy computations should be done in one system. The equivalents shown in Table 4.5 are used to bridge different measurement systems.

Liquid drug preparations, creams, and ointments are expressed as percentage concentrations. This simply means that a certain quantity of the drug or drugs is contained in the final quantity of the product. For instance, a 1% hydrocortisone cream contains 1 gram of the hydrocortisone drug in 100 grams of the final product (the drug plus the cream). A 5% sodium chloride (salt) solution contains 5 grams of sodium chloride in 100 milliliters of the final product (drug and distilled water). We already learned from our review of percents that 1 gram in 100 grams or 1/100 is equal to 0.01, or 1%. Similarly, 5 grams in 100 milliliters is equal to 5/100 or 0.05, or 5%.

In pharmacy, there are three ways of preparing a product that result in a percentage concentration. One method uses weight to weight (w/w) measurement. You

TABLE 4.5 COMMON CONVERSIONS

Linear Measure
1 meter (M.) = 39.37 inches
1 inch = 2.54 centimeters (cm.)
1 cm. = 0.39 inch
Fluid Measure
1 ml. = 16.23 minims (practical usage—rounded to 16 ♏.)
1 f℥ = 29.57 ml. (practical usage—rounded to 30 ml.)
1 pt. = 473 ml. (practical usage—rounded to 480 ml.)
Weight Measure
1 Gm. = 15.432 gr. (practical usage—rounded to 15 gr.)
1 Kg. = 2.2 lbs.
1 gr. = 0.065 Gm. or 65 mg.
1 oz. (avoirdupois) = 28.35 Gm. (practical usage—rounded to 30 Gm.)
1℥ (apothecary) = 31.1 Gm. (practical usage—rounded to 30 Gm.)
1 lb. = 454 Gm.
1 oz. = 437.5 gr. (avoirdupois)
1℥ = 480 gr. (apothecary)

can derive w/w percentage by dissolving a given quantity of ingredient (called the *solute*) in a liquid (called the *solvent*) measured in grams. W/w is also used in making creams and ointments with specific quantities of active ingredients. Percentage concentrations indicate the amount of active ingredient found in 100 grams of the solvent or cream. However, not every solution, cream, or ointment is 100 grams. As we learned, percentages can be established using any quantities. Consider the previous hydrocortisone (abbreviated HC) 1% cream example. Use 1 gram of HC and mix it thoroughly in 99 grams of cream. The result is a final preparation of 1 gram HC per 100 grams of total product. Note that any part of the HC 1% cream final product contains 1% HC. If you use 10 grams of a 100 gram jar, the 10 grams amount is a 1% HC preparation and the remaining 90 grams in the jar is a 1% HC cream. However, you will not usually be asked to make preparations in quantities convenient to the percentage system based on 100. HC 1% is usually prepared in 30-gram sizes.

How do you determine the necessary quantities of each ingredient for a 1% HC preparation?

Remember, 1% is also written as 0.01, HC is part of the entire product, and the entire product is 30 grams. The equation becomes:

$$\frac{\text{HC quantity}}{\text{30 grams}} = 0.01$$

Solution:

$$\text{HC quantity} = \text{30 grams} \times 0.01 = \text{0.3 grams}$$

You now know that you need 0.3 grams (or 300 mg.) of HC in 29.7 grams of cream to make 30 grams of HC 1% cream.

This simple example indicates the use of w/w in some product formulations. As a rule, however, w/w is uncommon for liquid product formulations.

Weight to volume, designated w/v, is the method commonly applied to solution percentage concentrations. As in the w/w methodology, the active ingredient or solute is measured in grams. A sufficient quantity or volume of solvent, measured in milliliters, is added to make the required solution. Observe that w/v is not applicable to creams and ointments.

Using our previous sodium chloride 5% example, theoretically 5 grams of sodium chloride is measured and placed in a beaker, cone graduate, or cylindrical graduate (laboratory pieces of equipment containing imprinted calibrated lines and used for measuring). Enough solvent (e.g., distilled water) is added to the sodium chloride to bring the level of the solution up to 100 ml. The 5 grams are dissolved in 100 ml. of finished product, making a 5% solution. The weight part of w/v is measured in grams and the volume part of w/v is measured in milliliters. Because not all solutions are premeasured as 100 ml., the quantity of solute used to prepare any volume is easily computed using the same steps discussed for the w/w method of percentage concentrations.

Most sodium chloride solutions are prepared in liter sizes. Because 1 liter is equal to 1,000 ml., calculate the amount of sodium chloride that will be needed to make 1 L. of 5% sodium chloride (sodium chloride is abbreviated NaCl). Following the same steps under the w/w method, you get:

$$\frac{\text{sodium chloride quantity}}{\text{1,000 ml.}} = 0.05$$

Solution:

$$\text{amount of NaCl needed} = 0.05 \times \text{1,000 ml.} = \text{50 grams}$$

Therefore, 50 grams of sodium chloride is placed in a graduate beaker, and solvent is added to the 1,000 ml. level. You have prepared a 5% sodium chloride solution.

Finally, there is the volume to volume, v/v, method used to determine a percentage concentration for liquid solutes dissolved in liquid solvents. This method measures the milliliters of an active ingredient (liquids are usually measured in terms of volume) to be incorporated in a total volume of the solution measured in milliliters. The percentage concentration is based on the milliliters of solute per 100 ml. of finished product. The mathematical operations are the same as those in the two previous examples.

A physician writes an order for a 5% solution of wintergreen oil in isopropyl alcohol. How much wintergreen oil will be needed to prepare 4 fluid ounces of the preparation?

You know:

1. You want a 5% solution of wintergreen oil.
2. You want a final amount of 4 fluid ounces.
3. Four fluid ounces equals 120 ml.

You need to know how much wintergreen oil is required to make the product.

The solution is:

$$\frac{\text{amount of solute}}{\text{quantity of finished product}} = 5\% = 0.05$$

Substituting where appropriate, you have

$$\frac{x}{120 \text{ ml.}} = 0.05$$

$$x = 0.05 \times 120 \text{ ml.} = 6 \text{ ml. of wintergreen oil}$$

Proceed to place 6 ml. of wintergreen oil in a beaker or graduate and stir in isopropyl alcohol until 120 ml. is attained.

Regardless of how you solve any percentage concentration problem, you must remember to express the relationship between the solute and solvent in the appropriate denomination, as shown in Tables 4.6 and 4.7.

In this chapter we discussed conversion, or the translation of quantities into forms that are workable for pharmacy computations. We discussed the various types of percentage concentrations and how each applies to pharmacy preparations.

One final conversion is often used in pharmacy and should be known. This is the temperature conversion from Fahrenheit to Celsius and vice versa. Sometimes the need to do so arises in bulk product manufacturing. Occasionally a patient may ask about a body temperature stated in Celsius. The following simple formula can be used to convert temperature either way by merely inserting the correct temperature:

$$(\tfrac{9}{5} \times {}^\circ\text{C}) + 32 = {}^\circ\text{F}$$

TABLE 4.6 METRIC CONCENTRATION RELATIONSHIPS

Methodology	Solute	Solvent
w/w	grams	grams
w/v	grams	milliliters
v/v	milliliters	milliliters

TABLE 4.7 APOTHECARY CONCENTRATION RELATIONSHIPS

Methodology	Solute	Solvent
w/w	grains	grains
w/v	grains	minims
v/v	minims or f℥	minims or f℥

Examine the following example using body temperature. You know that normal body temperature is 98.6 measured in degrees Fahrenheit (°F). How would it be written in degrees Celsius (°C) (which is usually the case in the hospital setting)?

$$(\tfrac{9}{5} \times °C) + 32 = 98.6$$
$$(\tfrac{9}{5} \times °C) = 98.6 - 32$$
$$\tfrac{9}{5}°C = 66.6$$
$$°C = 66.6 \text{ divided by } \tfrac{9}{5}$$
$$°C = 37$$

Therefore, 37 °C = 98.6 °F.

A doctor tells a patient that she is to call if her temperature goes above 38 °C. The patient realizes later that her thermometer is calibrated in Fahrenheit. She asks you to convert the Celsius temperature to Fahrenheit. What is 38 °C equivalent to in °F?

$$(\tfrac{9}{5} \times °C + 32 = °F$$
$$(\tfrac{9}{5} \times 38) + 32 = °F$$
$$68.4 + 32 = °F$$
$$100.4 = °F$$

Therefore, 38 °C = 100.4 °F.

EXERCISES

1. Complete the following chart:

Fraction	Decimal
1/64	
1/16	
	0.125
	0.25
4/16	
3/8	
	0.5
5/8	
	0.75
	1.000

2. How do you read 0.135?
3. How do you read 4.25?
4. Fill in the chart by completing the column labeled "Read as."

Decimal	Read as
0.1	
0.5	
0.0008	
0.2341	
18.451	

5. Write the following numbers as decimals.
   (a) 7/10
   (b) 6/100
   (c) 324/1000
   (d) 14 1/100
   (e) 4331/1000
   (f) 18 5/10
   (g) 301/1000
   (h) 146/100
   (i) 225/10
6. Write the following fractions to the nearest decimal thousandths.
   (a) 1/2
   (b) 3/4
   (c) 3/8
   (d) 5/16
   (e) 9/16
   (f) 17/32
   (g) 28/32
   (h) 14/16
   (i) 22/32
   (j) 56/64
7. Add $0.2 + 0.07 + 0.005 + 0.105 =$
8. Add $3.6 + 23.4 + 0.007 + 0.5 =$
9. Add $22.8 + 42.2 + 37.6 + 9.4 =$
10. Subtract $1.431 - 0.562 =$
11. Subtract $93.8 - 16.4327 - 20.009 =$
12. Subtract $0.005 - 0.0005 =$
13. Complete the necessary operations for this example:
    $27.65 + 18.402 - 2.39 + 7.63 - 1.1 =$
14. Multiply (0.021)(0.204).
15. Multiply (0.601)(1.73).
16. Multiply (9.06)(2.74).
17. Divide 497.865 by 1000.

18. Divide 0.724 by 1000.

19. Divide 12.24 by 7.31.

20. Divide 18.73 by 0.33.

21. Write the result of 6% + 8% in a decimal notation.

22. Write the percent equivalents of these fractions:
(a) 5/6
(b) 2/3
(c) 1/3
(d) 1/6
(e) 1/12
(f) 7/8
(g) 5/8
(h) 3/8
(i) 1/8

23. Write the fractional equivalents of these percents:
(a) 10%
(b) 20%
(c) 25%
(d) 40%
(e) 50%
(f) 60%

24. Change ½% to a fraction.

25. Change 3⅓ to a decimal.

26. Change 0.75 to a percent.

27. Change 0.0075 to a percent.

28. Change 75.00 to a percent.

29. If 4% of a cough medicine is an active ingredient, how much active ingredient is in 4 fluid ounces or 120 milliliters?

(*Note:* The answer is expressed in grams.)

30. Find 35% of 625 gallons.

31. A recent study showed, of 192 prescription errors, 8 were due to drug interactions and 9 were due to patient allergies. What does this translate into as percentage of total errors?
(a) drug interactions ______________________%
(b) patient allergies ______________________%

32. The same study also showed that an incorrect drug was dispensed six times. What percent of the total errors was this?

33. Again, reviewing the same study, we found that prescription deficiencies such as poor legibility, vague directions, and incomplete forms accounted for 50.6% of the errors. How many errors were there?

34. The directions for preparing a topical antiseptic solution state, "Add the contents of one bottle of oxychlorosene to 1,000 milliliters of saline." Each bottle contains 2 grams of powder, which dissolves completely in saline. What percentage concentration does this antiseptic solution have?

35. The package states the following information for nystatin oral suspension:

nystatin 100,000 units per milliliter
methylparaben 0.12%
propylparaben 0.03%

The total preparation contains 60 milliliters. How much methylparaben and propylparaben are in the preparation?
(*Note:* Express the answer in grams.)

36. A mixture requires two parts of water to four parts of alcohol. What percentage of the mixture is water?

37. If we were to take the mixture in question 36 and increase an amount of alcohol from 10 milliliters to 20 milliliters, how much water would we need?

38. A pole 10 feet high casts a shadow that is 25 feet long. If the pole were 15 feet high, how long a shadow would be cast?

39. We need 2,000 milligrams of a substance to make 20 capsules. How much of the substance will be needed to make 50 capsules?

40. If a cromolyn inhaler contains 200 metered sprays, how long will the inhaler last if the patient uses two sprays twice a day?

41. An albuterol solution contains 5 milligrams of active ingredient in each milliliter of solution. How many milligrams of active ingredient are in 120 milliliters?

42. A study found that of the 65 subjects tested, 10.7% of them suffered from insomnia after taking a certain drug. How many subjects had insomnia? If the drug is being taken by 53,000 people, how many of them can be expected to suffer from insomnia?

43. A physician writes a prescription that requires 1 grain of a sedative. How many 5 milligram tablets are needed to fill the prescription?
(*Note:* 1 grain = 65 milligrams)

44. A prescription calls for the following:

Rx

thiamine HCl	1.5 grams
folic acid	0.03 grams
ferrous sulfate	9.75 grams

Total quantity for 30 capsules

What do the contents of each capsule weigh?

45. What is the weight of the contents of one capsule of the following prescription?

Rx

phenobarbital	1⅗ grains
belladonna extract	2 grains
thyroid	1 grain

Contents for 10 capsules

46. If an alkaloid costs $4.75/gram, how much would 15 grams cost?

47. How much silver nitrate is required to prepare 30 milliliters of a 2.5% solution?

48. How much additional sodium chloride must be added to 25 grams to make 100 milliliters of a 50% solution?

49. A flask of alcohol containing 4,000 milliliters costs $18. Prescription A uses 1,000 milliliters, prescription B uses 500 milliliters, prescription C uses 250 milliliters, prescriptions D and E each use 125 milliliters, and prescription F uses 2,000 milliliters. How much of the cost for the original 4,000 milliliters is attributable to each prescription?

prescription A $____________________

prescription B $____________________

prescription C $____________________

prescription D $____________________

prescription E $____________________

prescription F $____________________

50. Calculate:

$$8 - 7 + 0.3 \div 11 \times 4.7 + \frac{1}{8} - 4\frac{2}{3} \div 9 \times 10 =$$

51. Define:

metrology

posology

52. List four systems of measurements.
(a)
(b)
(c)
(d)

53. Name the two systems accepted for drug measurement.
(a)
(b)

54. Fill in the blanks in the following chart for common equivalents.

Household Measure	Apothecaries' Measure	Metric Measure
1 drop		0.06 ml.
	1 fluid dram	4–5 ml.
1 tablespoonful	4 fluid drams	

55. Fill in the blanks.

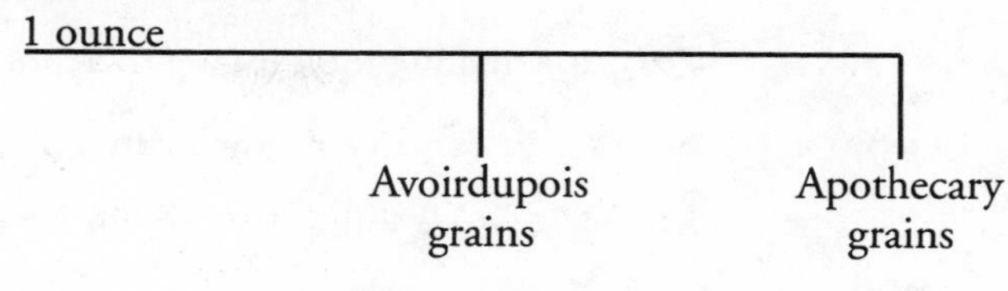

56. How many milliliters are there in a standard teaspoonful?
57. How many drops are there in a standard teaspoonful?
58. One tablespoonful contains ______________________________ teaspoonsful.
59. What is the standard unit of weight measure in the apothecaries' system?
60. What is the standard unit of fluid measure in the apothecaries' system?
61. Complete the following chart of common symbols.

Symbol	Meaning
	minim
	dram
	fluid dram
	ounce
	fluid ounce
	grain

62. How many grains are there in an apothecary dram?
63. How many grains are there in an apothecary ounce?
64. What does the Latin prefix *milli-* mean?
65. What does the Latin prefix *kilo-* mean?
66. What does the Latin prefix *centi-* mean?
67. How many grains are there in a kilogram?
68. How many grains are there in a milligram?
69. To what do *kilos* refer?
70. What is the unit of measure for length in the metric system?
71. How many centimeters are there in an inch?
72. What is the unit of volume or capacity in the metric system?
73. What is the abbreviation for milliliters?
74. What is the abbreviation for cubic centimeters?
75. How many cubic centimeters are there in 1 milliliter?
76. What is the metric unit of weight?
77. How many grams are there in a kilogram?

78. How many grams are there in a milligram?

79. How many milliliters are there in a fluid ounce?

80. A pint consists of how many milliliters?

81. How many milligrams are there in a grain?

82. How many grains are there in an apothecary ounce?

83. What are the three types of measurements that constitute percentage concentrations?
(a)
(b)
(c)

84. Write the formula used to convert Fahrenheit and Celsius temperatures.

85. Add the following weights and express the answer in total grams:

2.3 Kg.
125 mg.
10 Gm.

86. Add the following volumes and express the answer in total milliliters.

500 ml.
1.3 L.
0.25 L.

87. You receive a prescription requiring compounding. The script contains the following amounts of each ingredient to be prepared for each capsule. The physician wants the patient to have 30 capsules. What is the total amount of medication needed for 30 capsules? How much does each capsule weigh?

Per capsule:
medication Z = 500 mcg.
medication Y = 125 mg.
medication X = 0.075 Gm.
medication W = 300 mg.
medication V = 0.12 Gm.

88. A preparation contains 1.75 Gm. of filler and 250 mg. of active ingredient. What is the percentage concentration of the active ingredient?

89. Subtract 333 mg. from the 1.75 Gm. of filler in question 88. Using the same amount of active ingredient, prepare a 15% final product.

90. A physician wants a dozen pints of liquid disinfectant prepared by your pharmacy. How many liters of this disinfectant does he want?

91. A prescription calls for phenobarbital to be made up in powder packets for a child. The physician wants each dose to contain ⅛ gr. You are requested to prepare 24 doses. How many milligrams of phenobarbital will you need?

92. You receive a prescription for 500 minims of a nasal solution. The directions for the patient are to instill three drops to each nostril four times a day. How long will the bottle of nose drops last?

93. If a drug costs $1.50 per ounce, what is the cost of 2 drams?

94. Complete the following chart.
Reduce:

Quantity	To
180 minims	fluid drams
240 fluid drams	fluid ounces
32 fluid ounces	pints
32 fluid ounces	quarts
32 fluid ounces	gallons

95. How many grams of aspirin are contained in one bottle of 100 5-gr. tablets?

96. Fill in the blanks in the following charts (Figures 4.1 to 4.3).

Inches	Millimeters	Centimeters	Meters	Kilometers
1		2.54		0.0000254
39,370	1,000,000			1
0.3937		1		0.00001
0.03937				0.000001
39.37	1,000		1	

FIGURE 4.1

Grams	Milligrams	Micrograms	Pounds
1	1,000		0.0022
	1	1,000	
0.000001		1	
	454,000		1

FIGURE 4.2

Metric % Concentration Relationships	Solute	Solvent
w/w	grams	
w/v		milliliters
	milliliters	milliliters

FIGURE 4.3

CHAPTER 5

The Distributive Process

OBJECTIVES

When you have completed this chapter, you will be able to:

1. define the fundamental principles of distributive pharmacy
2. describe the pathway of distributive pharmacy
3. list the elements that comprise distributive pharmacy

This chapter of the unit introduces you to the traditional backbone of pharmacy known as *distributive pharmacy.* Much of what we discussed in the preceding chapters is tied together in this chapter. The fundamental distributive pharmacy system that currently exists is the same system we have had since pharmacy's beginnings. The medication scheme is classic. The doctor-patient relationship produces a diagnosis and, where needed, an order for a drug is written. This order or prescription is delivered to the pharmacy where the process continues with a pharmacist-patient-drug relationship. Therefore, in the typical drug distribution setting, the delivery process involves the physician, patient, pharmacist, and product (the 4 Ps).

Although changes to health-care delivery such as third-party payers, managed care, pharmacy benefit managers, and other pharmacy settings (e.g., infusion, assisted living, hospice) have evolved over the years, the classic system of pharmacy distribution remains intact. The drug products and the requirement that these drugs be accurately and appropriately dispensed is the ultimate reason that makes the job of the pharmacy technician so vitally important during the evolution of pharmacy from a product-oriented to a service- or information-oriented profession.

The field of pharmacy is based on tenets that support the practice of pharmacy. Tenets are principles or doctrines. These tenets contribute to the standards established for the practice of pharmacy.

As noted, pharmacy is evolving into both a medication-oriented or product part and a knowledge-based service or cognitive part. The facet of pharmacy dealing with the movement of the drug product from the pharmacy to the patient is becoming more the jurisdiction of the pharmacy technician as an adjunct to the licensed pharmacist, who is shifting to cognitive (i.e., information) services. Fundamental to the distributive pharmacy practice, which is a "manipulative" (e.g., hands-on product), is the classic tenet of *the right drug, to the right patient, at the right time.* In order to accomplish this requirement, the pharmacy technician assumes responsibilities that include patient contact, computer skills, phone poise, product inventory selection, drug stocking, and much more. The technician must greet the patient, gather information, clarify ambiguities, answer nonjudgmental questions, refer to the pharmacist questions and concerns where appropriate, and dispense the final product to the patient. The goal of each pharmacy technician is to make the pharmacy distribution system work as efficiently and effectively as possible.

THE DRUG DELIVERY PROCESS

The process of drug delivery from the time a prescription is written until you actually dispense the drug to the patient is part of a larger continuum of care. Patient care usually encompasses a variety of health-care needs including nutrition, lifestyle, and exercise. Health-care practitioners use drug products as part of their choices to deal with the complexities of abnormal health conditions.

Pharmacy technicians should have an overall concept of the needs for various health conditions. Knowing general care paths provides you with an expanded competence to be a significant resource while also enhancing your own confidence. A typical abbreviated care path for a patient with high blood pressure, for instance, addresses the need for proper nutrition that is low in sodium, a lifestyle that incorporates ways to deal with stress, stopping smoking as indicated, therapeutic walks, and compliance with a medication regimen. From this brief example, we see how you can be instrumental in providing guidance, structure, and support to improve a patient's quality of life. You are probably saying that this activity goes beyond dispensing a drug. That is true. However, always remember that health care is a continuum and the role of the pharmacy technician is becoming ever so important.

DRUG TRANSFERRAL

Drug distribution requires the transfer of an order from the prescriber to the pharmacy where the order is read, interpreted, and filled by a pharmacist or pharmacy technician. This order may be in the hardcopy form of a prescription written by the doctor, a facsimile (fax) sent by the doctor or his or her office personnel, a telephone order, or through electronic media such as electronic mail (e-mail) between computers. Orders that are transmitted electronically must be transcribed to a hard-copy form for pharmacy records.

Within the scheme of the prescription order "in" (i.e., received) to the drug and instructions "out" (i.e., delivery) are the important elements of medication management and clinical management. The pharmacy technician, within the activities comprising medication management, has the responsibility to assure that the right quantity of the medication is dispensed with the appropriate instructions to take the medication correctly (i.e., compliance—defined fundamentally as taking the medication the right way, at the right time, during the entire course of treatment). The pharmacy technician has a decisive role in patient medication management. I call this "first inquiry," in which the correct information is gathered, and "last dose tickler," which is ideally a follow-up to establish the patient compliance and medication effect.

The clinical management remains the responsibility of the pharmacist. That is not to say, however, that the pharmacy technician has no role in assisting the pharmacist in the clinical aspects of pharmacy. As part of these activities, the pharmacist utilizes the knowledge-based service or cognitive part of pharmacy by applying his or her knowledge about drug side effects, contraindications, and additional instructions to the patient to sharpen awareness for potentially adverse drug reactions (ADRs). Clinical management further includes medication treatment outcome and follow-up through tools such as lab tests and communication between the patient and the pharmacist.

DRUG DISTRIBUTION

Now that we have a concept of the distributive pharmacy practice, we are able to address the heart of drug product pharmacy called dispensing. *Dispensing* is the pharmacy activity that is initiated with the receipt by the "pharmacy" of a drug order. The subsequent events in dispensing include data entry, product selection, filling the prescription, checking, and, finally, delivery.

Community Settings The receipt of the drug order varies according to the different type of pharmacy settings. For instance, in the community setting, which is perhaps the predominant setting, the prescription is typically written by the prescribing doctor and delivered to the pharmacy by the patient or patient's caregiver, or the prescriber's office may call a prescription into the pharmacy. There are rules that govern special prescriptions such as controlled substances, narcotics, and special compounding.

Other retail pharmacy settings such as pharmacies that specialize in infusion medications (intravenous route of drug administration), parenteral nutrition formulas, nebulizer drugs (inhalation drug therapy), and others may be subject to different mechanisms of ordering and delivery of the drugs prescribed. Nebulizer drugs, for instance, may be ordered from a pharmacy by a supplier who specializes in oxygen delivery or other inhalation drug preparations such as albuterol, metaproteranol, ipratropium, and the like, which are used in a piece of equipment called a nebulizer. Note that nebulizers, infusion pumps, and the poles used to hold these devices are known categorically as durable medical equipment and often referred to as DME.

Institutional Settings These settings include hospitals, nursing homes (NH), skilled nursing facilities (SNF, pronounced "snifs"), and other long-term care (LTC) facilities. Depending on the arrangement for drug delivery, whether in-house or supplied by a source contracted outside the institution, the transmission of the drug may vary. More will be discussed in a later unit on distributive pharmacy practice in institutions, especially hospitals.

Entry of Prescription Drug Order Information For now, however, our general focus is on the data entry of information that we receive on the order. The information contained on the prescription or drug order must be interpreted and evaluated for clarity, completeness, and legality. (*Note:* I use the term *prescription* in the context of the ambulatory setting where the patient or a caregiver conveys the medication needs through this means, and the *drug order* in the institutional setting whereby the list of medications may be part of the entire requirements listed on a patient's record by the doctor.) You should look for three basic areas. They are the *prescriber,* the *patient,* and the *drug.* You should be able to answer the following questions in order to assure the health and safety of the patient.

- Could you identify the physician ordering the medication?
- Is the physician licensed to prescribe legend drugs? (Legend drugs are drugs approved by the FDA that are labeled with "Caution: Federal law prohibits dispensing without a prescription.")
- Does the prescription look legitimate? That is, is there any indication of fraud, forgery, or tampering on the prescription? This can readily be determined by differences in the shades of ink color, the width of lines of the letters, or the shape of specific letters. Tampering is often covered up by deliberate smudges or mutilation of the prescription blank. Examine dates, drug quantities, and

strengths that have been written over. Be especially cautious of prescriptions for controlled drug substances and narcotics.

Other items to check include:

- Is the date of the prescription within legal or clinical time frames? You would not routinely fill, without justification, a prescription over a year old. Legal parameters limit the period for which a prescription for narcotics may be filled.
- Is the patient's name clear? With common names, especially those names common to your geographic area, be specific with the patient and note on the prescription any special identifying information that may prevent dispensing the medication to the wrong patient.
- Is the patient's age noted?
- Is the patient's address listed and is it correct?

This information must be collected in order to assure the basic tenet of *the right drug, to the right person, at the right time.* Also, the correct information is important in the current environment because payment by third-party payers such as insurance companies rely on the correct patient-identifying information to properly process and pay for submitted drug claims.

DISTRIBUTION BEGINS

The patient has handed you a prescription, or the hospital pharmacist has read the patient's orders written by the doctor and reviewed them for medications. The required needs are now directed to you, the pharmacy technician. *Dispensing* has begun. In the ambulatory setting pharmacy technicians often enter the date into the patient profile by hand or electronically. The hospital setting may vary, but in most cases, the pharmacist will enter the drug information on the patient's profile and the drug requirement is transmitted to the pharmacy technician.

An entire set of events is set in motion. You are aware of the products available for dispensing. This may be influenced by who is paying the bill; the formulary that may drive the product selection; the requirement for brand name drug versus a generic form of the drug; the bioequivalence between the drug entities; patient information such as age or drug sensitivities; drug packaging, whether it is bulk, unit dose, or unit of use; or the need to compound a drug. Your decision and the subsequent product choice are the part of dispensing known as *product selection.*

The next step in the distributive process is to type a label containing the instructions on how to take the medication. Make the label as explicit as possible using short command sentences with "YOU" understood. For example, a label typed for eyedrops used BID (i.e., twice a day) would read, *Instill two (2) drops into each eye twice a day.* Embellishing this direction with more specificity such as ". . . twice a day at 8 A.M. and 8 P.M." would be a progressive step toward helping the patient comply with the medication regimen; however, unfortunately, unless stated on the prescription order or drug order, you do not have the authority to add information on the label beyond what the order states. The pharmacist, however, upon delivering the finished medication product to the patient or caregiver may mention that the usual BID schedule is based on every 12 hours, or may suggest that an 8 A.M./8 P.M. schedule would best fit the patient's work schedule or sleep patterns. Chronotherapy is becoming more significant as we learn more about the best times for drugs to be given for greatest effect. In time, best times for taking the drug will be part of the labeled instructions.

AUXILIARY LABELING

Auxiliary labels are necessary to inform the patient of some unique property or situation involving the medication. For example, a drug may change the color of urine. This can be alarming to a patient without an auxiliary label noting the property of the drug to change urine color.

Perhaps the medication will make the patient sensitive to sunlight, or some medications must be taken with food or a full glass of water. I cannot overemphasize the importance of informing the patient of special requirements to enhance the effectiveness of a drug or to prevent the patient from having unnecessary or harmful side effects.

Auxiliary labeling is a very important part of providing information that will help the patient take the medication appropriately. Auxiliary labels, also referred to as *strip labels,* may contain general, instructional, warning, or route of administration information. There are companies that print entire arrays of labels. Most pharmacies limit their label selection to those most commonly used. The following labels are examples of commonly used strip labels. Remember that the examples given are only representative.

Prepare a list of the drugs most often dispensed from your pharmacy. Include the auxiliary labels appropriate for those drugs and refer to your list when dispensing the specific drug. This uniformity and consistency is very important to both you and the patient.

General Information Labels

"MAY CAUSE DISCOLORATION OF THE URINE OR FECES"
(e.g., urinary anesthetics such as phenazopyridine)

"PROTECT FROM LIGHT"
(e.g., light-sensitive drugs such as sodium nitroprusside)

"SHAKE WELL BEFORE USING"
(e.g., suspensions such as reconstituted liquid antibiotics)

"KEEP IN REFRIGERATOR"
or
"KEEP IN REFRIGERATOR; DO NOT FREEZE"
(e.g., most reconstituted antibiotics, suppositories such as promethazine rectal suppositories, insulin)

"THIS IS THE SAME MEDICATION YOU HAVE BEEN GETTING. COLOR, SIZE, OR SHAPE MAY APPEAR DIFFERENT"
(*Note:* Many generic drug manufacturers market the same generic form of a drug. There are variations in the physical appearance among the products.)

"THIS PRESCRIPTION MAY BE REFILLED ____________ TIMES"
(Refill strip labels vary in wording. The general information enables the patient to make plans for subsequent refills in a timely manner.)

Instructional Labels

"CHEW TABLETS BEFORE SWALLOWING"
(e.g., tablets designed for chewing such as isosorbide dinitrate chewable tablets)

"DO NOT CHEW OR CRUSH; SWALLOW WHOLE"
(e.g., omeprazole delayed-release capsules)

"TAKE WITH FOOD OR MILK"
(e.g., A number of drug classes such as nonsteroidal anti-inflammatory agents and corticosteroids, require this strip label to minimize gastrointestinal irritation.)

"IMPORTANT: FINISH ALL THIS MEDICATION UNLESS OTHERWISE DIRECTED BY PRESCRIBER"
(e.g., Antibiotics and anti-infective agents must be taken for specific periods of time to prevent the development of resistant pathogenic bacteria.)

"DO NOT TAKE DAIRY PRODUCTS, ANTACIDS, OR IRON PREPARATIONS WITHIN ONE HOUR OF THIS MEDICATION"
(e.g., Tetracyclines, generally, require this strip label. Ciprofloxacin is another example of a drug that requires this strip label. However, references advise that the drug not be given within 4 hours of antacids or iron preparations.)

"TAKE MEDICATION ON AN EMPTY STOMACH 1 HOUR BEFORE OR 2 TO 3 HOURS AFTER A MEAL UNLESS OTHERWISE DIRECTED BY YOUR DOCTOR"
(e.g., Foods stimulate the production of gastric juices such as hydrochloric acid. Some drugs such as penicillin are inactivated in an acidic environment.)

"MEDICATION SHOULD BE TAKEN WITH PLENTY OF WATER"
(e.g., Drugs containing sulfonamides such as sulfamethoxazole/trimethoprim require plenty of water to prevent crystallization in the kidney.)

Warning Labels

"AVOID PROLONGED EXPOSURE TO SUNLIGHT WHILE TAKING THIS MEDICATION"
(e.g., Use this strip label for drugs that have potential for photosensitivity such as ciprofloxacin and tetracycline. Other drug compounds such as antifungals distribute in the skin. Sunlight reacts with these drugs.)

"MAY CAUSE DROWSINESS. ALCOHOL MAY INTENSIFY THIS EFFECT. USE CARE WHEN OPERATING A CAR OR DANGEROUS MACHINERY"
(e.g., There are many drug classes with specific drugs that require this strip label. They include analgesics, anxiolytics, antihistamines, muscle relaxants, and many more.)

"DO NOT DRINK ALCOHOLIC BEVERAGES WHEN TAKING THIS MEDICATION"
(e.g., Metronidazole is an example of a drug that requires this labeling.)

"NOT TO BE TAKEN BY MOUTH"
(e.g., Use this strip label for external preparations such as ointments, creams, and suppositories.)

"DO NOT TAKE ASPIRIN WITHOUT THE KNOWLEDGE AND CONSENT OF YOUR PHYSICIAN"
(e.g., This strip label is often used with oral hypoglycemic drugs and oral anticoagulant medication.)

"DO NOT USE AFTER DATE ______________________________"
(e.g., This label is used most often for drugs that are reconstituted and have a short subsequent duration of activity. For example, powdered penicillin is reconstituted to a liquid form. Once reconstituted, the activity lasts for 14 days if the product is stored in the refrigerator. This label may also be used to inform the patient of a medication that is expiring on a certain date.)

"DO NOT TAKE THIS DRUG IF YOU BECOME PREGNANT"
(e.g., Use this strip label for drugs included in FDA Pregnancy Category X such as folic acid antagonists and some central nervous system drugs.)

"CAUTION: FEDERAL LAW PROHIBITS THE TRANSFER OF THIS DRUG TO ANY PERSON OTHER THAN THE PATIENT FOR WHOM IT WAS PRESCRIBED"
(e.g., Use this strip label for narcotic medications. The specific citation is found in the Controlled Substances Act, Section 290.05, which states, "The label of any drug listed as a 'controlled substance' in schedule II, III, or IV of the Federal Controlled Substances Act shall, when dispensed to or for a patient, contain the following warning: [wording contained in the strip label].")

Route of Administration

"FOR THE NOSE"

"FOR THE EAR"

"FOR THE EYE"

"FOR RECTAL USE ONLY"

"FOR VAGINAL USE ONLY"

"FOR EXTERNAL USE ONLY"

"USE AS A GARGLE"

Common Hospital Strip Labels

"NOTE DOSAGE STRENGTH"
(Hospital pharmacy departments often are limited to a drug formulary that specifies the drug and strength that is in inventory. For example, a formulary may list ampicillin 250 mg. If a medication order requires ampicillin 500 mg., we double the quantity dispensed and provide this strip label to alert the nurse or medication technician that we have dispensed half the strength ordered. The caregiver then knows to double the ampicillin 250 mg. to get the 500 mg. ordered.)

"RTS" or "RETURN TO STOCK"
(Hospitals have a limited number of drugs that are located and inventoried on each floor. This is known as *floor stock.* When the floor uses floor stock, they request a replacement with an RTS notation. We deliver the required stock to the floor with this strip to notify floor personnel that the stock is to be replaced in inventory and not given to a patient.)

"STAT"
(The STAT label alerts the pharmacy delivery personnel to deliver the drug immediately.)

CONTAINER SELECTION

We are at the point in the process where we have selected the drug; typed the label with the patient's name, the date, the identifying prescription number, the directions for taking the drug, the name and strength of the medication, the prescriber's name; and you have chosen the necessary information auxiliary labels. Now the pharmacy technician selects the appropriate container.

Although we most often use the plastic drachm (pronounced "dram") vial for solid oral medications (pills, tablets, capsules) and glass or plastic bottles called "ovals" for liquid preparations, sometimes a drug has a need for special packaging. Nitroglycerin oral capsules and tablets must be placed in an amber glass container to prevent premature deterioration of the drug. Medications that deteriorate when exposed to sunlight must be placed in an amber or other colored container instead of clear glass that allows the ultraviolet rays from sunlight to penetrate the container and affect the sensitive drug. Nitroprusside sodium, a drug used for hypertensive emergencies, upon reconstitution must be protected from light by promptly wrapping the container with an opaque sleeve such as aluminum foil.

Fortunately, overall there are few medications with special container needs. You should be aware that compounded ointments go into ointment jars or ointment tubes. Rectal ointments in a tube should be accompanied by an attachment that enables the patient to insert the ointment rectally. Sterile preparations such as eyedrops and injectable testing antigens must be placed in sterile containers. Also be sure to use the appropriate size container for the medication. An excessively large size container for a product looks poorly, and a too-small container can be destructive to the contents if the drug is forced into the container.

Now we are ready to put the medication, container, label, and auxiliary label together to produce the final product. This activity entails measuring the medication by counting, pouring, or weighing as necessary, and affixing the proper labels to the container. Look to dispense a "pharmaceutically elegant" product.

FINAL REVIEW

Patient Review The product is ready for delivery, but the dispensing is not complete. Upon delivery the pharmacist should review with the patient or caregiver the instructions for taking the medication and any other pertinent information that will assure the effectiveness of the drug and the safety and comfort of the patient. You can assist the pharmacist by providing essential handouts to the patient or in other capacities as delegated by the pharmacist.

Drug Review Remember, your function as the pharmacy technician does not end when you affix the labels to the container. You must do a final validation check. Read the bulk bottle label from which you selected the drug, noting the drug name, strength, and form. Also check the expiration date and, finally, you should ideally look at the manufacturer's lot number, which becomes important if your pharmacy maintains a list of drug recalls by lot number.

Inventory Review You have completed your tasks as a pharmacy technician when you check the inventory for the drugs you have used. The pharmacy may have specific reorder levels. If not, a good rule to use for ordering is to have at least one or two quantities that constitute a usual regimen. For example, if ampicillin 250 mg. capsules are used for a prescription, the usual dose is one capsule four times a day for 10 days. Therefore, one regimen equates to 40 capsules (i.e., four capsules per day, times 10 days). We should not be left with fewer than 40 capsules to fill another prescription. Also consider the frequency of use for drugs. Ampicillin 250 mg. capsules may be a fast mover in your area. If that is the case, you should have at least a full backup bottle of 100 or 1000 capsules and still list the drug in the reorder book.

Record Review Finally, complete whatever record keeping and signatures are required by your practice setting or the pharmacy's policy. I find that entering a brief description of the drug often comes to good use, especially in an environment of multi-source generic drugs. Patients become very concerned when the refills do not look the same as the originally filled prescription. You are prepared to assure the patient that the refill is correct by providing information about the manufacturer and drug description. This knowledge establishes a wonderful rapport between you (and you as a representative of your pharmacy) and the patient.

SAFE MEDICATION PRACTICES

Another tenet of pharmacy practice is, *pharmacy personnel strive to comply with safe medication practices.* Patients trust pharmacy personnel to provide accurate and competent service, safe and effective medications, and information that includes an awareness of the potential hazards or side effects associated with the prescribed medication.

Safe medication practices extend beyond the right drug, for the right person, at the right time. These practices mean that you must be familiar with common side effects, contraindications, and drug or food reactions with medications. The specific information for each drug is beyond the scope of this textbook. I offer you the following advice: Know the adverse drug reactions, side effects, contraindications, drug/food interactions, and the safe/effective dosage ranges, at minimum, for those drugs most commonly used in your practice setting or geographical location. As a general rule, 20 percent of the drugs used in your practice will account for 80 percent of the drugs used. For example, if your practice uses 100 different drugs, the top 20 drugs (20% = 20 out of 100 drugs) will account for 80 percent of these drugs dispensed in your practice activity. This theory enables you to be a good resource for both the patient and the pharmacist by providing you with a solid base of knowledge, even if it is for a limited number of drugs. You will be on target at least 80 percent of the time. The remaining 20 percent can be lookups with little strain on your time.

HANDLING REFILLS

Safe medication practices also include reviewing *refills* for the number of refills and the drug selection. Since a substantial number of generic drugs are currently available, a variety of drug descriptions are likely. What may have been dispensed as an oval white tablet for the initial prescription may now be stocked as a salmon-colored round tablet manufactured by another company. You would certainly put the patient at ease by volunteering the information about the differences in drug description. Always check the label on your bulk bottle to be sure of the drug and strength.

As a general rule, keep in mind the most common types of medication errors. These include:

- Errors of omission (i.e., information that is missing about the patient or the drug)
- Wrong drug prescribed, or wrong drug dispensed as a consequence of poor legibility
- Wrong dose (i.e., either the strength is nonexistent for the product ordered, or the dose is wrong for the regimen required by the patient's condition)
- Wrong dosage form or route of administration (e.g., tablets for a one-year-old child, or suppositories prescribed for oral use)
- Wrong directions (e.g., Q.I.D. dosing for a long-acting drug)

- Drug with an expired "expiration date"
- Drug abbreviations (e.g., *DPH—diphenhydramine*, the antihistamine, or *diphenylhydantoin*, the anti-seizure medication?)

Safe medication practices are key to competent pharmacy practices. Your goal as a pharmacy technician is to adhere to another pharmacy tenet, which is *minimize errors and maximize medication therapy outcome.* You can do this by knowledge of usual dosages, dosage forms, and most-likely regimens for specific drugs. Check and double-check the drug order, your drug selection, and the label. Question all strange and unfamiliar abbreviations used in the directions. NEVER DISPENSE GUESSWORK.

The number of refills is a good indicator of noncompliance, misuse, or abuse. Whatever the reason, significantly early or late refills indicate a potentially unsafe medication practice. You can intervene by making the pharmacist aware of the situation.

STORAGE OF MEDICATIONS

Proper storage of drugs is another part of safe medication practice. Drugs should be kept in the container in which they were dispensed, although daily doses are often removed and placed in devices that assure the patient is taking the drug as directed. Drugs should also be kept free from humid environments such as bathrooms. Refrigerated medications should be stored in the refrigerator and not in the freezer. Medications, even in colored containers, should never be placed in direct sunlight such as on windowsills. Remember, a deteriorated drug is ineffective, and may even be a hazard if the condition is not being treated appropriately. When necessary, use auxiliary labels with proper storage instructions on the container. This will present a constant reminder to the patient.

Where children are concerned, safety (or childproof) caps should be provided. Patients with conditions (i.e., arthritic conditions, fractures, coordination/strength problems) that make opening prescription containers difficult may request easy pop-off tops. Have these patients sign a form or the prescription blank documenting the nature of the problem and the need for a non-safety cap container.

HIGH-RISK DRUGS

Institutional and infusion pharmacy practices are two types of pharmacy settings faced with the hazard of toxic drugs used to prepare intravenous products. These drugs primarily include the ones used in chemotherapy. Other drugs in themselves are not toxic but may be potentially hazardous to a technician who is sensitive or allergic to the drugs. Penicillin is such a drug. Handling or inhaling the drug may invoke an allergic response in the technician preparing the compound.

In particular, the pharmacy technician must be aware of high-risk, hazardous drugs. The technician should be able to recognize and acknowledge the need for prompt and decisive action. The emergency may require a needed drug, information, or cleanup. In the hospital setting and infusion pharmacy setting, preparation of products containing toxic materials is common.

Notably, chemotherapy preparations require special needs for protecting yourself. Use aprons or smocks, latex or vinyl gloves, masks, and goggles for protection. Preparation of toxic materials should be done under a laminar flow hood. The laminar flow hood will be discussed in another chapter of the textbook. You must also adhere to the facility's procedures for handling toxic materials. The operational procedures are a result of many reviews and experiences and are meant to protect you. Be sure the materials needed for cleanup and containment are readily available. You can never be careful enough.

HANDLING THE UNEXPECTED

As discussed, the distributive practice of pharmacy is basic and classic. The prescription is written, interpreted, filled, and delivered. However, in reality distributive pharmacy has elements that are associated with it and performed to assure that the process moves smoothly and efficiently. Some of these items include patient profiling, patient monitoring, controlled substances monitoring, special pharmacy needs for chronic care patients, billing and payment mechanisms, and more.

In the ambulatory setting, you may receive calls involving ingestion of the toxic substances or overdoses. Another tenet of pharmacy is *an able pharmacy practitioner (i.e., a pharmacist or pharmacy technician) is one who is prepared.* Have immediate access to the phone numbers for the nearest poison control center. Have an antidote chart readily available for interim emergency measures while the caller seeks help from the poison center, waits for the emergency response unit, or brings the victim to the emergency room. Be familiar with pharmacy references. I would even recommend you have a favorite reference with which you are very comfortable. By knowing the text format, you can go to information quickly and smoothly, thumbing through the material, highlighting pertinent information with ease and confidence.

Fortunately, emergencies that involve the pharmacy are not common. Nevertheless, we should not overlook potential emergencies that are associated with drug preparation or drug consumption. From this perspective we develop another tenet of pharmacy; that is, *in any pharmacy practice, expect the unexpected.*

PATIENT MONITORING

Other special activities that make the drug delivery process efficient include patient monitoring. Although the operational philosophy of your pharmacy setting may not support active follow-up with patients directly, you are able to determine patient compliance and medication outcome by simply reviewing a patient's refill schedule and asking the patient how he or she feels after taking the prescribed medicine. Premature refills, as discussed, indicate some inconsistency in the drug regimen. Perhaps the patient is taking the medication too often. Delayed refills, on the other hand, may show the possibility that the patient is missing doses. In either event, we have discovered a problem. We can have a vital role in helping the pharmacist intervene for the health and safety of the patient, thereby fulfilling another tenet of pharmacy. *Health and safety of the patient are primary goals for pharmacy practice.*

Asking the patient about how the drug is working can open up many doors about the patient and the drug. Often we can associate the patient's neglect for refills with the patient's negative assessment of the drug outcome. Discussion with the patient may disclose a problem with side effects being too uncomfortable to handle or the daily schedule of the drug being inconvenient. Maybe the drug was a poor selection for the ailment. Whatever the situation, you may identify a problem that you can present to the pharmacist for intervention, again fulfilling a tenet of pharmacy practice.

PATIENT PROFILING

Controlled substances, narcotics, poisons, syringes, and needles require special attention. Because they are regulated by federal and state regulating agencies, precise records covering purchase and dispensing must be kept. You must maintain accurate counts and do regular inventory checks to assure the counts balance.

A good distributive pharmacy operation has an effective patient profiling system. The information contained on a patient profile, whether electronic or hard copy, can protect the patient and you. A functional profile format contains the patient's *full* name and other identifying information such as a nickname, the home address, phone numbers (home and work), attending doctors and their specialties with addresses and phone numbers, allergies, contact persons, and other information that can save you time and the patient from discomfort before filling the prescription, by reviewing the profile for the right patient, allergies or sensitivities, duplicate prescription, and so forth. Promptly complete the profile from the available information soon after dispensing the medication. Do not place profiles on the side, with the intent of completing them later. This does not work and is prone to error.

INFORMATION KNOWLEDGE IS KEY

A pharmacy technician's first consideration is to ensure the health and safety of the patient. One way to accomplish this is by keeping updated with recalls, drugs withdrawn from the market, and new findings about a drug. Little time is needed to check the lot numbers in your stock with those numbers listed on direct mail recalls or listed in journals or other publications. You would be wise to make a notation on the bulk bottle identifying some new information that may be overlooked by the prescribing physician.

Today's health-care environment is driven by payers other than the patient. You should have some familiarity with billing parties and practices. Often referred to as third-party payers, these include insurance companies, unions, and government agencies such as Medicare and Medicaid. Each payer provides its enrollees with a plan that may or may not include a prescription benefit. Know what drugs are covered by each plan, the forms that must be submitted for processing and payment, and the actual payment formula (e.g., average wholesale price plus or minus an established percentage markup, or drug cost plus a dispensing fee, etc.). Medicare, for instance, does not cover drugs that are self-administered. These, obviously, are oral drugs and some injections. However, legislation was passed to cover *oral* anticancer drugs and oral immunosuppressive drugs. Keep up to date and be a resource to the patient. This establishes the premise for another pharmacy tenet. *Be current with all aspects impacting on pharmacy, which include clinical, reimbursement, and legislative issues.*

Although different plans may accept most forms, some plans may specifically require their own customized forms for submission. Other forms that are submitted may be subject to denial or rejection, which in either case means no payment. A basic knowledge about how drugs are paid for, by whom and when, can save you and your patient many agonizing phone calls looking for payment. The more information you have about payers makes you a relevant resource to both your customer and the physician. Ultimately, the more knowledge you have makes the entire distributive pharmacy process more efficient and effective.

EXERCISES

1. The fundamental principle of pharmacy is to prepare and deliver the right ____________________, to the right ____________________, at the right ____________________.
2. As part of a patient care continuum, the pharmacy technician can be involved in the patient's ____________________, ____________________, and ____________________.
3. Define compliance.
4. What are ADRs?
5. What is the meaning of the acronym DME?
6. How can we determine if a drug is a "legend" drug?
7. When do we use auxiliary labels?
8. What is the distributive pharmacy process?
9. What are some ways to determine if someone has tampered with a prescription?
10. What is the difference between the label and the auxiliary label?
11. What is another name for auxiliary labels?
12. Does the auxiliary label "PROTECT FROM LIGHT" refer to the drug, patient, or both?
13. What general groups of auxiliary labels are available?
14. What is another name for the container used to package solid oral medications such as capsules and tablets?
15. What are the bottles used for liquid preparations called?
16. What should you read on the bulk bottle to prevent medication error?
17. What other product information is helpful to know to prevent harmful medication management?
18. List five common types of medication errors.
19. What should you tell patients about storing drugs in the bathroom?
20. Are child-resistant containers used for all medications?
21. How would a pharmacy technician protect himself or herself while preparing toxic preparations?
22. What is needed to be prepared for a call about an overdose or ingestion of a toxic substance?
23. What is one way to determine a patient's compliance with his or her drug regimen?
24. List the basic elements on a functional patient profile.
25. What is the pharmacy technician's foremost consideration?

CHAPTER 6

Special Pharmacy Skills

OBJECTIVES

When you have completed this chapter, you will be able to:

1. explain the types and nature of special requirements in pharmacy
2. list references available to meet the needs of special pharmacy skills
3. discuss intravenous preparations as a special pharmacy sterile-compounding skill
4. describe the importance of good communication in health-care delivery
5. understand the laws as they pertain to dispensing various classes of drugs

COMPOUNDING

Drugs are primarily manufactured in dosages and forms ready for dispensing by the pharmacy and use by the patient. There are times, however, when special dosages, alternative forms, or modified formulations are necessary or requested by the doctor. Tailored product preparation is a special skill in pharmacy practice known as *compounding.* You may also hear the term *extemporaneous,* which refers to the type of formulation that is apart from the commonly manufactured drugs on the market. As an extemporaneous formulation, the preparation is tailor-made to comply with the doctor's order, which ultimately fulfills the needs of the patient.

Compounding is generally divided into two types. *Sterile* compounding is associated with preparing intravenous admixture products, prefilled syringes, irrigation solutions, and ophthalmologic preparations. The preparation of *non-sterile* formulations refers to specialty formulas (e.g., special ointments, solutions, capsules, etc.) and bulk compounding (in hospitals referred to as bulk manufacturing) of products that may be too expensive to purchase on the market or that are discontinued by the manufacturer. I also include unit dose repackaging and drug prepackaging within the compounding function of pharmacy technicians.

Sterile compounding requires strict measures to assure that the environment is free of pathogenic bacteria. Therefore, a laminar airflow hood is used to provide a "germ-free" environment for compounding eye preparations, intravenous admixture preparations, prefilled syringes, and irrigation solutions. The cardinal rule for sterile compounding is *aseptic technique* (i.e., "handling" methods used to assure a germ-free environment), which is accomplished by using clean handling techniques of drugs in a filtered air environment. The work is performed within a laminar airflow hood in an area designated as the "clean room."

Although non-sterile compounding does not require the same stringent rules within the principles of aseptic technique, cleanliness is vital. The compounding area should be clean and free of clutter. All equipment should be washed thoroughly with soap and water before and after compounding. AVOID CONTAMINATION OF YOUR PRODUCT.

GENERAL COMPOUNDING PROCEDURES

There are general procedures common to all types of compounding. We interpret the order, calculate the quantities, check references for compatibility, select ingredients, access appropriate equipment, check our steps, verify, compound, verify, package, label, record, and dispense.

Upon receipt of the order, check for the appropriateness of the compound. For example, we know that using a long-acting form of a drug to prepare a solution of the drug destroys the extended action of the drug. If we are assured that the compounding is sensible, we calculate the quantity of drug. If the order requires more than one drug, we should check with a reference to determine their compatibility. More of these responsibilities are falling to the pharmacy technician. Pharmacy technician certification supports many activities performed by technicians that would otherwise have been thought to be outside the scope of pharmacy technician responsibilities.

Select the correct quantity of drug, which often must be measured or weighed, and excipients (i.e., inert substances used as a filler, diluent, or vehicle), and clean the equipment you need and the preparation area. Check your steps, verify your calculations, and compound the product, combining the ingredients in an appropriate sequence. Verify your steps up to this point.

You must have adequate area to lie out the components of your compound and the equipment that will be used to prepare the compound. Be sure the area is clean before you start your compounding. If you are using a laminar airflow hood for sterile compounding, clean the work area within the "hood" with a germicidal detergent and rinse with 70% isopropyl alcohol. Clean the work surface with 70% isopropyl alcohol before each batch of work. A sink and refrigerator, which are usually in the general area of the hood, should also be kept clean to prevent contamination.

A basic selection of equipment and instruments needed to do compounding or to reconstitute (i.e., convert from a powder form to a liquid form by adding liquid, usually sterile water) drugs include the following:

1. A prescription balance (a torsion balance or digital balance) used to weigh ingredients
2. A set of metric (milligrams and grams) weights for the torsion balance
3. Mortars (nonporous glass and porous wedgewood types) and pestals made of associated material as the mortars
4. Spatulas (stainless steel and hard rubber) in various sizes
5. Graduates and cylinders (glass or plastic) in a variety of sizes
6. Beakers and flasks
7. Funnels and funnel filter papers
8. Thermometer
9. Glass stirring rods
10. Brushes for cleaning graduates, cylinders, beakers, and flasks

In addition to the equipment, the compounding area is complete with supplies that include parchment papers for levigating ointments (some pharmacies use a glass plate ointment slab to compound ointments), powder papers for weighing out powdered ingredients from bulk stock, containers for various types of products, and empty gelatine capsules that measure from smaller to larger in sizes 5, 4, 3, 2, 1, 0, 00, 000.

FOLLOWING THE PREPARATION

Transfer the preparation into the appropriate container. Label with the name and quantity of the ingredients, or strength (concentration) of the finished product. Give the product a compounding and expiration date, along with your initials. Include a control or batch number, which, in some cases, may be the lot number of the bulk active ingredient.

Record the information on a pharmacy manufacturing log. If the pharmacy does not have one, start a log that records the date, the drug compounded, a control number and expiration date, the compounder's initials, and the initials of the pharmacist who verified the compounding.

If the compound is prepared for the first time, complete a step-by-step compounding instructions book. This task assures compounding uniformity and consistency, while saving time for subsequent orders for the same formulation. A general uniform outline should include the ingredients; the quantity of each ingredient; the equipment needed; a stepwise instruction for preparing the formulation; the formula listing quantities to make a specific amount of final product; packaging instructions (i.e., type of container); and labeling instructions including auxiliary labels, storage requirements, and an expiration period or shelf life. You may want to allow space for additional comments.

Each final product must be labeled appropriately. At minimum, the label should contain the contents, quantities or percentages of each ingredient, the date of preparation, the preparer's initials, an expiration date, and a control number. Control numbers and expiration dates should be listed in one location for referral as needed. If the compounding is bulk, put a copy of the label in the book.

Whether the compounding is bulk, unit dose, special formulation, or intravenous admixture, follow the aforementioned requirements common to all types of compounding. Compliance with all the requirements assures the safety of each compound, consistency in preparing each formulation, and uniformity in the methodology for compounding each formula.

Intravenous Compounding

Intravenous admixture preparation is a facet of sterile compounding practice that requires special attention. Pharmacy technicians who specialize in a pharmacy department's intravenous admixture program are called *bottle techs.* Bottle techs perform a task that is associated with extensive responsibilities that include preparing the hood, stocking the drugs and supplies, evaluating returned unused formulations for possible reuse, assembling containers/additives/supplies/labels, preparing the products, and labeling.

Parenteral therapy is the term for a larger therapeutic modality that includes the IV route of drug administration. Parenteral therapy is characterized by drugs administered by the injectable route into tissue or blood vessels. See Figure 6.1 for the spectrum of parenteral therapy.

As a bottle tech, you must understand and respect the significance of parenteral therapy in order to minimize any potential harm to patients. Advantages of the injectable route of administration include:

1. Immediate drug effect—it is especially significant in conditions such as respiratory airway disease, cardiac arrest, and shock.
2. Avoids digestive secretions—some drugs (e.g., insulin and some antibiotics) are inactivated by enzymes in the gastrointestinal tract.

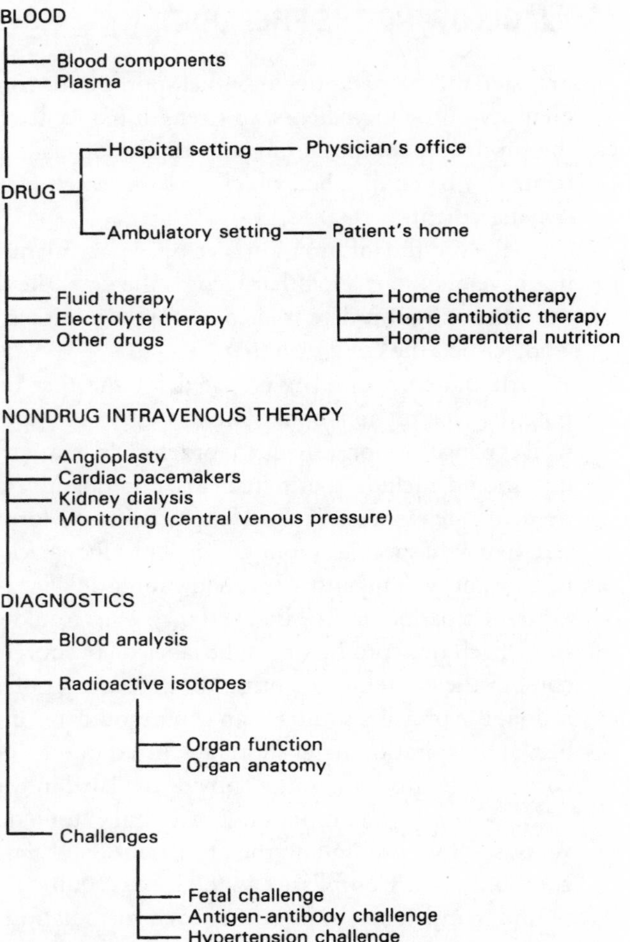

FIGURE 6.1 The spectrum of parenteral therapy.

3. Method of treating unreactive patients—it is often necessary to use a parenteral form of drug in patients who are uncooperative, unconscious, or unable to swallow.
4. Assure compliance in some ambulatory patients—all drugs require compliance with a dosage schedule for successful treatments. Some drugs (e.g., antibiotics) require absolute compliance for a successful outcome. In the case of some ambulatory patients, a practitioner may select a long-acting (sustained release) parenteral form of a drug to assure the correct amount of drug is used over a specific period of time. Injectable intramuscular penicillin suspensions are prime examples of long-acting parenteral formulations.
5. Localize treatment areas—there are times when a patient requires only a specific area to be treated. For example, a cortisone injection into a joint to relieve inflammation, an epinephrine injection into cardiac muscle to treat a cardiac arrest, or local nerve blocks with anesthetic drugs such as lidocaine.
6. Present as the sole treatment—intravenous therapy may be the only way to treat serious fluid and electrolyte imbalances, stubborn infections, or the only form in which some drugs are manufactured.
7. More predictable treatment—effective outcomes are more predictable as a result of a drug's rapid action. A practitioner has timely flexibility if a change of therapy is necessary.

Disadvantages of parenteral therapy are:

1. Requires trained personnel to administer drug
2. Requires strict aseptic technique
3. Rapid effects may be irreversible
4. Usually more expensive than oral formulations
5. Less drug stability than oral formulations
6. Increased risk of infection, septicemia, clinically significant drug interactions, clotting mishaps, and breakdown of tissue (necrosis) surrounding the injection site
7. Requires patient hospital stay for most intravenous therapies

As a result of the greater risks associated with IV therapy, legal responsibilities mandate total competence. Increased reliance on pharmacy technicians for many facets of pharmacy, including IV admixtures, requires learning as much as possible and adhering to hospital protocol.

This chapter deals with a generalized academic exposure to parenteral therapy. Specific guidelines for preparing IV admixtures, the specific products purchased by hospitals, in-house protocols, and so on, will be determined by the facility at which you are gaining valuable practical experience while providing significant services. IV therapy is a highly dynamic area of medicine. It is continuously subject to change due to the many ongoing improvements in medical practice, drugs, and equipment.

The parts of the human anatomy that impact most significantly on IV drug administration are the skin, muscle, and circulatory system. Figure 6.2 shows the configuration of the layers comprising the skin portion of the integumentary system. The various routes of drug injection administration are also noted for each layer.

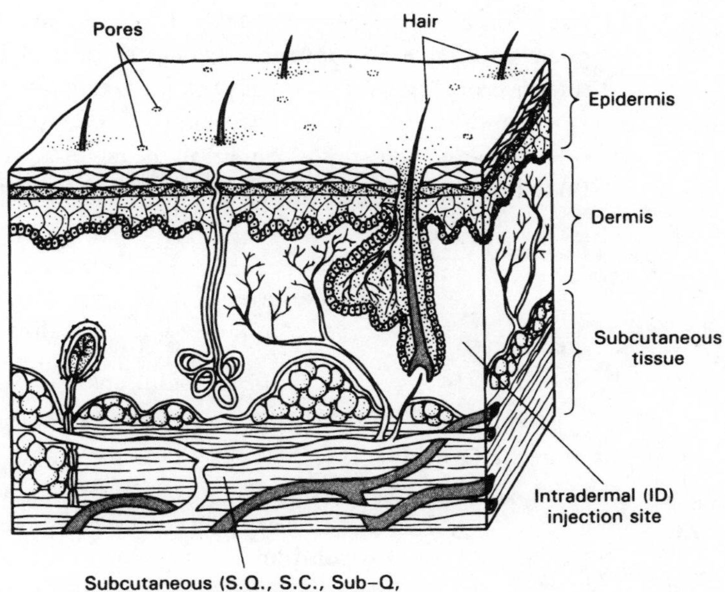

FIGURE 6.2 Cross section of cutaneous layers.

Figure 6.3 indicates additional layers below the subcutaneous tissue layer and the identification of specific routes of drug administration. Note the location of veins surrounded by muscle. Some drugs are manufactured specifically for intramuscular

(IM) use. Practitioners administering parenteral medications must exercise extreme caution and avoid injecting IM preparations into a vein.

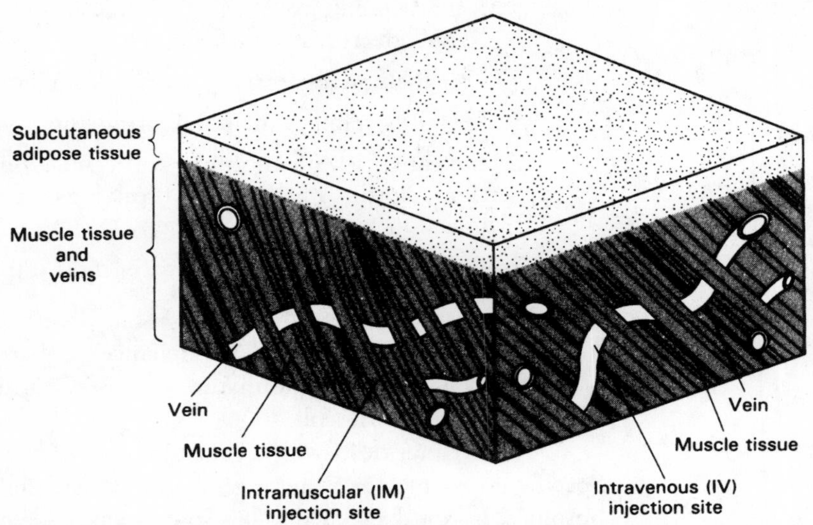

FIGURE 6.3 Cross section of subcutaneous layer and muscle tissue.

The circulatory system includes blood, lymph fluid, and the vessels through which they pass. The lymphatic system functions to return tissue fluid (called lymph fluid upon return to the lymphatic vessels) to the blood. Currently, there are no drugs that are indicated for specific injection directly into the lymph vessels. Blood serves to dilute parenteral drugs and transport these drugs throughout the body.

All drugs administered by commonly used injection sites will eventually find their way to the bloodstream where they will be carried along to exert their effects at the appropriate sites. Table 6.1 summarizes parenteral drug injection sites. Review Table 6.2 for a summary of the anatomy and physiology used in intravenous therapy.

An organism in perfect working order has proper balance, or homeostasis. This means that the body fluids contain all the essential elements in the correct proportions. Body fluids are comprised mostly of water and electrolytes ("lytes"), as follows:

Essential Vitamins

Water-soluble

thiamine (B_1)
riboflavin (B_2)
niacin or nicotinic acid (B_5)
pantothenic acid
pyridoxine (B_6)
biotin
folic acid
cyanocobalamine (B_{12})
ascorbic acid (vitamin C)

Fat-soluble

vitamin A
vitamin D
vitamin E
vitamin K

Trace Elements

zinc (Zn)
copper (Cu)
selenium (Se)
molybdenum (Mo)

TABLE 6.1 PARENTERAL DRUG ROUTES

Route	Abbreviation	Notes
Intradermal	ID	Small drug volumes (0.1 ml.) are administered into the dermal layer of skin.
Subcutaneous, hypodermic	S.Q., S.C., Sub-Q, subcut., hypo	Small drug volumes are administered into the subcutaneous layer of the outer surface of the arm or thigh.
Intramuscular	IM	Up to 2 ml. volumes of drug may be administered into the muscle of the upper arm. Up to 5 ml. volumes may be administered into the muscle of the buttocks.
Intravenous	IV	Injection into the vein. Volume of drug is not a major factor. Drug effect, predictability, and dosage requirement impact on volume.
(Less frequently used routes)		
Intra-arterial		Into an artery ending at a specific site in a target organ.
Intracardiac		Into the heart.
Intra-articular		Into a joint.
Intraspinal		Into the spine.
Peridural		Into the area around the spine.
Intrathecal		Into the spinal fluid.
Intrasynovial		Into the fluid surrounding a joint.
Hypodermoclysis		Large volume of fluid into the subcutaneous tissue layer.

TABLE 6.2 ANATOMY AND PHYSIOLOGY INVOLVED IN INTRAVENOUS THERAPY

Structure	Function
Skin	Protects, maintains moisture, responds to stimuli, eliminates waste, regulates body temperature
Blood vessels	Carry blood throughout the body; arteries carry blood away from the heart, while veins carry blood toward (into) the heart
Blood	Supplies body cells with oxygen, nutrients, and chemicals, which regulate body functions; carries waste products to organs, which eliminate wastes
Cells	Basic building blocks for each type of body organ

chromium (Cr)　　cobalt (Co)
manganese (Mn)　　iodine (I)

The FDA acceptable standards for multiple trace element solution additives are:

zinc	4 mg.
copper	0.5 mg.
chromium	10 mcg.
manganese	0.15 mg.

The ideal total body water content is approximately 70 percent of body weight. The body fluids can be further divided into the fluid inside the cells (intracellular), at 50 percent, and outside the cells (extracellular), amounting to 20 percent. Extracellular fluid is comprised of fluid located in the spaces between the tissues (interstitial) and intravascular fluid in the blood (plasma).

The normal body fluid distribution may be upset by infection, age, environmental trauma, or genetic-related disorders. A fluid/electrolyte imbalance can cause a number of abnormal body states.

Common States of Body Fluid/Electrolyte Imbalance

sodium excess (hypernatremia)

sodium deficit (hyponatremia)

water loss (dehydration)

acid-base imbalance (acidosis/alkalosis)

potassium deficit (hypokalemia)

potassium excess (hyperkalemia)

magnesium deficit (hypomagnesemia)

magnesium excess (hypermagnesemia)

The physician is trained to evaluate imbalances in a patient. He or she must consider many factors before selecting the appropriate therapeutic defense action (e.g., intravenous antibiotic, chemotherapy), regulating action (e.g., antiulcer, anti-inflammatory, fluid/electrolyte therapy), or nutritional support (e.g., total parenteral nutrition or partial parenteral nutrition). The physician, with the aid of pharmacy technology, will select a treatment to correct profound alterations in anatomical or physiological derangements in fluid balance. See Figure 6.4.

Modern technology has provided a variety of therapeutic tools in the form of fluids, drugs, and equipment. Inasmuch as the scope of this text is to develop an understanding of the parenteral components and their functions, we will review fluid therapy generically.

Since the seventeenth century, the parenteral/intravenous modality evolved from blood transfusions, going through stages which included the instillation of drugs, diagnostic techniques, and intravenous feeding. Associated with this increasing and ad-

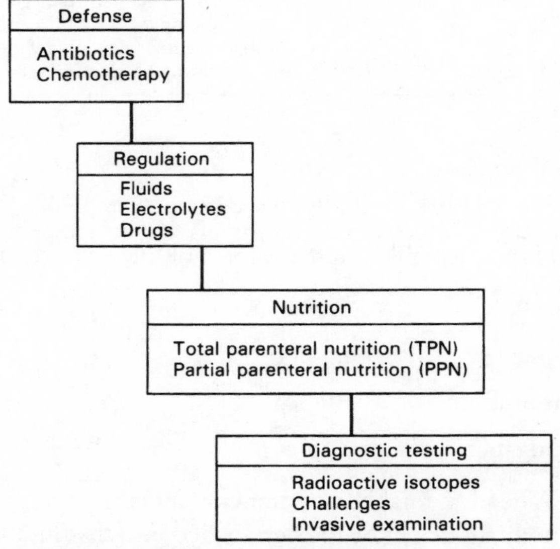

FIGURE 6.4 Intravenous therapy selection.

vancing spectrum of intravenous tools are improvements in technology—from the historical silver tubes to today's modern computerized volumetric IV pumps.

There are a multitude of solutions used for IV therapy, which vary enormously in contents, volumes, and use. The basic large-volume fluids include solutions of dextrose, sodium chloride, electrolytes, fats, and amino acids. Small-volume drugs are also available commercially. They include vitamins, trace elements, and many drugs for different treatments. Many drugs must be added to large-volume solutions for dilution. The resulting product is known as an admixture. The drug added to the large-volume solution is called an additive or "ad."

SELECTION OF THERAPY

FLUIDS: Restore and maintain homeostatic body fluid balance.

Examples:

Plasma expanders:

dextran
hetastarch
lactated Ringer's injection
plasma
normal human serum albumin

DRUGS: Restore regulatory processes, defend against invading pathogens, and relieve symptoms associated with disorders.

Examples:

antimicrobial drugs
analgesics
anticonvulsants
general anesthetics
respiratory drugs
cardiovascular drugs
anticoagulant agents
steroid agents
antihypertensive drugs
diuretics
thrombolytic drugs
hormones
antiulcer drugs
antineoplastic (oncolytic) drugs

NUTRIENTS: Sustain body processes while patient is unable to ingest and/or use traditional foods.

Examples:

dextrose
minerals/electrolytes
trace elements
amino acids

The number of commercially available intravenous solutions is enormous. Note the following sample of commonly used intravenous fluids.

Single electrolyte solutions:

- sodium chloride 0.45%, $\frac{1}{2}$NS, 0.5NS (*Note:* NS may appear as S) (also called half-normal saline or hypotonic saline)
- sodium chloride 0.9%, NS (also called normal saline or physiological saline or isotonic saline)
- sodium chloride 3%
- sodium chloride 5%
  (*Note:* any sodium chloride [salt] concentration greater than normal saline solution is a *hypertonic* solution.)

- sodium lactate
- sodium bicarbonate 5%

Dextrose solutions:

- dextrose 5% in water, D5W
- dextrose 10% in water, D10W
- dextrose 20% in water, D20W

Combination dextrose and electrolyte solutions:

- dextrose 2.5% and sodium chloride 0.45%, D2.5 $\frac{1}{2}$S
- dextrose 5% and sodium chloride 0.2%, D5 $\frac{1}{4}$S
- dextrose 5% and sodium chloride 0.45%, D5 $\frac{1}{2}$S, D5 0.5S
- dextrose 5% and sodium chloride 0.9%, D5S, D5NS
- dextrose 5% plus potassium chloride (KCl) in a variety of concentrations
- dextrose 5% plus $\frac{1}{2}$NS plus KCl

Other preparations are commercially formulated to include other concentrations of dextrose, sodium chloride, and other electrolytes (for example, dextrose 5% in Ringer's solution or lactated Ringer's solution).

Multiple electrolyte solutions:

- lactated Ringer's solution (Hartmann's solution)
- Ringer's solution

Amino acid solutions:

- amino acid solutions
- amino acids plus dextrose
- amino acids plus dextrose plus electrolytes

Fat emulsions for intravenous use:

- products are available in 10% and 20% concentrations

Other available fluids:

- invert sugar in water
- invert sugar and electrolytes
- fructose in water
- fructose and electrolytes
- dextran in dextrose solution
- dextrain in sodium chloride solution
- sodium lactate $\frac{1}{6}$M (M = molar)
- sterile water for injection
- water for injection
- bacteriostatic water for injection

Electrolyte preparations are also available in single small quantities. For example, you will usually find potassium chloride (KCl) in 10 ml. or 20 ml. vials containing 20, 30, or 40 mEq. These products must be diluted before use. They allow the physician greater flexibility in adjusting concentrations for specific electrolytes. See Figure 6.5 for commonly used electrolytes.

Anions / Cations	HCO_3	Cl	PO_4	SO_4	gluconate	acetate	lactate
Na	$NaHCO_3$	NaCl				Na acetate	Na lactate
K		KCl	*				
Ca		CaCl			Ca gluconate		
Mg				$MgSO_4$			
NH_4		NH_4Cl					

*Commercial preparations of potassium phosphate injections contain a mixture of monobasic potassium phosphate (KH_2PO_4) and dibasic potassium phosphate (K_2HPO_4).

FIGURE 6.5 Commonly used electrolyte additives. These electrolyte preparations are available in small quantities and may be used in varying amounts, giving the physician greater flexibility in adjusting concentrations of commercially available preparations.

NUTRITIONAL SUPPORT

Nutrient solutions are used in patients who are unable to ingest, digest, or absorb nutrients from the gastrointestinal tract. Patients who have undergone surgery usually require a short-term intravenous feeding. In these cases the objective is to supply enough carbohydrates (approximately 150 grams/day) to prevent protein breakdown, maintain brain metabolic activities, and assure erythrocyte metabolism. Dextrose solutions in low concentrations of 5% or 10% with sodium chloride in concentrations of 0.25% or 0.45% (i.e., D5 $\frac{1}{4}$ S, D5 $\frac{1}{2}$S, D10 $\frac{1}{4}$S, or D10 $\frac{1}{2}$S) are the usual fluid selections. These solutions are infused through a peripheral vein.

Patients may require a modified parenteral feeding for a short time in order to sustain the body's metabolic functions. This modified nutritional support program is called *partial parenteral nutrition (PPN).* A PPN therapy requires an amino acid solution (a nitrogen source) with a low dextrose concentration (up to 10%) optional. Some practitioners may prescribe a fat emulsion to be added to the PPN regimen. The PPN is infused through a peripheral vein.

PARTIAL PARENTERAL NUTRITIONAL REGIMENS

- amino acid (supplies nitrogen) and dextrose (supplies carbohydrate)
- amino acid, dextrose, and fat emulsion (supplies calories)
- amino acid solution alone

Long-term intravenous total nutritional support is indicated for patients with excessive protein deficits. *Parenteral hyperalimentation* or *total parenteral nutrition (TPN)* is a therapy that provides the patient with all the nutritional requirements to support the functions of life. TPN is comprised of amino acids and a high-concentration dextrose as a fundamental solution, and is infused through a central venous route. The central venous route is necessary because the blood flow is greater, thereby diluting the concentrated TPN solution rapidly. The practitioner, after a thorough assessment of the patient and laboratory values, prescribes specific concentrations or quantities of electrolytes, vitamins, minerals, and trace elements to be added to the TPN solution. See Figure 6.6.

Fat emulsions are also available and are used as a nonprotein source of calories in addition to the dextrose. Fat emulsions are given intravenously through a separate intravenous line.

Intravenous preparations present a part of pharmacy that is vast and constantly changing. The knowledge you acquire, the techniques you learn, and familiarity with the products you use will develop from experience. Regardless of the changes and advancements you encounter, some rules never change.

RULES FOR PROPER MIXING

Aseptic Technique Always follow the rules of aseptic technique. Use alcohol to cleanse and sterilize diaphragm tops of vials, laminar airflow hood work spaces, and so on. Take every precaution to assure purity, safety, and sterility by preventing contamination. Intravenous solutions should always be prepared under a clean laminar flow hood. *Nothing can be substituted for cleanliness, care, and caution.*

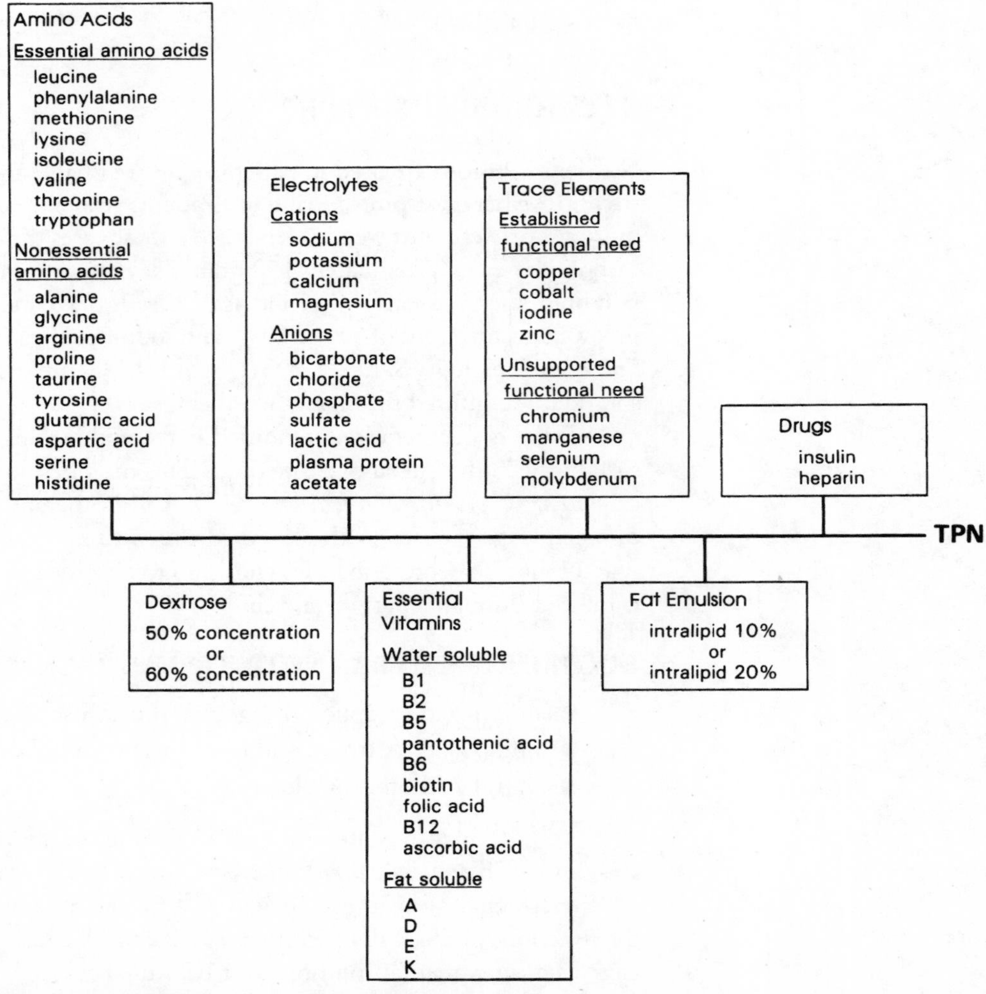

FIGURE 6.6 Elements of total parenteral nutrition.

Proper Mechanics There is only one right way to prepare IV solutions and mixtures. Never substitute convenience and shortcuts for good judgment and accepted admixture preparation techniques. *Haste makes waste.*

Noncongested Work Area Make only your needed accessories available under the laminar airflow hood. Too many items invite confusion and error. *A cluttered space is a cluttered mind.*

Uniform Products You must guarantee product integrity to the best of your ability. Concern yourself with uniformity in your techniques. Consistency in your approved methods of admixture preparation is a sure approach toward freedom from pyrogens, microbes, and particulate matter. *Patient safety is basic to the practice of pharmacy.*

Interpretive Orders You must interpret IV orders properly. Avoid the slightest misinterpretation with a call to the prescribing physician for clarification. *Never dispense guesswork.*

Accurate Compounding You must know your mathematics and double-check your calculations. Always keep in mind that the IV route of administration is the most dangerous route. *Knowledge is the precursor to competence.*

Acceptable Product The final properly prepared product is complete only when the appropriate label is affixed to the bottle. Acceptable admixture solutions should be made only at the time of need. Total parenteral nutrition solutions should be discarded 48 hours after their preparation. *Safety is first.*

Current Knowledge You have an obligation to be current with information. You must remain constant with the state of the art. There are many references containing information on safety, incompatibilities, and dosages. *Competence is the precursor to confidence.*

Hospital Policy You must always be aware of hospital policy and hospital intravenous protocols. Protocols are usually the result of intense research and investigation used by pharmacy therapeutics committees. *What is proven is true.*

Self-protection You should take every precaution to protect yourself from highly toxic drugs (i.e., chemotherapeutic agents). Wear surgical gloves, masks, and proper smocks. Carefully change surgical gloves within each half hour. Properly dispose of used supplies. *Caution is an IV technician's best friend.*

Compounding processes most often require some type of mathematical calculation. The mathematics for calculating the necessary ingredients of an IV solution is fundamental. Ratio, proportion, and percentages are the essential areas of mathematics for providing safe and effective admixtures to patients.

In addition to patient safety, correct calculations assure product economy by minimizing product waste. You should start early to train yourself to be accurate, and assure your accuracy by always rechecking your numbers, calculations, and mathematical processes. If necessary, consult with the pharmacist or ask another technician to review your calculations. Be sure a pharmacist checks your final calculations and product.

Review the sample TPN solution order shown in Figure 6.7. Cover the answer. Using the available information, calculate the necessary volumes of each electrolyte, insulin, and heparin to be used.

Specific IV hardware is used to prepare large-volume infusion solutions. Likewise, additives used in admixtures and the reconstitution of many drugs require IV hardware.

Needles. Vary in diameter size (gauge) and length. The larger the gauge, the smaller the diameter. An 18-gauge needle has a smaller diameter than a 16-gauge needle.

Syringes. Vary in size and calibrations. Some syringes are specific for drugs given in small amounts or requiring specific calibrations such as insulin ("insulin" syringe) and tuberculin ("tuberculin" syringe).

PATIENT: John Doe
AGE: 47
SEX: M
RACE: Cauc.
CHART NO. 009876D

MEMORIAL HOSPITAL
BALTIMORE, MARYLAND
PHYSICIAN'S ORDER RECORD

BEAR DOWN ON HARD SURFACE WITH BALL POINT PEN

GENERIC EQUIVALENT IS AUTHORIZED UNLESS CHECKED IN THIS COLUMN

ALLERGY OR SENSITIVITY TO NKDA
DIAGNOSIS S/P TUR
NONE KNOWN ☐ SIGNED: [signature]

DATE	TIME	ORDERS	PHYSICIAN'S SIG.

TOTAL PARENTERAL NUTRITION (TPN) SOLUTION ORDERS—CENTRAL

AMINOSYN 10% 500 ml Final Concentration 5%
DEXTROSE 50% WATER 500 ml Final Concentration 25%
Rate 100 ml/hour

Bottle # 9
POTASSIUM PHOSPHATE 10 mEq — OTHER ____
SODIUM CHLORIDE 40 mEq — OTHER ____
SODIUM ACETATE 20 mEq — HEPARIN 1000 UNITS
POTASSIUM CHLORIDE 40 mEq — TRACE ELEMENTS *see below
REGULAR HUMULIN 10 units — VITAMINS *see below

AMINOSYN 10% 500 ml Final Concentration 5%
DEXTROSE 50% 500 ml Final Concentration 25%
Rate 100 ml/hour

Bottle # 10 MULTI-ELECTROLYTE CONCENTRATE CONSISTING OF:
SODIUM 25 mEq CALCIUM 5 mEq CHLORIDE 30 mEq
POTASSIUM 20 mEq MAGNESIUM 5 mEq ACETATE 25 mEq
HEPARIN 1000 units
REGULAR HUMULIN 8 units
OTHER APPROVED ADDITIVE ____

20% FAT EMULSION IS TO RUN CONTINUOUSLY THROUGH THE PROXIMAL MEDICINAL ENTRY AT 20 ml/hour (PHARMACY WILL SEQUENTIALLY LETTER BEGINNING WITH A)

NOTE: VITAMINS AND TRACE ELEMENTS WILL BE ADDED AS DESCRIBED IN PROTOCOL
Hang all bottles in consecutive order. RECORD the EXACT TIME hung as well as the bottle number and total volume. Maintain a constant rate. DO NOT catch up or slow down the infusion. Orders must be rewritten DAILY. THE TPN LINE SHOULD NOT BE USED FOR ANY OTHER PURPOSE.

PATIENTS ON TPN ARE TO RECEIVE:

1. CBC, BUN, LYTES, CREATININE, GLUCOSE every day for five days then MONDAYS and THURSDAYS.
2. SGOT, Ca, ALK PHOS, Mg, SGPT, BILIRUBIN, ALBUMIN, GLOBULIN, PO_4, PROTHROMBIN TIME, PARTIAL THROMBOPLASTIN TIME Monday, Thursday for the first week, then weekly.
3. Urine Acetone and Glucose and Specific Gravity every four hours for the first week then four times a day.
4. Weigh daily.
5. Serum transferrin level once per week.
6. In depleted patients and patients on prolonged hyperalimentation trace element levels should be requested.
7. Weekly twenty-four hour urine with an ALIQUOT for CREATININE and UREA NITROGEN.
8. DIETARY CONSULT.

PHARMACY COPY

FIGURE 6.7a Sample TPN order and calculations.

SUPPLIES:

Electrolyte/Drug	*Abbreviation*	*How Supplied*
potassium phosphate	KPO_4	10 ml. vial containing 4.4 mEq./ml.
sodium chloride	NaCl	30 ml. vial containing 4 mEq./ml.
sodium acetate	Na Acet.	20 ml. vial containing 40 mEq.
potassium chloride	KCl	10 ml. vial containing 20 mEq.
insulin		10 ml. vial containing 100 u/ml.
heparin		4 ml. vial containing 10,000 u/ml.

CALCULATIONS FOR BOTTLE #9:

Ingredient	*Required Amount*
KPO_4	10 mEq.

Solution: Each ml. of KPO_4 contains 4.4 mEq. Therefore, use 10 mEq./4.4 mEq. = 2.27 ml. 2.27 ml. provides 10 mEq.

Ingredient	*Required Amount*
NaCl	40 mEq.

Solution: Each ml. of NaCl contains 4 mEq. Therefore, use 40 mEq./4 mEq. = 10 ml. 10 ml. provides 40 mEq.

Ingredient	*Required Amount*
Na Acet.	20 mEq.

Solution: Each vial of Na Acet. contains 40 mEq. Therefore, use 20 mEq./40 mEq. = $\frac{1}{2}$ vial. $\frac{1}{2}$ of the 20 ml. vial is 10 ml. 10 ml. will contain 20 mEq. required.

Ingredient	*Required Amount*
KCl	40 mEq.

Solution: Each vial contains 20 mEq. Therefore, use 40 mEq./20 mEq. = 2 vials. Two vials will provide 40 mEq. of KCl required.

Ingredient	*Required Amount*
insulin	10 units

Solution: Each vial contains 100 u per milliliter. Therefore, use 10 u/100 u = 0.1 ml. 0.1 ml. provides 10 units of insulin.

Ingredient	*Required Amount*
heparin	1,000 units

Solution: Each vial contains 10,000 u/ml. Therefore, use 1,000 u/10,000 u = 0.1 ml. 0.1 ml. provides 1,000 units of heparin.

FIGURE 6.7 *(continued)*

Catheters. Must be sterile for the preparation of IV products. They vary in length and style (straight or "Y"-shaped).

Filters. Are necessary to filter particulate matter and materials usually greater than 0.22 microns in size.

Containers. Vary widely in composition (glass or plastic); content (drug, solution, evacuated, partial fill, frozen); and purpose (receptacle for admixture preparation, "piggyback," small-volume drugs such as antibiotics, ready-for-use solutions).

Pump infusions. Deliver accurate quantities and volumes of drugs in a rapid fashion. They usually require a syringe into which a solution is drawn.

Transfer spikes. Enable the transfer of drugs reconstituted in a small vial to be added to large-volume solutions. They are double-ended piercing pins. Some spikes are specialized, such as the *chemo dispensing pin,* used for chemotherapeutic medications.

Connectors. Used to assure proper closure between a catheter end and a syringe, needle, or another catheter. The most commonly used lock is known as the Luer lock.

Administration sets. Used to transfer the many components (drugs, fluids, etc.) that often make up a final product. Sets include general sets, piggyback sets, filter sets, extension sets, transfer sets, and more.

Tips

- Solutions should be clear (including colored solutions).
- Always check expiration dates of products being used.
- Follow IV protocols explicitly.
- Dextrose supplies 3.4 calories per gram.
- Fat supplies 9 calories per gram.
- Protein supplies 4 calories per gram.
- The formula for *osmolarity* is:

$$\text{mOsm/L} = 100(\text{AA\%}) + 50(\text{dextrose \%}) + \text{mEq./L.}$$

- Complete a preparation before leaving the workstation.
- Work well inside the laminar airflow hood.
- Run the laminar airflow hood for at least 30 minutes before preparing IV products.
- Rotate supplies to assure orderly flow of expiration dates.
- Have supplies readily available.
- Label, date, and properly store partially used vials.
- Know key abbreviations used in IV admixture programs and add to this list when necessary. See Table 6.3.

Intravenous pharmacy is perhaps the most challenging, demanding, and critical area of pharmacy. If you adhere to the proper principles associated with preparing IV products, you will easily meet the challenge and demand, thereby assuring your ultimate goal—safety to the patient and effectiveness of the therapy.

Review the following practice TPN orders (Figures 6.8 to 6.11). Complete the calculations for each practice problem using the same format as in the sample order in Figure 6-7. Solutions may be found at the end of the practice orders.

TABLE 6.3 IMPORTANT ABBREVIATIONS USED IN INTRAVENOUS ADMIXTURE PROGRAMS

Abbreviation	Meaning
AA	amino acids
IV or I.V.	intravenous
mEq.	milliequivalent
IVPB	intravenous piggyback
NS	normal saline
R	Ringer's solution
LR	lactated Ringer's solution
LVP	large-volume parenteral
Na Bicarb	sodium bicarbonate
Na lact	sodium lactate
PCA	patient-controlled analgesia
SVP	small-volume parenteral

PATIENT: Jane Doe
AGE: 38
SEX: F
RACE: N
CHART NO. 002346J

MEMORIAL HOSPITAL
BALTIMORE, MARYLAND
PHYSICIAN'S ORDER RECORD

BEAR DOWN ON HARD SURFACE WITH BALL POINT PEN

GENERIC EQUIVALENT IS AUTHORIZED UNLESS CHECKED IN THIS COLUMN

ALLERGY OR SENSITIVITY TO ASA
NONE KNOWN ☐ SIGNED: [signature]

DIAGNOSIS S/P remove mass (R) lung

DATE	TIME	ORDERS	PHYSICIAN'S SIG.

TOTAL PARENTERAL NUTRITION (TPN) SOLUTION ORDERS—CENTRAL

AMINOSYN 10% 500 ml Final Concentration 5%
DEXTROSE 50% WATER 500 ml Final Concentration 25%
Rate 100 ml/hour

Bottle # 12
POTASSIUM PHOSPHATE 10 mEq
SODIUM CHLORIDE 40 mEq
SODIUM ACETATE ____ mEq
POTASSIUM CHLORIDE 50 mEq
REGULAR HUMULIN ____ units
OTHER ____
OTHER ____
HEPARIN 1000 UNITS
TRACE ELEMENTS *see below
VITAMINS *see below

AMINOSYN 10% 500 ml Final Concentration 5%
DEXTROSE 50% 500 ml Final Concentration 25%
Rate 100 ml/hour

Bottle # 13 MULTI-ELECTROLYTE CONCENTRATE CONSISTING OF:
SODIUM 25 mEq CALCIUM 5 mEq CHLORIDE 30 mEq
POTASSIUM 20 mEq MAGNESIUM 5 mEq ACETATE 25 mEq
HEPARIN 1000 units
REGULAR HUMULIN 10 units
OTHER APPROVED ADDITIVE ____

20% FAT EMULSION IS TO RUN CONTINUOUSLY THROUGH THE PROXIMAL MEDICINAL ENTRY AT 20 ml/hour (PHARMACY WILL SEQUENTIALLY LETTER BEGINNING WITH A)

NOTE: VITAMINS AND TRACE ELEMENTS WILL BE ADDED AS DESCRIBED IN PROTOCOL
Hang all bottles in consecutive order. RECORD the EXACT TIME hung as well as the bottle number and total volume. Maintain a constant rate. DO NOT catch up or slow down the infusion. Orders must be rewritten DAILY. THE TPN LINE SHOULD NOT BE USED FOR ANY OTHER PURPOSE.
PATIENTS ON TPN ARE TO RECEIVE:

1. CBC, BUN, LYTES, CREATININE, GLUCOSE every day for five days then MONDAYS and THURSDAYS.
2. SGOT, Ca, ALK PHOS, Mg, SGPT, BILIRUBIN, ALBUMIN, GLOBULIN, PO_4, PROTHROMBIN TIME, PARTIAL THROMBOPLASTIN TIME Monday, Thursday for the first week, then weekly.
3. Urine Acetone and Glucose and Specific Gravity every four hours for the first week then four times a day.
4. Weigh daily.
5. Serum transferrin level once per week.
6. In depleted patients and patients on prolonged hyperalimentation trace element levels should be requested.
7. Weekly twenty-four hour urine with an ALIQUOT for CREATININE and UREA NITROGEN.
8. DIETARY CONSULT.

PHARMACY COPY

FIGURE 6.8

PATIENT: Jim Doe
AGE: 53
SEX: M
RACE: Cauc.
CHART NO. 001357JD

MEMORIAL HOSPITAL
BALTIMORE, MARYLAND
PHYSICIAN'S ORDER RECORD

BEAR DOWN ON HARD SURFACE WITH BALL POINT PEN

GENERIC EQUIVALENT IS AUTHORIZED UNLESS CHECKED IN THIS COLUMN

ALLERGY OR SENSITIVITY TO: Ø
NONE KNOWN ☐ SIGNED: [signature]

DIAGNOSIS: Intestinal Obstruction

DATE	TIME	ORDERS	PHYSICIAN'S SIG.

TOTAL PARENTERAL NUTRITION (TPN) SOLUTION ORDERS—CENTRAL
AMINOSYN 10% 500 ml Final Concentration 5%
DEXTROSE 50% WATER 500 ml Final Concentration 25%
Rate 100 ml/hour
Bottle # 4 POTASSIUM PHOSPHATE 10 mEq OTHER
SODIUM CHLORIDE 40 mEq OTHER
SODIUM ACETATE 40 mEq HEPARIN 1000 UNITS
POTASSIUM CHLORIDE ____ mEq TRACE ELEMENTS *see below
REGULAR HUMULIN ____ units VITAMINS *see below

AMINOSYN 10% 500 ml Final Concentration 5%
DEXTROSE 50% 500 ml Final Concentration 25%
Rate 100 ml/hour
Bottle # 5 MULTI-ELECTROLYTE CONCENTRATE CONSISTING OF:
SODIUM 25 mEq CALCIUM 5 mEq CHLORIDE 30 mEq
POTASSIUM 20 mEq MAGNESIUM 5 mEq ACETATE 25 mEq
HEPARIN 1000 units
REGULAR HUMULIN 8 units
OTHER APPROVED ADDITIVE ____

20% FAT EMULSION IS TO RUN CONTINUOUSLY THROUGH THE PROXIMAL MEDICINAL ENTRY AT 20 ml/hour (PHARMACY WILL SEQUENTIALLY LETTER BEGINNING WITH A)

NOTE: VITAMINS AND TRACE ELEMENTS WILL BE ADDED AS DESCRIBED IN PROTOCOL
Hang all bottles in consecutive order. RECORD the EXACT TIME hung as well as the bottle number and total volume. Maintain a constant rate. DO NOT catch up or slow down the infusion. Orders must be rewritten DAILY. THE TPN LINE SHOULD NOT BE USED FOR ANY OTHER PURPOSE.
PATIENTS ON TPN ARE TO RECEIVE:

1. CBC, BUN, LYTES, CREATININE, GLUCOSE every day for five days then MONDAYS and THURSDAYS.
2. SGOT, Ca, ALK PHOS, Mg, SGPT, BILIRUBIN, ALBUMIN, GLOBULIN, PO_4, PROTHROMBIN TIME, PARTIAL THROMBOPLASTIN TIME Monday, Thursday for the first week, then weekly.
3. Urine Acetone and Glucose and Specific Gravity every four hours for the first week then four times a day.
4. Weigh daily.
5. Serum transferrin level once per week.
6. In depleted patients and patients on prolonged hyperalimentation trace element levels should be requested.
7. Weekly twenty-four hour urine with an ALIQUOT for CREATININE and UREA NITROGEN.
8. DIETARY CONSULT.

PHARMACY COPY

FIGURE 6.9

PATIENT: Liu Doe
AGE: 60
SEX: M
RACE: Oriental
CHART NO. 002468DL

MEMORIAL HOSPITAL
BALTIMORE, MARYLAND
PHYSICIAN'S ORDER RECORD

BEAR DOWN ON HARD SURFACE WITH BALL POINT PEN

GENERIC EQUIVALENT IS AUTHORIZED UNLESS CHECKED IN THIS COLUMN

ALLERGY OR SENSITIVITY TO: Ragweed, fish
NONE KNOWN ☐ SIGNED:

DIAGNOSIS: ABD. CA.

DATE	TIME	ORDERS	PHYSICIAN'S SIG.

TOTAL PARENTERAL NUTRITION (TPN) SOLUTION ORDERS—CENTRAL

AMINOSYN 10% 500 ml Final Concentration 5%
DEXTROSE 50% WATER 500 ml Final Concentration 25%
Rate 100 ml/hour

Bottle # 11 POTASSIUM PHOSPHATE 10 mEq OTHER ______
SODIUM CHLORIDE 80 mEq OTHER ______
SODIUM ACETATE ______ mEq HEPARIN 1000 UNITS
POTASSIUM CHLORIDE ______ mEq TRACE ELEMENTS *see below
REGULAR HUMULIN ______ units VITAMINS *see below

AMINOSYN 10% 500 ml Final Concentration 5%
DEXTROSE 50% 500 ml Final Concentration 25%
Rate 100 ml/hour

Bottle # 12 MULTI-ELECTROLYTE CONCENTRATE CONSISTING OF:
SODIUM 25 mEq CALCIUM 5 mEq CHLORIDE 30 mEq
POTASSIUM 20 mEq MAGNESIUM 5 mEq ACETATE 25 mEq
HEPARIN 1000 units
REGULAR HUMULIN ______ units
OTHER APPROVED ADDITIVE ______

20% FAT EMULSION IS TO RUN CONTINUOUSLY THROUGH THE PROXIMAL MEDICINAL ENTRY AT 20 ml/hour (PHARMACY WILL SEQUENTIALLY LETTER BEGINNING WITH A)

NOTE: VITAMINS AND TRACE ELEMENTS WILL BE ADDED AS DESCRIBED IN PROTOCOL
Hang all bottles in consecutive order. RECORD the EXACT TIME hung as well as the bottle number and total volume. Maintain a constant rate. DO NOT catch up or slow down the infusion. Orders must be rewritten DAILY. THE TPN LINE SHOULD NOT BE USED FOR ANY OTHER PURPOSE.

PATIENTS ON TPN ARE TO RECEIVE:

1. CBC, BUN, LYTES, CREATININE, GLUCOSE every day for five days then MONDAYS and THURSDAYS.
2. SGOT, Ca, ALK PHOS, Mg, SGPT, BILIRUBIN, ALBUMIN, GLOBULIN, PO_4, PROTHROMBIN TIME, PARTIAL THROMBOPLASTIN TIME Monday, Thursday for the first week, then weekly.
3. Urine Acetone and Glucose and Specific Gravity every four hours for the first week then four times a day.
4. Weigh daily.
5. Serum transferrin level once per week.
6. In depleted patients and patients on prolonged hyperalimentation trace element levels should be requested.
7. Weekly twenty-four hour urine with an ALIQUOT for CREATININE and UREA NITROGEN.
8. DIETARY CONSULT.

PHARMACY COPY

FIGURE 6.10

PATIENT: Jennifer Doe
AGE: 33
SEX: F
RACE: Cauc.
CHART NO. 009753DJ

MEMORIAL HOSPITAL
BALTIMORE, MARYLAND
PHYSICIAN'S ORDER RECORD

BEAR DOWN ON HARD SURFACE WITH BALL POINT PEN

GENERIC EQUIVALENT IS AUTHORIZED UNLESS CHECKED IN THIS COLUMN

ALLERGY OR SENSITIVITY
TO_____
NONE KNOWN [X] SIGNED: [signature]

DIAGNOSIS
Toxic Colitis
s/p colectomy

DATE	TIME	ORDERS	PHYSICIAN'S SIG.
	••		••

TOTAL PARENTERAL NUTRITION (TPN) SOLUTION ORDERS—CENTRAL

AMINOSYN 10% 500 ml Final Concentration 5%
DEXTROSE 50% WATER 500 ml Final Concentration 25%
Rate 100 ml/hour

Bottle # 14
POTASSIUM PHOSPHATE 10 mEq — OTHER_____
SODIUM CHLORIDE 40 mEq — OTHER_____
SODIUM ACETATE 20 mEq — HEPARIN 1000 UNITS
POTASSIUM CHLORIDE 20 mEq — TRACE ELEMENTS *see below
REGULAR HUMULIN _____ units — VITAMINS *see below

AMINOSYN 10% 500 ml Final Concentration 5%
DEXTROSE 50% 500 ml Final Concentration 25%
Rate 100 ml/hour

Bottle # 15 MULTI-ELECTROLYTE CONCENTRATE CONSISTING OF:
SODIUM 25 mEq CALCIUM 5 mEq CHLORIDE 30 mEq
POTASSIUM 20 mEq MAGNESIUM 5 mEq ACETATE 25 mEq
HEPARIN 1000 units
REGULAR HUMULIN _____ units
OTHER APPROVED ADDITIVE _____

20% FAT EMULSION IS TO RUN CONTINUOUSLY THROUGH THE PROXIMAL MEDICINAL ENTRY AT 20 ml/hour (PHARMACY WILL SEQUENTIALLY LETTER BEGINNING WITH A)

NOTE: VITAMINS AND TRACE ELEMENTS WILL BE ADDED AS DESCRIBED IN PROTOCOL
Hang all bottles in consecutive order. RECORD the EXACT TIME hung as well as the bottle number and total volume. Maintain a constant rate. DO NOT catch up or slow down the infusion. Orders must be rewritten DAILY. THE TPN LINE SHOULD NOT BE USED FOR ANY OTHER PURPOSE.

PATIENTS ON TPN ARE TO RECEIVE:

1. CBC, BUN, LYTES, CREATININE, GLUCOSE every day for five days then MONDAYS and THURSDAYS.
2. SGOT, Ca, ALK PHOS, Mg, SGPT, BILIRUBIN, ALBUMIN, GLOBULIN, PO_4, PROTHROMBIN TIME, PARTIAL THROMBOPLASTIN TIME Monday, Thursday for the first week, then weekly.
3. Urine Acetone and Glucose and Specific Gravity every four hours for the first week then four times a day.
4. Weigh daily.
5. Serum transferrin level once per week.
6. In depleted patients and patients on prolonged hyperalimentation trace element levels should be requested.
7. Weekly twenty-four hour urine with an ALIQUOT for CREATININE and UREA NITROGEN.
8. DIETARY CONSULT.

PHARMACY COPY

FIGURE 6.11

SOLUTIONS

The SUPPLIES are the same for all the practice TPN orders:

Electrolyte/Drug	Abbreviation	How Supplied
potassium phosphate	KPO_4	10 ml. vial containing 4.4 mEq./ml.
sodium chloride	NaCl	30 ml. vial containing 4 mEq./ml.
sodium acetate	Na Acet.	20 ml. vial containing 40 mEq.
potassium chloride	KCl	10 ml. vial containing 20 mEq.
insulin		10 ml. vial containing 100 u/ml.
heparin		4 ml. vial containing 10,000 u/ml.

Figure 6-8

CALCULATIONS FOR BOTTLE #12:

Ingredient	Required Amount	Solution
KPO_4	10 mEq.	10 mEq./4.4 mEq. = x ml./1 ml. x = 2.27 ml.
NaCl	40 mEq.	40 mEq./4 mEq. = x ml./1 ml. x = 10.0 ml. ($\frac{1}{3}$ of the vial)
KCl	50 mEq.	50 mEq./20 mEq. = x ml./10 ml. x = 25.0 ml. ($2\frac{1}{2}$ vials)

CALCULATIONS FOR BOTTLE #13:

Ingredient	Required Amount	Solution
insulin	10 u	10 u/100 u = x ml./1 ml. x = 0.1 ml.

Figure 6-9

CALCULATIONS FOR BOTTLE #4:

Ingredient	Required Amount	Solution
KPO_4	10 mEq.	10 mEq./4.4 mEq. = x ml./1 ml. x = 2.27 ml.
NaCl	40 mEq.	40 mEq./4 mEq. = x ml./1 ml. x = 10 ml. ($\frac{1}{3}$ of the vial)
Na Acet.	40 mEq.	40 mEq./40 mEq. = x ml./20 ml. x = 20 ml. (1 vial)

CALCULATIONS FOR BOTTLE #5:

Ingredient	Required Amount	Solution
insulin	8 u	8 u/100u = x ml./1 ml. x = 0.08 ml.

Figure 6-10

CALCULATIONS FOR BOTTLE #11:

Ingredient	Required Amount	Solution
KPO_4	10 mEq.	10 mEq./4.4 mEq. = x ml./1 ml. $x = 2.27$ ml.
NaCl	80 mEq.	80 mEq./4 mEq. = x ml./1 ml. $x = 20$ ml. ($\frac{2}{3}$ of the vial)

CALCULATIONS FOR BOTTLE #12:

No calculations are required.

Figure 6-11

CALCULATIONS FOR BOTTLE #14:

Ingredient	Required Amount	Solution
KPO_4	10 mEq.	10 mEq./4.4 mEq. = x ml./1 ml. $x = 2.27$ ml.
NaCl	40 mEq.	40 mEq./4 mEq. = x ml./1 ml. $x = 10$ ml. ($\frac{1}{3}$ of the vial)
NaAcet.	20 mEq.	20 mEq./40 mEq. = x ml./20 ml. $x = 10$ ml. ($\frac{1}{2}$ of the vial)
KC1	20 mEq.	20 mEq./20 mEq. = x ml./10 ml. $x = 10$ ml. (1 vial)

CALCULATIONS FOR BOTTLE #15:

No calculations are required.

What we have covered in IV pharmacy so far indicates the complexity and importance of the subject. Therefore, because IV pharmacy is such an intricate and specialized part of pharmacy practice, and so much responsibility is attached to the tasks involved in preparing parenteral formulation, I am convinced that the following expanded synopsis is warranted, albeit there is some duplication. Intravenous admixture techniques and procedures are learned and developed primarily through hands-on experience. An in-depth basic knowledge base will assist you in learning IV pharmacy comprehensively and competently.

In summary, therefore, IV pharmacy is concerned with the facility or workroom area, the needs of the IV personnel, the primary equipment required, the supplies used for preparation, and the handling of all components used in parenteral product formulation. As a technician, your responsibilities are always present even in a less-than-ideal environment. Therefore, practice good pharmacy by using aseptic techniques, by following principles of self-protection when using cytotoxic drugs, and by using good judgment.

THE IV PHARMACY ENVIRONMENT

The IV pharmacy ideally is a separate room that has been prepared to provide a clean environment. This room is defined as the "clean room." Efforts must be taken to keep the room clean. This means the room is off-limits to food, drink, newspapers, smoking, and unnecessary traffic. Tacky mats placed in front of the entry to the clean room assure that impurities are removed from the bottom of footwear before anybody enters the room. The room should be designed to be free from dust by using wire baskets that do not foster dust collection because of the limited surface area, continuous floor-to-wall moldings, and open space to avoid the many little spaces popular for dust.

IV PERSONNEL ATTIRE

There are some important requirements for IV personnel. Your attire in the clean room is of major concern because clothing is potentially a major source of contamination. You should exercise good hygiene habits by washing your hands, making sure your hair is covered to avoid distributing particles, and using cosmetics such as nail polish and face powder prudently. A full clean-room outfit, which includes a one-piece jumpsuit or coverall, shoe covers, gloves, mask, goggles, and head cover, is not necessary for the majority of tasks you perform. For most activities, a smock that opens in the back, a head cover, a mask, gloves, and shoe covers are sufficient. Depending on the type of laminar airflow hood used, goggles may be optional. Although some practitioners do not support the need for a mask when working in a vertical hood (i.e., the hood has a window that slides down to separate the preparer from the work area), I recommend using a mask to prevent potential contamination from sneezing or coughing.

Note: Unpowdered gloves should be used to prevent particle contamination common with talcum powder often used in gloves.

Special Attire. Special attire is mandatory when working with cytotoxic material (e.g., chemotherapeutic agents), or if you are allergic to specific drugs used in the formulation. Because the goal here is to assure self-protection, permit NO shortcuts.

The primary requirement for achieving self-protection is through the use of protective apparel. A disposable coverall or solid-front gown should be made from lint-free fabric and woven or made from a material that allows very little permeability. Unpowdered latex gloves are essential in all processing of sterile products; however, a high-quality latex or vinyl (if sensitive to latex) glove is mandatory for handling cytotoxic drugs. The cuffs of the gloves should be tucked over or under the gown to prevent any skin exposure. Chemotherapy sleeves that provide extra impervious protection are also available. Although double gloving with routine latex gloves is common when preparing cytotoxic chemotherapy preparations, there are protective gloves specifically designed for handling antineoplastic drugs.

Hair and shoe covers minimize the potential for contaminating your product and for picking up unwanted particles in your hair and on your shoes. Wear goggles to protect your eyes, and use a dust and mist respirator when the need arises.

SPILL PROTECTION

Protecting yourself includes being prepared to handle spills of toxic drugs. A satisfactory spill kit should contain:

- Protective eyewear
- Utility gloves

- Absorbent toweling
- A non-permeable gown
- A respirator
- Absorbable spill pads
- Shoe covers
- Disposable bag(s)

Handle spills in accordance with hazardous materials guidelines established by your employment organization or an accredited professional agency.

THE LAMINAR AIRFLOW HOOD

The most important piece of equipment needed to provide a microscopically clean environment for product formulation is the laminar airflow cabinet, or the "hood." There are three types of hoods that we may encounter in practice. The horizontal hood is used for most routine IV activities. The vertical hood is commonly used for the preparation of toxic and hazardous drugs, such as cytotoxic neoplastic agents. The vertical hood has a window that can slide down between you and the work area, thereby providing an added measure of safety. The vector hood is not commonly used.

Regardless of the type of hood, the purpose is to achieve a microscopically clean environment in which to prepare sterile preparations. To accomplish this, hoods are fitted with a high-efficiency particulate air (HEPA) filter, which filters out nearly 100 percent of micron-sized particles as small as 0.3 microns. Filters are changed routinely in accordance with a maintenance schedule recommended by the manufacturer.

IV PREPARATION SUPPLIES

The supplies you need to prepare your formulations should be in the clean room. These include containers, transfer sets, spikes, filters, syringes, and needles. All supplies should be conveniently available for your needs.

Empty containers that are required as a receptacle for combining multiple fluid drug components are made of either glass or plastic. Glass containers are fitted with a hard rubber stopper covered with a latex diaphragm. Plastic containers are provided with appendage-like tubing called *portals,* each with a specific function—a transfer set portal to deliver the component drug fluids, an injection portal to introduce small-volume drugs such as most electrolytes and vitamins, and an administration portal used to deliver the final formulation to the patient.

Transfer sets are a series of tubing connected to spikes and needles at the ends. These are used to transfer multiple drug components into a single receiving container that ultimately contains a single formulation comprised of the multiple drugs. For example, a parenteral nutrition mixture would be prepared by using stock solutions of dextrose and amino acids, and a stock emulsion of lipids. This is sometimes called a 3-in-1 solution.

Many types and sizes of syringes are used in the preparation of IV admixtures. Syringes provide accurate measurement and administration, via needles, into the admixtures. Each syringe consists of a barrel with precisely graduated markings, and a plunger. The syringes used in extemporaneous compounding are made of plastic and intended for single use. The syringes are available with or without a needle. Glass syringes are available and used when an incompatibility between the drug and the plastic components in a plastic syringe may occur.

Tuberculin syringes have a 1 ml. capacity and are used to measure small drug volumes. Hypodermic syringes are larger in size and may range from 2 ml. to more than 60 ml. capacity. You must select an appropriate size syringe for the volume you are using. As a rule for accuracy, the volume you are measuring must never be less than 20 percent of the rated capacity of the syringe. That is, for example, 2 ml. cannot be measured accurately in a syringe with a capacity greater than 10 ml. (*Calculation:* 2 ml. divided by 10 ml. equals 20 percent. Therefore, any capacity greater than 10 ml. reduces the 20 percent.)

Needles vary in length, thickness of the walls and the inside opening. Consider the need for the needle in your selection. A thicker walled needle is necessary to penetrate the hard rubber stopper of vials, whereas a thin-walled needle is adequate to withdraw the contents from an opened ampule. The length of the needle will depend on the size of the vial or ampule. A longer needle obviously will be needed to remove the contents of long ampules.

There are various types of needles. Vented needles permit the release of pressure that may build up in some containers. Filter needles ensure the removal of particles that may be present after opening an ampule or penetrating a vial's rubber stopper. (Referred to as coring, these minute pieces of rubber stoppers become particles that must be removed.) When using a filter needle, be sure to use one filter needle for withdrawing a drug from a vial into the syringe and a different filter needle when you introduce the syringe contents into your next solution. That is, do not use the same filter needle for more than one direction of fluid flow.

The final segment of IV admixture and parenteral formulation addresses the overall handling in the compounding process. There are steps to follow to prepare for compounding. These include the cleaning of the hood, as already discussed, lining up the drugs that will be used in the formulation, and placing your required supplies for easy availability.

ENVIRONMENTAL PROCEDURES

The procedures you use may depend on department policy and the state-of-the-art compounding procedures at the time. However, some techniques and procedures are based on practical sense regardless of where you perform your duties. For example, after you have prepared a mixture that results in filling an empty plastic container, squeeze the container to remove any air present before clamping the portal. Remember, AIR IS OUT. Air is a detriment to the patient, and whether the air bubble is in the final large-volume bag or in the syringe after drawing up fluid from a vial or ampule, it must be removed. Also always be sure to swab the *critical areas* (defined as the areas at the point of entry into an ampule or vial) before introducing the needle to withdraw the fluid. Finally, work aseptically and close to the hood filter.

The bottle technician must always be cognizant of physical incompatibilities. Combining fluids for admixtures always presents a chance for a chemical or physical incompatibility. The result is usually an observable clouding, flocculation, or precipitation. Report to the pharmacist any questionable preparation. Remember, NEVER DISPENSE GUESSWORK.

"COMPUTILIZATION"

If you are to function in society, you must have at least a minimal amount of knowledge about electronic technology and computer literacy. Regardless of where you are or what your activities may be, electronic technology is out there influencing you and being influenced by you. We should approach electronic technology, or "electech," as an all-encompassing field of managing, maintaining, and manipulating data through state-of-the-art hardware and software.

Electronic technology and computers have a very important place in our work lives and private lives. Computers are important instruments that have the attributes of being present, penetrating, versatile, and controlling. We need to know about them, to work with them, and to not fear them.

Computer systems are comprised of hardware and software. Hardware designates the equipment such as the central processing unit (CPU), the keyboard, the monitor (CRT or cathode ray tube), scanners, and other associated equipment. The instructions that direct the computer what to do are called software, applications software, or programs. Generally, software programs perform word processing, spreadsheet functions, database management, publishing activities, and communications. The intelligence, known as the operating system, constitutes the "environment," which is the basis for operating the computer. Two of the more utilized operating systems are the disk operating system (DOS) and Windows (developed by Microsoft).

Computers can be stand-alone units, joined to other stand-alone units in a local area network (LAN), or they can be hooked into massive mainframes with almost limitless storage capacity. They can sit on a desk or you can carry them in a briefcase. However the equipment is situated, the computer and its function is a presence we must recognize and use.

Information called *data* is handled through four primary operations. *Input* is data that is entered into the computer. The program that is being used determines the type of *processing* of the data that will be done. An *output* is provided after the processing operations are completed. The output may be reviewed on the monitor or printed out on the printer in what is known as "hard copy." The final area of operations is *storage.* The capability of the hardware to store information (i.e., memory) depends on the capacity of the storage equipment, usually referred to as the hard drive or hard disk (*Note:* there also are other media such as tapes).

Pharmacy practice is notably influenced by computerization; hence, the subject term *computilization* to signify the *use* of computers in pharmacy, and not how to operate a computer. Dispensing is automated through the use of robotics. Parenteral formulations and IV admixtures are formulated and prepared by computerized equipment called *compounders.* Unit dose packaging and drug repackaging and labeling are driven by computers. Equipment is available to pick, pack/fill, and label. Bar codes are read by scanners and drug information processed by computers. We use computers clinically to collect drug data, analyze them, and store the data for future retrieval or processing. The technology is used to provide clinical and business information used to assist practitioners and management in making decisions.

SPECIALIZED PHARMACY NEEDS

Special pharmacy software has been developed to calculate formulas for IV solutions, analyze the peak and trough measurements of gentamicin, prepare medication schedules, solve problems, and much more. In addition to accurate calculations, very fast processing, and enormous memory, software enables pharmacy practitioners to practice pharmacy with enhanced safety, accuracy, uniformity, and consistency.

The amount of pharmacy information is staggering and always growing. The computer makes prescription ordering (i.e., prescriber to pharmacy) and drug information storage, retrieval, and transmission possible through communications software and hardware linkages. Prescriptions and drug orders are transmitted electronically by a variety of media such as facsimiles (fax), electronic mail on the computer, and voice mail on the telephone.

Networks of databases provide many online resources (accessible by the computer through a modem hooked up to a telephone line) for information in all areas of practice. For example, ONCOlink provides cancer information, trials, and research. There are sites for clinical trials, disease management, and scientific information. Organizations such as the American Medical Association (AMA) and the Food and Drug Administration (FDA) have accessible sites for the latest medical news and drug information, respectively. The sources and subjects seem to be endless.

Computers (i.e., specialized software packages) help us to reduce medication errors by alerting us to interactions, contraindications, patient allergies and cross-allergies, special warnings, dose limits, duplications, and more. Databases maintain patient profiles that can be easily updated and reviewed for irregularities. Computers provide consistent patient education and assist pharmacists in counseling patients. They enable managers to control budgets by controlling inventory. Purchasing is made convenient and efficient by online ordering. Billing third-party payers through electronic means supports a cost-saving paperless environment in addition to faster reimbursement.

As a technician you will be dealing with lots of data. The data you encounter will cover drugs, reimbursement, and contain information about the patient. Laws exist to protect the privacy and confidentiality of patient information. Therefore, patient information should be discussed with the pharmacist only. Maintain your ethical and professional obligation to protect the patient's rights to his or her confidentiality and privacy.

Electronic technology is what you make it. State of the art electech can assist you in your pharmacy tasks. A discussion of specific systems is beyond the scope of this textbook. Each system requires your interactivity and attention. This section covered the rudiments of computers, the components of a system, and how computerization interfaces with the multiple facets of pharmacy. We looked at what a computer was capable of accomplishing in pharmacy. You have the responsibility as a pharmacy technician to stay current with technological advancements.

REFERENCE SOURCES

Every pharmacy setting should have a reference library. Every pharmacy technician should have his or her own favorite resources, which may include textbooks, desktop references, newsletters, or journals. Some references are mandated by law or regulation as part of being a licensed pharmacy.

The pharmacy's reference resources may be in print form or electronic media. The references are important to pharmacy technicians and also to pharmacists, pharmacy clerical support staff, employees learning on the job, and to other health-care professionals. Therefore, as a basic rule, each reference should be complete (especially if you have texts about specific areas of pharmacy such as IV admixture, pediatric dosing, etc.), reliable, current, and easy to use.

Text references should be in a location that is accessible and available to all. Multiple copies should be available of some texts that pharmacy staff frequently uses. Ideally, the references should be near a telephone and computer work area (if appropriate), with appropriate lighting and ample desk space available for writing. Many references are bulky and cumbersome, thereby making their use less than convenient unless a specified area has been designated for their use.

Reference sources should also be updatable. If the reference does not have monthly updates, the most current copyright of these texts should be part of the pharmacy reference resources. Only current information can accommodate your needs in pharmacy's constantly changing environment.

The pharmacy's selection of texts meets a number of needs. The vast amount of drug and pharmacy information is beyond the knowledge capabilities of any pharmacy practitioner; therefore, references are essential. Most pharmacy settings do some sort of on-the-job training or continuing education effort. Continuous quality improvement (CQI), a given philosophy for all pharmacy practices, is also served best by current, reliable, complete, and easy-to-use references. You want to be sure that reference texts for drugs contain information about the product contents, how it is available (i.e., by prescription or over-the-counter), the dosage and dosaging, interactions with other drugs/nutrients, side effects, use during pregnancy and lactation, and indications for use.

Pharmacy practice is regulated by state boards of pharmacy, which govern the safety of the patient and the propriety of the profession. As part of these requirements, the boards standardize the legitimate drugs by recognizing an "official compendia" in which they are listed. *The United States Pharmacopoeia and National Formulary* is designated as the official compendium, which lists drugs appropriate for packaging and labeling.

Other than official compendia stated by the state board of pharmacy, the choices of references are enormous. In a general approach, the pharmacy's references may be divided into subject-matter orientations such as drug-product, pharmacy practice, disease and pharmaceutical management, desktop references such as medical dictionaries, and administrative issues and activities.

There are many drug-product texts. They may contain information about the profile of a product or clinical data. These texts, at a minimum, should contain information about labeled indications, dosing and administration, side effects, storage and handling, and drug interactions. Additional information about cost, packaging availability, reimbursement, manufacturers, and formulary issues may be helpful, but not directly pertinent to your activities. *Some* examples of these texts include:

Clinical Information

- *Physicians' Desk Reference (PDR)*
- *Facts and Comparisons*
- *American Hospital Formulary Service (AHFS) Drug Information*
- *United States Pharmacopoeia Dispensing Information (USPDI)*
- *American Medical Association (AMA) Drug Evaluations*
- *Martindale's The Extra Pharmacopoeia*
- *Drug Information Handbook for the Allied Health Profession*
- *The Pharmacologic Basis of Therapeutics*

Product Information

- *First Data Bank*
- *Red Book*
- *American Drug Index*

Pharmacy Practice

- *Remington's Pharmaceutical Sciences*
- *Handbook of Institutional Pharmacy Practice*

- *Pharmaceutical Calculations*
- Various catalogs for ordering drugs and supplies
- Professional journals and newsletters

Pharmacy Specialties

- *Handbook of Injectable Drugs*
- *Guide to Parenteral Admixtures*
- *Cancer Chemotherapy Handbook*

Disease and Pharmaceutical Management

- *The Merck Manual*
- *Conn's Current Therapy*
- *Manual of Medical Therapeutics*
- *Applied Therapeutics: The Clinical Use of Drugs*

Desktop References

- *Dorland, Gould, or Stedman's Medical Dictionary*
- *Hansten's Drug Interactions*
- *Drug Interaction Facts*
- *Textbook of Adverse Drug Reactions*
- *Basic Skills in Interpreting Laboratory Data*
- *Drugs in Pregnancy and Lactation*
- *Stedman's Specialty Word Books*

Administrative References

- *Practice Standards of the American Society of Health-Systems Pharmacists*
- State board of pharmacy handbook on pharmacy practice or regulations governing pharmacy practice
- Joint Commission on Accreditation of Healthcare

Organizations

- Pharmaceutical manufacturers directory
- *Coding and Reimbursement Guide for Pharmacists*

Not every reference text is needed to competently operate a pharmacy department, whether ambulatory or institutional. Also, the reference sources used will depend on the type of pharmacy in which you are practicing. Finally, be selective in your personal choices of reference sources. They should be complete, reliable, current, and easily referenced.

COMMUNICATION

Defined by one dictionary, *communication* is "giving or exchanging information, signals, or messages by talk, gestures, or writing." We communicate personally or through technology via telephone, facsimile, and computer. The process of communicating is one that, regardless of its complexity, follows a common sequence. Much of this sequence is influenced by perception. Make a good impression and you will provide the basis for a positive perception.

Health care is at a point where patients insist on participating in their own health management during sickness and health. Pharmacy is at a point where the role of the pharmacist has expanded to providing informational service to patients, thereby leaving much of the distributive/manipulative pharmacy tasks to the pharmacy technician. However, depending on the pharmacy environment and legal interpretations, the extent of pharmacy technician activities varies. Your role in the communication process is significant, whether the communication is with the pharmacist, doctor, other health-care professional, vendors, caregivers, third-party payers, patient, or public.

As a provider of information, many factors influence communication and the effectiveness of the delivery of your message to the receiver. Factors include cultural background, level of education, attitudes, and more. The effectiveness of your communication depends on your knowledge of basic tenets of communication, and reacting to reverse communication called "feedback" from the receiver.

Effective communication is based on practical elements that you should apply to yourself. Patients are ill and, hence, usually not personable; time becomes critical to them. Therefore, make the best use of time with the patient. Understanding the patient's feelings helps you to respond positively to objections, complaints, and other forms of venting.

Other important principles to support effective communication include:

- Deal with barriers such as level of education, ethnic background, and bias
- Streamline communication by organizing questions
- Be attentive to detail in the receiver's verbal and nonverbal communications (i.e., be a good listener and observer)
- Show empathy and support to patients and interest to other receivers of information
- Listen with a focused ear
- Always be prepared and have alternatives available
- Show respect for the patient
- Be cognizant of a severely ill patient's stages of adjustment: denial, bargaining, anger, depression, and acceptance
- Always maintain confidentiality and a patient's privacy
- Live by the credo, "The Patient Is Primary"

After a short period of adhering to these principles of effective communication, getting your message across in a concise, timely, responsive, and friendly way becomes second nature.

In health-care delivery, effective communication between you and the receiver is vital for the safety and well-being of the patient, who is the primary reason for our existence. The wrong message, or the right message communicated improperly, can result in inconvenience and potential harm to the patient. Although the information about communication that follows may focus on the patient, the basic tenets of communicating is left up to you to apply as needed, regardless of the type of pharmacy setting or the receiver of information.

Effective communication is a challenge that is founded on both art and science. The science of communication includes techniques of communication and the dynamics of people. The art is in the implementation of our knowledge about people and the principles of communicating.

As a resource person you must possess a knowledge base that assures competence. The way you present your knowledge provides the perception that follows. Obviously, the pharmacy environment plays an important role in the way you present information and to the receiver of information. In an institutional setting such as the hospital where you have little contact with patients, your primary receiver of information is the pharmacist, followed by other health-care staff. You may have encounters with physicians also to clarify illegible writing, discuss a third-party payer's policy regarding generic drugs, or duplicate medications from multiple doctors. Your knowledge base in this environment focuses primarily on product profile and clinical information.

You may have significant interactions with patrons in the retail community pharmacy environment. In this setting, you encounter healthy and sick customers. Questions often arise in the community pharmacy about over-the-counter drugs, the prescription drug filled or refilled for the patient, health and beauty aids products, durable medical equipment (i.e., canes, commodes, wheelchairs, etc.), and supplies. There may be times when you will be the focal point in recommending lifestyle changes (i.e., non-pharmacologic therapy changes such as smoking cessation) to enhance a patient's quality of life. You may be called upon to provide nonjudgmental information in response to questions about any of these issues. You may also have the responsibility to interact with physicians, vendors, and third-party payers. You can meet the challenge of effective communication by being competent (especially about drug products) and designating yourself as a resource person. You are an active part in the continuity of care in health-care delivery.

As a communicator, your job in the pharmacy realm is to explain, support, reinforce, and focus. Customers and patients want explanations for what they do not understand. Support your position by showing your concern for the ill patient and interest in the healthy customer. Reinforce your support by using the knowledge you have to explain the directions on the label or to answer questions. Focus on the patient and patient care. Reassure the patient that the pharmacy is there when needed.

Effective communication requires a comfort level between the sender and the receiver. The age, gender, professional role, and environment each play a significant part in the success of getting the information across to the patient.

Establish part of the comfort level through your professional role by showing intent. The primary concern for both you and the patient is the well-being of the patient. The customer also responds well to feeling that there is a rapport and his or her concerns are being met, whether the information is about insulin supplies or suntanning lotion.

Make it known that you share the interest and concern of the patient. This commonality, as the shared interest is called, differs among the various receivers of information. If you are communicating with the patient, show interest in the illness and drug management for the illness by knowing about the illness (even in generalities following a basic format such as the name[s] of the illness, the observable symptoms, the path it follows from start to finish, and the drug and nondrug management). You may have the opportunity to talk with the doctor. Again, have a basic concept about the illness, know the patient information, and be prepared to offer information on drug products. Be prepared by planning.

As mentioned, perception significantly influences the outcome of communication. Show competence, and the impression that follows builds credibility. Therefore, the drug information you provide must be concise (i.e., do not impress by "dumping" all the information you have about a product) and accurate. If you are unsure about an answer, explain that you want to check into the answer further. People respect honesty and the effort to provide the correct information.

Competence is further fostered by having complete patient information. This includes the health profile of the patient, the medications, and notes that may be helpful about him or her.

Finally, your presentation solidifies the perception you make. Assess your customer or patient and communicate with an appropriate rate of speech and tone. For instance, elderly people may require that you speak a little louder and slower. You can easily access this from feedback.

In summary, your role is as a resource person for drugs and ancillaries. You understand ill-person dynamics and respond accordingly in an informative and supportive way. Follow the principles of effective communication, and guide your dialog such that you listen to learn, gather information to guide, and assimilate facts to assist.

LAW

Laws are rules enacted by legislatures at the federal and state levels. Pharmacy rules govern the conduct of the profession and are enforceable in court with penalties for not adhering to the laws. In pharmacy, these laws are used to enforce minimal standards established for the profession in its quest to protect the health, safety, and welfare of the patient/customer.

As laws are rules that mandate how pharmacy practitioners must practice pharmacy, professional ethics is another set of rules established by the profession. A code of ethics is comprised of standards based on moral values that guide pharmacy practitioners in the way pharmacy should be practiced. These latter rules are nonenforceable and designed to regulate the profession through social custom.

A number of facets of pharmacy that are regulated include pharmacy practice (i.e., the distributive and clinical activities); drugs, controlled substances, and narcotics; and manufacturing. Generally, state boards of pharmacy through regulations (administrative interpretation of the law) and professional associations through a code of ethics and standards regulate pharmacy practice; state and federal regulatory agencies regulate drugs, controlled substances, and narcotics; and federal agencies regulate drug manufacturers.

Pharmacy is governed by the Federal Food, Drug, and Cosmetic Act (FDCA), the Controlled Substances Act (CSA), the Poison Prevention Packaging Act (PPPA), which requires the use of child-resistant safety containers, and the Omnibus Budget Reconciliation Act of 1990 (OBRA 90). In addition to the federal laws, states have their own statutes to regulate pharmacy practice and controlled substances. Pharmacies must also meet strict standards in order to be accredited by the Joint Commission on Accreditation of Healthcare Organizations (JCAHO). Although voluntary, accreditation is important if an organization wants to do business with third-party payers who require certification through the accreditation process.

The FDCA was enacted to regulate the purity, quality, effectiveness, and safety of drug products. The drug was defined to be used in the diagnosis, cure, mitigation, prevention, or treatment of disease, or to alter a bodily function. The act recognizes as the official drug compendia the *United States Pharmacopoeia,* the *National Formulary,* and the *Homeopathic Pharmacopoeia of the United States.* Drugs that can be filled only by prescription bear a statement on the bulk packaging: "Caution—Federal Law Prohibits Dispensing Without a Prescription." This phrase is called a *legend* and, therefore, the drug is often referred to as a legend drug.

The CSA regulates the manufacture, distribution, and dispensing of controlled substances. The impact of this act on pharmacy practice focuses on the requirements for keeping accurate records for inventory and dispensing of controlled substances, and verifying the legitimacy of the prescriptions for these drugs.

Controlled substances are categorized according to their potential for being abused. Drugs regulated by CSA are divided into five schedules designated as follows:

- Schedule I or C-I—high potential for abuse and no currently accepted medical use (e.g., heroin). These drugs are not likely to be found in a pharmacy practice.
- Schedule II or C-II—high abuse potential with severe psychological or physical dependence possible, and accepted medical use (e.g., morphine). *Note:* Keep records for Schedule II drugs separate from other records.
- Schedule III or C-III—abuse potential may lead to low physical dependence or high psychological dependence, and accepted medical use (e.g., acetaminophen and codeine combination). Schedule III records may be combined with noncontrolled prescription records and identified with a red "C" on the lower right corner of the prescription or filed separately with Schedules IV and V prescriptions.
- Schedule IV or C-IV—limited psychological and physical dependence relative to Schedule III, and accepted medical use (e.g., phenobarbital). Schedule IV records follow the same scenario as Schedule III record keeping.
- Schedule V or C-V—low abuse potential relative to Schedule IV, and accepted medical use (e.g., usually over-the-counter preparations containing limited quantities of narcotic drugs such as guaifenesin with codeine). Schedule V record keeping for legend drugs follows the same scenario as for Schedule III. States vary in their record keeping requirements for OTC-Schedule V drugs.

Check the pharmacy regulations for the state in which you are practicing to determine if there are more restrictive requirements for retail and hospital pharmacy practice.

In 1970, the Poison Prevention Packaging Act (PPPA) was enacted in part to protect children from accidentally ingesting medications by making the container of the drug difficult for children to open. We often refer to this packaging as child-resistant containers. All oral prescription drugs must be dispensed in a child-resistant container. However, there are a few exemptions, which include such prescription drugs as follows:

- Sublingual nitroglycerin
- Sublingual and chewable isosorbide dinitrate 10 mg. or less
- Oral suspensions of erythromycin ethylsuccinate containing no more than 8 grams of erythromycin
- Oral solid forms of erythromycin ethylsuccinate in packages containing up to 16 grams of erythromycin
- Powdered anhydrous cholestyramine
- Unit dose of potassium supplements not exceeding 50 milli-equivalents in each unit dose
- Liquid and solid forms of sodium fluoride in packages containing up to 264 mg. of sodium fluoride
- Manufacturer's dispenser packages of betamethasone tablets containing up to 12.6 mg. of betamethasone
- Tablets of methylprednisolone in packages containing up to 84 mg.
- Powdered colestipol in packages of up to 5 grams
- Solid forms (i.e., tablets, capsules, or powder) of pancrelipase preparations
- Oral contraceptive preparations packaged in the manufacturer's memory-aid dispenser package
- Tablets of prednisone in packages containing up to 105 mg. of prednisone

- Manufacturer's memory-aid dispenser packaging of conjugated estrogen tablets containing up to 26.5 mg. of conjugated estrogens
- Manufacturer's memory-aid dispenser packages of norethindrone acetate tablets containing up to 50 mg. of norethindrone
- Medroxyprogesterone acetate tablets

The PPPA permits the prescriber or the patient to request a container that is NOT child-resistant. Although the PPPA does not require the request to be in writing, you would be prudent to have the patient sign a statement requesting a noncomplying container.

The enactment of the OBRA 90 included an expanded role for pharmacists. OBRA 90 mandates pharmacists to offer to discuss with each Medicaid recipient (i.e., patient) or caregiver information about new and refill prescriptions. Most states have adopted this for all (i.e., *not* Medicaid-only) patients. The elements of the discussion or counseling with the patient or caregiver depend on the pharmacist and may include the following information:

- The name and description of the drug
- The route, dosage form, and route of administration, and duration of therapy
- Special directions, precautions, and use by the patient
- Common severe side effects, adverse effects, interactions (drug, food, etc.), and therapeutic contraindications
- The actions required to respond to the side effects, adverse effects, and so forth
- How to monitor the therapy
- Proper storage
- Refill information
- What to do in the event of a missed dose

The law also requires that a record for the patient be established and maintained. This record should include information about the patient's demography (i.e., address, telephone number, date of birth, gender, etc.), known allergies and drug reactions, list of medications, and comments/notes about the drug therapy.

A pharmacist or his or her designee may offer to counsel a patient or the caregiver. Individual state pharmacy regulations may limit this activity to pharmacists. However, some states permit a pharmacist designee such as a pharmacy technician to offer counseling, thereby making the pharmacy technician's role more substantial. The same is true for collecting patient medication and medical history information pursuant to OBRA 90.

The supervising pharmacist is responsible and, thereby, liable for violations committed by the pharmacy technician. Therefore, the pharmacy technician has a responsibility and obligation to comply with the federal and state laws and regulations governing pharmacy.

The federal law establishes the rules for safe and effective drugs by regulating the manufacture of drugs according to strict standards. Once met, these drugs can post the "CAUTION" legend and be dispensed only by prescription, written by a practitioner licensed to practice medicine and write for legend drugs. Note that non-prescription (over-the-counter—"OTC") drugs must also conform to requirements that assure they have been manufactured according to the good manufacturing practices standards of the FDA.

State pharmacy rules dictate protection for the patient by establishing who can dispense drugs, how drugs are dispensed, and when drugs can be dispensed, which impacts on the time frames for new prescriptions and refills. The scope of this textbook is to generalize laws that govern everyday pharmacy practice. Because individual states have variations to the federal law as well as state laws appropriate to local pharmacy practice, request from your state board of pharmacy the rules that govern your practice. This information should be a part of your resource information previously discussed.

The following points constitute a short course in pharmacy law that will be used in your daily practice. Remember that individual state laws may differ. Therefore, check with the pharmacist or request from your state board of pharmacy the regulations that regulate pharmacy practice.

- All prescriptions for controlled substances must have the full name and address of the patient, date written, and the name, address, DEA number, and signature (in ink) of the practitioner.
- An emergency dose of a Schedule II drug may be dispensed on an oral authorization provided a written prescription is postmarked to the pharmacy within 72 hours of the oral order, and is attached to the oral order transcribed by the pharmacy. The phrase "Authorization for Emergency Dispensing" and the date of the oral order should be written on the prescription.
- Controlled substances listed in Schedules III, IV, and V may be dispensed pursuant to either a written prescription or a telephoned order.
- Refills of prescriptions for Schedule II drugs are prohibited.
- Schedule II drugs may be partially filled if the full quantity is not available, but the balance must be provided with 72 hours or the balance is voided. If the patient requests only a partial filling, the balance is voided.
- The label of the drug listed in Schedules II, III, and IV must bear the warning that it is a crime to transfer the drug to any person other than the patient. The "transfer warning statement" reads, *"Caution: Federal law prohibits the transfer of this drug to any person other than the patient for whom it was prescribed."*
- The prescription label for a controlled substance requires:
  - The name and address of the pharmacy
  - The patient's name
  - The prescription serial number
  - The date of dispensing
  - The name of the prescriber
  - The directions for use
- Authorized refills for Schedules III and IV drugs may not exceed 6 months after the date of issue and may not be refilled more than five times. Individual states' drug control laws may be more restrictive.
- Legend drugs require refill authorization. Prescriptions written for OTC drugs follow the same requirements as for legend drugs.
- Generally, prescriptions must be filled within 6 months of the date written, and authorized refills filled within 1 year from the date of issuance.
- Each authorized refill must be recorded with the date dispensed, the quantity dispensed, and the pharmacist's initials on the back of the prescription.
- Referring to "PRN" or "ad lib" refill authorization: "The FDA does not regard any such designation that puts no limit on the frequency of refilling, or the length of time that a prescription may be refilled, as a valid authorization for refilling a prescription."
- Facsimile transmission of all prescriptions (including Schedule drugs) is permitted if state law provides for it.
- Pharmacy technicians may dispense controlled drugs under the supervision of a pharmacist in accordance with state law.
- The prescription label on the drug dispensed must contain the following minimum information:
  - The name and address of the pharmacy
  - The serial number of the prescription

- The date of the prescription is written, filled, or refilled (check state regulations)
- The name of the prescriber
- The name of the patient
- Directions for use, including precautions, if indicated
- Expiration date

Check state regulations for additional information that may be required.

- Check state drug laws regarding filling out-of-state prescriptions.
- Affix labels to containers.
- The expiration date should not exceed 1 year from the date dispensed.
- Schedule V drugs permitted by state law to be sold over the counter at retail outlets must be recorded in a log or record book containing the:
    - Name and quantity (i.e., there are quantity limitations) of the item purchased
    - Name and address of the purchaser
    - Date of the purchase
    - Initials of the pharmacist (some states may require the signature of the pharmacist) who sold the item
    - Signature of the purchaser (some states)
    - Name and address of the pharmacy on the Schedule V product (some states)
- Hospital pharmacies require control sheets that indicate administration of each dose for all Schedule II controlled drugs.

Briefly, pharmacy ethics regulate the conduct and character of pharmacy practitioners according to what is right. The pharmacy technician has the professional obligation, for instance, to protect the confidentiality of the patient. The preamble to the Code of Ethics for Pharmacy Technicians states, "Pharmacy Technicians are healthcare professionals who assist pharmacists in providing the best possible care for their patients. The principals of this code, which apply to pharmacy technicians working in any and all settings, are based on the application and support of the moral obligations that guide the pharmacy profession in relationships with patients, healthcare professionals, and the society at large."

EXERCISES

1. Intravenous therapy is a therapeutic approach using a route directly into ______________________________.

2. Parenteral therapy is a therapeutic approach using routes directly or indirectly into __________________________.

3. The parenteral route of administration is appropriate for _________________, __________________________, and __________________________.

4. List the advantages and disadvantages of IV therapy.

Advantages	**Disadvantages**
a.	**a.**
b.	**b.**
c.	**c.**
d.	**d.**
e.	**e.**
f.	**f.**
g.	**g.**

5. True or False: Intramuscular and intravenous formulations are interchangeable.
6. What is the role of blood for most of the drugs used intravenously?
7. Why are IM formulations considered parenteral therapy?
8. List the essential water-soluble vitamins:
   a. f.
   b. g.
   c. h.
   d. i.
   e.

9. List the essential fat-soluble vitamins:
   a.
   b.
   c.
   d.

10. What is the difference between arteries and veins?
11. For which trace elements has the FDA set acceptable dosage standards? (List trace element and dosage amount.)
   a.
   b.
   c.
   d.

12. Complete the states of body fluid and electrolyte imbalances by filling in the blanks.

This State	Is Also Known As
	hypernatremia
sodium deficit	
	dehydration
acid imbalance	
	alkalosis
potassium deficit	
	hyperkalemia
magnesium deficit	
	hypermagnesemia

13. What are the four common therapeutic needs for selecting an IV modality?
14. What is an admixture?
15. What is an accepted abbreviation for an additive?
16. What is the use of fluids in IV therapy?
17. When are nutrients used intravenously?

18. What is Hartmann's solution?

19. What are the common KCL concentrations?

20. What does PPN therapy require?

21. Give four examples of anions.

a.
b.
c.
d.

22. Give three examples of cautions.

a.
b.
c.

23. Translate the following notations:

HCO_3

PO_4

SO_4

Mg

NH_4

24. Which therapy is used for long-term IV nutritional support?

25. What is the fundamental generic formulation for TPN?

26. How do the sites of administration differ for PPN and TPN?

27. Why must a central venous route be used for TPNs?

28. What is the use of fat emulsions?

29. True or False: Fat emulsions and amino acid/dextrose solutions can be delivered through the same IV line.

30. Why is it so important to exercise aseptic technique when preparing IV solutions?

31. What does a laminar airflow hood do?

32. True or False: With experience, it is safe to interpret slightly questionable IV orders.

33. True or False: It is necessary to recheck all calculations used for preparing IV solutions.

34. What is needle gauge?

35. True or False: Larger gauge needles have smaller diameters, while small gauge needles have larger diameters.

36. Why are filters necessary when preparing IV solutions?

37. Why is it important to always check expiration dates of drugs and solutions being used?

38. What method assures an orderly flow of expiration dates?

39. What do the following abbreviations mean?

    AA

    mEq

    IVPB

    NS

    LR

40. True or False: The IV admixture function requires competence, total aseptic technique, and extreme mental concentration.
41. What are the two general types of compounding?
42. Why should all equipment used in compounding be washed thoroughly?
43. What are excipients?
44. Why should you complete in a compounding book a stepwise approach for a first-time extemporaneous preparation?
45. List the contents of a satisfactory spill kit.
46. What is computer hardware?
47. What is computer software?
48. How are computers used in pharmacy?
49. Which are the official compendia for pharmacy?
50. Maintaining ______________________________ is the most important aspect in the pharmacy-patient relationship.
51. A good communicator learns by ______________________________, uses the information he or she collects to ______________________________; and with the facts assimilated, a good communicator is able to ________________________ the patient.
52. What federal laws regulate pharmacy?
53. What is a legend drug?
54. How is a legend drug identified on the bulk packaging label?
55. What are the categories designated by the CSA?
56. How are Schedules III and IV (C-III and C-IV) prescriptions that are mixed with noncontrolled prescriptions identified?
57. What does the PPPA require pharmacy practitioners to do?
58. Are refills for Schedule II (C-II) drugs permitted?
59. What limits are placed on refills for Schedules III and IV (C-III and C-IV) drugs?
60. How are authorized refills recorded?

UNIT 2

Drugs

CHAPTER 7

Basics of Human Functioning and Pharmacokinetics

OBJECTIVES

When you have completed this chapter, you will be able to:

1. understand how drugs work in relation to basic anatomy and physiology
2. describe the nature and importance of the cell as an anatomical building block
3. describe basic physiological processes
4. associate various anatomical systems with their make-up, functions, and disorders
5. describe the basis of pharmacokinetics

This section is intended to briefly guide the reader through the anatomy, physiology, and kinetics that are associated with the way drugs work. As you gain an understanding of the complexity of how drugs work, you will appreciate and respect the potency of drugs, what they can do, and how they do it. Hopefully, this understanding will instill and keep viable the tenet of NEVER DISPENSE GUESSWORK.

AN OVERVIEW OF HUMAN ANATOMY AND PHYSIOLOGY

You may have heard some stories of an individual living in a location highlighted by some outstanding landmark, such as the Empire State Building or the Golden Gate Bridge, who never avails himself or herself of the opportunity to see the famous structure that attracts so many. The same situation is true of our own bodies. Very few of us are familiar with our own body structure (anatomy) and the function of our systems (physiology). As a pharmacy technician, you should be familiar with this battery of knowledge about human anatomy and physiology, in order to appreciate where and how a drug works on a specific region of the body. Familiarity with anatomy and function will help you to communicate and answer many questions patients ask. In addition, this information will help you achieve and maintain a professional position, credibility, and a working relationship with other members of the health-care team, such a nurses, respiratory therapists, medical technicians, and so on.

A text of this dimension is intended to highlight the areas of anatomy and physiology that are useful to you as a pharmacy technician in your daily application to drug activities. If your interest and curiosity warrant further exploration of this area, many excellent texts are available.

By textbook definition, human anatomy is comprised of 10 systems. Each system is composed of special parts or components. The role each system plays in maintaining functions and processes is referred to as *physiology.* When an abnormality occurs within a system or systems, the resulting condition is a disease state or disorder.

CELLS: THE BUILDING BLOCKS

The primary structural building block of any anatomical system is the cell. Therefore, we will begin by briefly discussing the structure and physiology of the cell.

The branch of anatomy that deals with the study of cell structure and function is known as *cytology* (*cyt.-* = cell, *-ology* = study of). Cells are the smallest units of living matter. They vary in size from those that can be seen only with the aid of an electron microscope, to those which can be seen with the naked eye. In addition to the variety of sizes, their shapes also differ.

All cells contain protein, carbohydrate, fat, nucleic acid (DNA and RNA), and other materials. Each cell is surrounded by a membrane called the *cell membrane.* This membrane assures that the cell remains intact. The cell membrane is made of a lipid (fat) layer surrounded by a protein layer. This composition of the cell membrane allows only certain substances to pass into the cell. This process of selective passage through the cell membrane is referred to as the *permeability* of a cell.

Inside the cell there are two major parts. The *nucleus* is the component responsible for cell activities and is considered the control center. The second major part is the living substance that surrounds the nucleus and is contained by the cell membrane. This material is known as *cytoplasm.* There are other structures in the cell, each having specialized functions in the cell's activities.

Groups of like cells form tissues, which form the organs. Therefore, all muscle cells are specific, all heart cells are specific, and so on. Reactions that are due to disease or drugs occur at the cell level. A drug being used to treat an abnormally functioning heart, for instance, passes through the heart cell membrane in order to create a response in the heart.

Two organs of particular importance in drug activities are the liver ("hepatic" . . .) and kidney ("renal" . . .). These organs have significant effect on the disposition of drugs. The role of the liver is primarily to detoxify or reduce drugs to a usable form, which enables them to reach the systemic circulation from where they can then reach specific receptor sites. The kidneys' primary function is to excrete liquid waste, which includes soluble drug waste.

These masses of like cells form any of five basic tissues: epithelial (e.g., skin), connective (e.g., cartilage, bone), muscle, nerve, and blood. Tissues combine in specific arrangements to form organs (e.g,. heart, stomach, liver, brain). Finally, a group of organs join in a specialized manner, called a *system,* to perform a major function in the body.

Through physiologic processes, each system performs a role in maintaining a body balance, called *homeostasis.* When the balance is upset, problems occur. For example, note the effects when an imbalance occurs in the electrolyte-water balance. Hypertension, congestive heart failure, and a host of other problems ensue. When the balance of blood components is lost, diseases such as leukemia may be diagnosed. The essence of physiology is to assure that the body's functions are maintained in a state of balance. Each body system is governed by principles of physiology.

BASIC PHYSIOLOGIC PROCESSES

Three mechanisms are used to move substances (nutrients, drugs, and wastes) across cell membranes.

1. FILTRATION
   a. Depends on differences in pressure on each side of membrane
   b. Involves the passage of water and dissolved substances

   c. Filters out large materials such as blood proteins, and occurs most often in the capillary network (tiny blood vessels) in the body. Importance to pharmacy: Drugs will pass through the blood-brain barrier or into the milk of nursing mothers. (*Note:* The blood-brain barrier refers to the barriers separating the circulating blood from the brain cells and permitting selective passage of certain substances into the brain at specific rates.)

2. DIFFUSION
   a. Depends on molecules being in constant motion
   b. Results in molecules automatically distributing themselves equally in an available space. For example: Open a bottle of ammonia in a room. Eventually the entire room fills with the permeating smell of ammonia. The molecules have diffused into the air and distributed themselves equally throughout the room.
   c. Occurs most readily in our lungs, between the air in the lungs (which contains oxygen and carbon dioxide among other things) and the blood vessels passing through the lungs
   d. Is important to pharmacy because inhalers are used to diffuse a drug into the lungs

3. OSMOSIS is a certain type of diffusion that relies on a special membrane (called a semipermeable membrane) separating two solutions of unequal concentration. This membrane allows only water to pass. Water will pass from the side having a smaller concentration (fewer particles in the solution) to the side of greater concentration (more particles in the solution) until the concentration of both sides of the semipermeable membrane are equal (i.e., the number of particles in the same amount of water on each side of the semipermeable membrane is equal). When equal concentration is achieved, equilibrium and homeostasis are attained. In pharmacy, drugs can disrupt this equilibrium by introducing particles such as sodium to the body, forcing water to move to the area of greater concentration (more particles). This situation can result in fluid buildup, called edema, or water retention.

   Sodium chloride (salt) is very important to the body system. The concentration of the salt in blood is 0.9% (0.009 Gm. or 9 mg. of salt per every 100 ml. of blood). Changing the concentration elicits an immediate physiologic response to remedy the change by either diluting a higher concentration or making a low concentration more concentrated. In pharmacy, electrolyte concentrations are especially important when dealing with intravenous solutions of various concentrations.

AN OVERVIEW OF ANATOMICAL SYSTEMS

(*Note:* Drugs listed for each drug class are only illustrative examples of drugs that may be used for associated disorders.)

SYSTEM: INTEGUMENTARY

Branch of Anatomy: Dermatology

Medical Specialist: Dermatologist

Components

1. Skin
2. Hair
3. Nails

4. Sweat glands
5. Oil glands
6. Hair follicles

Function/Responsibility

- Protects against bacterial invasion
- Maintains proper moisture in tissues
- Regulates body heat and temperature
- Conducts stimuli such as heat, cold, pain, and touch
- Eliminates water and waste products

Additional Information Sweat glands regulate body temperature by means of water elimination through evaporation. Oil glands (sebaceous glands) keep skin pliable by secreting oils. Hair helps to retain body heat and amplify the sense of touch. Skin color can be indicative of a variety of conditions:

- Bluish (cyanotic)—inadequate supply of oxygen is being transported
- Yellowish (jaundice)—malfunctioning liver
- Paleness (pallor)—indicates possible shock, fright, or anemia
- Redness (flush)—indicates fever

Associated Disorders

Bacterial infections

Fungal infections

Viral infections

Pruritus

Dermatitis

Inflammation

Malignancies

Drug Classes/Drugs

Antibiotics: penicillins, tetracyclines, erythromycin, bacitracin, neomycin, ciprofloxacin, clindamycin, metronidazole, vancomycin

Antifungals: amphotericin B, nystatin, clotrimazole, haloprogin, miconazole, tolfanate, zinc undecylanate

Antivirals: acyclovir

Steroids: prednisone, triamcinolone, hydrocortisone

Tranquilizers: diazepam, clordiazepoxide, hydroxyzine, lorazepam

Antihistamines: diphenhydramine, chlorpheniramine, brompheniramine, terfenidine

Antineoplastics: fluorouracil, methotrexate, hydroxyurea, etoposide

Terms and Definitions

Dermis: deep layer of skin

Desquamation: process by which the dead cell layer is eventually sloughed off and replaced by a new keratin layer

Epidermis: top layer of skin

Intradermal: within the skin

Keratin: layer of dead cells that forms as the outermost part of the epidermis. This layer acts as a protective covering.

Lesion: a structural skin alteration

a. *Macule:* flat discolored spot, such as a freckle or flat mole
b. *Papule:* a solid, elevated lesion, such as a pimple
c. *Nodule:* a palpable solid lesion, such as a cyst
d. *Vesicle:* a circumscribed elevated lesion, such as a blister
e. *Pustule:* a superficial, elevated lesion containing pus, such as seen in acne
f. *Wheal:* an elevated, itching, swollen lesion, such as seen in insect bites
g. *Telangiectasia:* dilation of superficial blood vessels that form elevated, dark red spots as seen in certain warts

Sebaceous: oil glands

Subcutaneous: subQ or SQ, under the skin

SYSTEM: SKELETAL

Branch of Anatomy: Osteology
Medical Specialist: Orthopedist

Components

1. Bones
2. Ligaments
3. Cartilage
4. Tendons
5. Joints

Function/Responsibility

- Framework of the body
- Support of the body
- Protect vital organs (e.g., ribs protect the heart and lungs, the skull protects the brain)
- Store calcium and phosphorous
- Manufacture red blood cells

Additional Information The body contains a total of 206 bones. The skeleton is divided into the axial skeleton (spine, skull, chest), containing 80 bones, and the appendicular skeleton (upper and lower extremities), which is comprised of 126 bones. Bones serve as a site for attachment for skeletal muscles. The vertebral column (spine) is composed of bones called vertebrae, separated from each other by cartilage pieces called intervertebral discs or "discs." The vertebral column has five sections extending from the neck to the base of the spine:

1. Cervical
2. Thoracic

3. Lumbar
4. Sacrum
5. Coccyx

Associated Disorders

Arthritis

Gout

Chondrocalcinosis

Bursitis

Osteoarthritis

Paget's Disease (osteities deformans)

Osteoporosis

Osteomyelitis

Bone and joint neoplasms

Drug Classes/Drugs

Analgesics: narcotics (codeine, meperidine), salicylates (aspirin), nonsalicylates (acetaminophen, ibuprofen, propoxyphene)

Gold compounds: gold sodium thiomalate, aurothioglucose

Chelating agents: penicillamine

Nonsteroidal anti-inflammatory agents (NSAIA): indomethacin, naproxen, ibuprofen, fenoprofen, tolmetin, sulindac, phenylbutazone

Steroids: prednisone, hydrocortisone, cortisone

Uricosuric agents: colchicine, allopurinol, probenecid, sulfinpyrazone

Nerve blocking agents: procaine

Muscle relaxants: diazepam

Antihypercalcemic agents: calcitonin

Nutritional agents: calcium

Hormones: estrogen, oxandrolone, testosterone

Antibiotics: methicillin, oxacillin, nafcillin, penicillin, erythromycin, lincomycin, cephalosporins

Immunosuppressive drugs: cyclophosphamide, azathioprine

Terms and Definitions

Appendicular skeleton: skeleton of the arms and legs

Articulations: joints

Axial skeleton: skeleton of the head and trunk

Cartilage: elastic, supporting tissue at joints that protects joints against shock

Cranium: part of skull that encloses the brain

Crepitation: crackling of joints

Crush fractures: fractures that occur without trauma. For example, in osteoporosis, the bones become so weak that the weight of the person alone causes the vertebrae to collapse and crush.

Erythropoiesis: manufacture of red blood cells by red bone marrow

Ligament: tissue structure that holds bones together at their joints

Ossification: bone formation

Osteoarthritis: degenerative joint disease

Sternum: breast bone

Tendons: connective tissue that attaches muscles to bone

SYSTEM: MUSCULAR

Branch of Anatomy: Myology

Medical Specialist: Orthopedist

Components

1. Muscles
2. Tendons

Function/Responsibility

- Voluntary movements of body parts (e.g., lifting an arm)
- Involuntary movements of body organs (e.g., beating of the heart)

Additional Information There are approximately 656 muscles in the body. Muscle tissue may be categorized as:

1. Involuntary
   a. smooth muscle (nonstriated or visceral muscle)
      (1) digestive tract
      (2) blood vessels
      (3) gallbladder
      (4) urinary bladder
      (5) lungs
   b. cardiac muscle
      (1) heart
2. Voluntary
   a. striated or skeletal muscle
      (1) arms
      (2) legs
      (3) tongue
      (4) abdomen

Associated Disorders

Rheumatism
Myalgia
Spasms
Myositis
Polymyositis

Fibromyositis
Torticollis (wryneck)
Myasthenia gravis
Myotonic myopathies
Drug-induced muscle blocks

Drug Classes/Drugs

Muscle relaxants: diazepam, meprobamate, orphenadrine, quinine

Analgesics: aspirin, acetaminophen

Nerve-blocking agents: procaine, lidocaine

Steroids: hydrocortisone, prednisone

Immunosuppressants: methotrexate, cyclophosphamide

Cholinergic drugs: neostigmine, pyridostigmine

Anticonvulssants: phenytoin

Cholinesterase reactivators: pralidoxime

Anticholinergics: atropine

Nutritional supplements: potassium

Nonsteroidal anti-inflammatory agents (NSAIA): indomethacin, naproxen, ibuprofen, fenoprofen, tolmetin, sulindac, phenylbutazone

Terms and Definitions

Atrophy: decreased growth or wasting away

Hypertrophy: increased growth

Intramuscular: within the muscle tissue

Muscle tone: state of continued partial muscle contraction

Rigor mortis: permanent state of muscle contraction after death

Tendons: connective tissue that attaches muscles to bone

Tetany: muscular cramps and twitching caused by a decrease in serum calcium

SYSTEM: NERVOUS

Branch of Anatomy: Neurology

Medical Specialist: Neurologist

Components

1. Brain
2. Spinal cord
3. Sense organs
   a. eyes
   b. ears
   c. tongue
   d. nose

Function/Responsibility Coordinate activities of all the body parts by means of a "stimulus-response" mechanism and a collection of data that is stored in memory.

Additional Information The brain and spinal cord form the *central nervous system (CNS)*. The sense organs, those structures outside the CNS, comprise the *peripheral nervous system (PNS)*.

Built into the nervous system are two process-oriented nervous systems. The *autonomic nervous system (ANS)* controls involuntary processes such as breathing and eye blinking. The *somatic nervous system (SNS)* operates under conscious control and responds only to conscious or voluntary commands to initiate such activities as walking and lifting objects.

The ANS is divided further into the *sympathetic nervous system* and *parasympathetic nervous system*. The sympathetic nervous system, also referred to as "fight and flight," prepares the body for stress or emergency situations by increasing the heart rate, constricting blood vessels, and so on. Generally, the sympathetic nervous system is associated with increased activities.

The parasympathetic nervous system is also known by the phrase, "feed and breed." This part of the nervous system deals primarily with relaxing conditions and a quiet state of the body. The heart rate slows, blood is directed to the stomach for digestion, blood vessels dilate, and so on. The parasympathetic is primarily concerned with digestion and storage of substances required for the body's well-being.

Nerve endings or receptors are specialized. They are affected by specific stimuli. Receptors can be *interoreceptors* (visceral receptors), which are stimulated by sensations from the internal organs or viscera:

1. Hunger
2. Thirst
3. Visceral pain

Proprioreceptors respond to sensations from muscles, tendons, and joints and inform of:

1. Position
2. Movement
3. Deep pressure
4. Balance

Exteroreceptors (somatic receptors) are concerned with sensations from outside the body:

1. Touch
2. Pain
3. Temperature
4. Vision
5. Hearing

The responding motor activities are carried out by structures called *effectors*. Somatic effectors are located in the skeletal muscles and the visceral effectors are found in smooth muscles, cardiac muscle, and secretory glands.

Nerve pathways are connected by junctions called *synapses.* In order for nerve impulses to cross a synapse, chemical substances called neurotransmitters are required to carry the impulse. The neurotransmitters are specific for the type of response elicited:

1. Excitatory neurotransmitters
   a. acetylcholine (Ach)
   b. epinephrine (Epi)
2. Inhibitory neurotransmitter
   a. gamma-aminobutyric acid (GABA)

Associated Disorders

Pain

Cephalalgia (headache)

Trigeminal neuralgia

Vertigo

Seizure disorders

Narcolepsy

Bacterial meningitis

Mycotic meningitis

Brain abscess

Multiple sclerosis

Tremors

Parkinsonism

Ballism

Hemiballism

Huntington's chorea

Drug Classes/Drugs

Analgesics: aspirin (ASA), acetaminophen (APAP), propoxyphene

Narcotic analgesics: codeine, meperidine, hydromorphone, methadone

Anticonvulsants: carbamazepine, phenytoin, primidone

Tranquilizers: chlorpromazine, meprobamate, diazepam, haloperidol

Sedatives: phenobarbital

Antiemetics: perphenazine, meclizine, dimenhydrinate

Stimulants: amphetamine, ephedrine, dextroamphetamine, methylphenidate

Antibiotics: chloramphenicol, penicillin G, ampicillin, kanamycin, gentamicin, carbenicillin, tetracycline

Antifungals: amphotericin B

Steroids: dexamethasone, prednisone

Antiparkinson agents: levodopa, carbidopa

Terms and Definitions

Afferent nerve cells: transmit sensory impulses to CNS

Axons: parts of nerve cell that carry impulses away from the cell

Connector nerve cells (interneurons): transmit impulses between afferent and efferent neurons

Dendrites: branches of a nerve cell; carry impulses to the nerve cell

Efferent nerve cells: transmit motor impulses away from CNS

Gustatory: refers to the sense of taste

Learning: a process by which the nervous system collects and stores information received from experiences

Neurons: the nerve cell

Neurotransmitters: chemical substances that facilitate the transmission of impulses across synapses

Olfactory: refers to the sense of smell

Ophthalmic: refers to the eye

Optic: refers to the sense of sight

Otic: refers to the sense of hearing

Synapse: junction between two neurons

Tactile: refers to the sense of touch

SYSTEM: CARDIOVASCULAR/CIRCULATORY

Branch of Anatomy: Cardiology (heart), Hematology (blood)

Medical Specialist: Cardiologist (heart), Vascular Surgeon (blood vessels), Hematologist (blood)

Components

1. Heart
2. Blood vessels
3. Lymph vessels
4. Lymph nodes
5. Spleen
6. Blood

Function/Responsibility Supplies the cells of the body with oxygen and nutrients, transports chemical body regulators (hormones), produces and transports body defenses (antibodies), transports cellular waste products for elimination, and regulates body temperature.

Additional Information The heart pumps blood through two main pathways in the body. The pulmonary circuit carries blood from the heart to the lungs by way of pulmonary veins and from the lungs back to the heart via pulmonary arteries. The much larger systemic circuit carries blood throughout the body by means of arteries that carry blood away from the heart, to capillaries throughout the body, and finally back to the heart by way of veins.

The lymph system passes lymph fluid through spaces between cells. This lymph fluid is filtered through lymph nodes, filtering out bacteria and other foreign particles, before emptying into veins.

The spleen is composed largely of the same material that makes up lymph nodes. The spleen filters out old, worn-out red blood cells and extracts the iron from them to be reused by bone marrow to make new red blood cells. Although the spleen has an important function, it is not essential to life.

Blood is composed of a liquid part and solid components. The liquid is called *plasma* and the solid elements consist of red blood cells, white blood cells, and platelets.

Arterial blood pressure (BP) measurement is the result of two readings using a blood pressure device called a *sphygmomanometer*. The reading is displayed as the systolic reading over the diastolic reading. The systolic reading is a measure of the force of blood pushing against arterial blood vessel walls when the ventricles (lower chambers of the heart) are contracting. The diastolic reading represents the force of blood pushing against the arteries when the ventricles are relaxed. Variations from normal blood pressure may indicate hypertension, heart disease, or hardening of the arteries. The average normal blood pressure varies with age. For example, the young adult male has an average BP of 120/80 (systolic/diastolic).

Associated Disorders

Anemia

Vitamin B-12 deficiency

Vitamin deficiencies

Allergic reactions

Leukemia

Coagulation disorders

Disseminated intravascular coagulation

Lymphoma (Hodgkin's Disease)

Hypertension

Shock

Congestive heart failure (CHF)

Tachycardia

Bradycardia

Hypertensive cardiovascular disease

Angina pectoris

Myocardial infarction (MI)

Bacterial endocarditis

Cardiovascular syphilis

Raynaud's disease

Phlebitis

Drug Classes/Drugs

Iron preparations: ferrous sulfate, ferrous gluconate

Vitamin B-12 preparations: cyanocobalamine, liver extract

Vitamin preparations: pyridoxine, thiamine, folic acid

Vitamin K preparations: phytonadione

Antihistamines: diphenhydramine

Steroids: dexamethasone, prednisone

Sympathomimetics: epinephrine

Antineoplastic agents: chlorambucil, cyclophosphamide, melphalan, vincristine, mechlorethamine, procarbazine, doxorubicin, bleomycin

Anticoagulants: heparin

Diuretics: hydrochlorothiazide, furosemide, spironolactone, triameterne

Antihypertensive agents (hypotensive agents): methyldopa, clonidine, reserpine, hydralazine, guanethidine

Vasopressors: isoproterenol, dopamine, metaraminol, levarterenol (norepinephrine)

Cardiac agents: digoxin, digitalis, digitoxin, nitroglycerin

Electrolyte replacements: potassium, potassium chloride

Beta-blocking agents: propranolol, metoprolol

Antiarrhythmic agents: procainamide, quinidine

Antibiotics: penicillin, tetracycline, erythromycin, methicillin, streptomycin, nafcillin

Vasodilators: nylidrin, isoxsuprine, papaverine, tolazoline

Terms and Definitions

Arteries: blood vessels that carry blood away from the heart

Capillaries: networks of minute blood vessels that connect arteries and veins

CBC: complete blood count, an analysis of RBCs, WBCs, and platelets

Differential white count: "differential" is a test used to count the amount of each type of white blood cell making up the total leukocyte (WBC) count

Edema: collection of fluid in body tissues

Embolus: a thrombus, blood clot, that breaks free and flows in a blood vessel

Erythropoiesis: process of forming RBCs

Hemoglobin: an iron-containing pigment in the red blood cell that carries oxygen in the blood

Hemostasis: the blood clotting mechanism

Hgb: hemoglobin

Platelets: an element in blood important in the clotting process of blood, thrombocytes (old term)

RBC: red blood cell, erythrocyte, carries oxygen

Serum: fluid portion of blood resulting after blood clots

Thrombus: abnormal clot that develops in a blood vessel

Veins: blood vessels that carry blood away from the heart

WBC: white blood cell, leukocyte, used in defense against infection

SYSTEM: RESPIRATORY/PULMONARY

Branch of Anatomy: Pulmonary
Medical Specialist: Pulmonologist
Components

1. Nose
2. Pharynx
3. Larynx
4. Trachea
5. Bronchi
6. Lungs
7. Sinuses

Function/Responsibility Supplies oxygen to the blood (oxygenation of the blood) and removes the carbon dioxide (a waste product resulting from metabolism).

Additional Information When you breathe, air passes through the nostrils, where it is moistened, warmed, and filtered through nasal hairs on its way to the lungs. Once inhaled, the oxygen is extracted from the air in the lungs and transported into the blood (attaches to the RBC in blood) for use by the cells. Carbon dioxide, a waste product of metabolism, is diffused into the air sac in the lung and exhaled out into the atmosphere.

The breathing activity is also responsible for speech production or phonation. The breathing process forces air from the lungs through the larynx upon exhaling, thereby producing sounds.

The lungs are referred to as lobes. Sections of the lung have definite locations:

1. Left upper lobe
2. Left lower lobe
3. Right upper lobe
4. Right middle lobe
5. Right lower lobe

Associated Disorders

Upper respiratory infection (URI)

Sinusitis

Rhinitis

Bronchitis

Asthma

Bronchiectasis

Lower respiratory infection

Pneumonia

Tuberculosis

Emphysema

Pleurisy

Drug Classes/Drugs

Analgesics: aspirin, acetaminophen

Antipyretics: aspirin

Antihistamines: diphenhydramine, chlorpheniramine, brompheniramine

Vasoconstrictors: phenylephrine, naphazoline, ephedrine, pseudoephedrine

Antitussives: hydrocodone, dextromethorphan, codeine

Antibiotics: penicillin, ampicillin, amoxicillin, erythromycin, tetracycline

Steroids: hydrocortisone, prednisone

Bronchodilator: theophylline, aminophylline, isoproterenol, epinephrine

Antitubercular agents: isoniazid, ethambutol, ethionamide, pyrazinamide, rifampin

Terms and Definitions

Alveolar ducts: tubes that carry air to the alveolar sacs

Alveolar sacs: air sacs found within the lungs

Apex: top of the lung

Apnea: breathing stops

Base: bottom of the lung

Breathing: the mechanical act of inhaling and exhaling

Bronchi: two branches of the trachea, each one extending into a lung

Bronchial tree: the air passageways consisting of a large tube, the trachea, and dividing into smaller passageways, called the bronchi, which divide into even smaller passageways called the bronchioles

Bronchioles: smaller divisions of the bronchi in the lungs

Dyspnea: labored or difficult breathing

Hypoxia: deficiency in the amount of utilization of oxygen by body tissues

Larynx: voice box

Metabolism: physical and chemical changes that nutrients undergo in order to become usable by the body

Pharynx: throat

Respiration: refers to the process of exchanging oxygen and carbon dioxide between body cells and the cell surroundings. Oxygen is transported to the cells, while carbon dioxide is transported away from the cells and out to the atmosphere.

Trachea: windpipe.

SYSTEM: Digestive

Branch of Anatomy: Gastroenterology
Medical Specialist: Gastroenterologist
Components

1. Mouth
2. Tongue
3. Teeth
4. Pharynx
5. Esophagus
6. Stomach
7. Small intestine
8. Large intestine
9. Accessory glands
   a. salivary glands
   b. liver
   c. gallbladder
   d. pancreas

Function/Responsibility Food that has been consumed is converted into a form that can be used by the body cells for growth, energy, and repair.

Additional Information Of all the systems comprising the human anatomy, the digestive system has the most profound effect on drugs consumed orally.

Drugs are sensitive to acid/base balance. In order for drugs to achieve their intended effect, the acidity of the stomach and alkalinity are considered.

The intestines contain bacterial and yeast organisms called flora, which keep each other in balance. An overgrowth of one or the other produces severe health complications.

The liver is a vital organ. It is responsible for controlling blood sugar levels, storing a reserve of nutrients (glycogen), producing blood clotting factors (prothrombin and fibrinogen), producing bile salts used to digest fat and aid in the absorption of vitamin K from the gastrointestinal (GI) tract, and detoxifying many substances, including drugs.

Food is composed of starches and sugars (collectively called carbohydrates), fats, and proteins. The digestive process breaks these complex compounds into their simplest elements.

1. Starches and sugars to monosaccharides
2. Proteins to amino acids
3. Fats to fatty acids and glycerol

The acid found in the stomach is hydrochloric acid (HCl). This acid is responsible for facilitating the action of digestive enzymes on the food entering the stomach.

Digestion of food begins in the mouth when the digestive enzyme, ptyalin, breaks down starch. The mouth is also responsible for mechanical digestion, called mastication (chewing). Absorption of digested food begins in the stomach to some degree, but almost all absorption occurs from the small intestinal walls.

Associated Disorders

Nausea and vomiting (often considered symptoms)

Hiccups (singultus)

Constipation

Gastrointestinal gas (flatulence)

Diarrhea

Candidiasis

Oral cancer

Glossitis

Leukoplakia

Reflux esophagitis

Gastritis

Peptic ulcer

Gastric ulcer

Duodenal ulcer

Jejunal ulcer

Stomach carcinoma

Enteritis

Colitis

Sprue

Jaundice

Hepatitis

Cirrosis

Cholecystitis

Cholelithiasis (gallstones)

Pancreatitis

Peritonitis

Drug Classes/Drugs

Antihistamines: dimenhydrinate

Antiemetics: prochlorperazine (phenothiazine)

Tranquilizers: prochlorperazine, metoclopramide

Sedatives: pentobarbital

Local anesthetics: viscous lidocaine

Antispasmodics: atropine sulfate

Laxatives: docusate sodium, cascara sagrada, bisacodyl, phenolphthalein, psyllium hydrophilic mucilloid, milk of magnesia, citrate of magnesia, lactulose

Antiflatulence medications: simethicone

Antidiarrheal agents: diphenoxylate with atropine, loperamide, paregoric

Analgesics: pentazocine, meperidine

Antimicrobials: ampicillin, clindamycin, "aminoglycosides," metronidazole, sulfasalazine, tetracycline, trimethoprim-sulfamethoxazole

Antifungal agents: nystatin, clotrimazole, ketoconazole

Antacids: aluminum hydroxide, magnesium hydroxide, magnesium carbonate, magnesium trisilicate, alginic acid

Histamine H_2-receptor blockers: cimetidine, ranitidine

Cholinergic agents: bethanechol chloride

Gastrointestinal stimulants: metaclopramide

Antiulcer agents: sucralfate

Antineoplastic agents: mitomycin C, 5-fluorouracil, adriamycin, cytarabine

Steroids: prednisone, cortisol, hydrocortisone

Diuretics: spironolactone, furosemide

Pancreatic supplements: trade name products; Cotazyme, Festal, Viokase, Ilozyme

Miscellaneous: chenodeoxycholic acid (dissolves some cholesterol stones)

Terms and Definitions

Absorption: passage of food from the digestive tract to the blood after the food has been broken down during the process of digestion

Anabolism: constructive metabolism or buildup of simple substances synthesized into complex substances that are used for body/protein rebuilding

Basal metabolic rate (BMR): the amount of energy used for metabolism when a body is at rest

Calories: measurement of the quantity of heat required to raise one gram of water, one degree Celsius (centrigrade). This unit is used to express the heat output of an organism or energy value given off by food.

Catabolism: destructive metabolism or breakdown of complex organic substances to simpler substances with energy being released

Defecation: elimination of feces from the rectum

Digestion: process of chemically breaking down complex food material into soluble material that can be absorbed by the body

Duodenum: the tube leading from the stomach to the small intestine; it is the first of three portions of the small intestine.

Electrolytes: a substance such as sodium or chloride that is capable of carrying an electrical charge

Esophagus: a collapsible tube that opens into the stomach

Feces: waste product resulting from digestion of food

Gallstones: hard, stone-like masses formed in the gallbladder

Insulin: a hormone produced by the pancreas, responsible for the breakdown of sugar

Metabolism: the total chemical processes of anabolism and catabolism

Minerals: inorganic chemical compounds required by body processes for appropriate functioning

Occult blood: blood, abnormally found in the stools

Peristalsis: wave-like movements resulting from contraction and relaxation of muscles, especially in the intestines

Pharynx: a passageway common to both the respiratory and digestive systems

Vitamins: group of organic compounds required for normal metabolism, growth, and maintenance of life in man

SYSTEM: ENDOCRINE

Branch of Anatomy: Endocrinology

Medical Specialist: Endocrinologist

Components

1. Glands
    a. pituitary
    b. thyroid
    c. parathyroid
    d. pancreas
    e. adrenal
    f. gonads
        (1) testicles
        (2) ovaries
    g. thymus
2. Hormones

Function/Responsibility Chemical control, unification, and coordination of the many complex activities of the whole body.

Additional Information Saliva, mucus, and pancreatic juice secretions produced by specific glands called *exocrine glands* are carried by tubes called ducts. *Endocrine glands* are ductless and pass their secretions, called *hormones,* directly into the blood. The blood circulation transports hormones to their target organs.

Both the endocrine and nervous systems control bodily functions. The effects of the endocrine system (via chemical mediators) take longer. The effects of the endocrine activities last longer than the effects of the nervous system, which uses electrical impulses.

Only minute amounts of hormones are required to elicit a physiological response. Hormones function to regulate the rate of existing body processes. Hormones do not initiate a process. Hormones may be associated with either metabolism or regulatory functions. For instance, insulin is a metabolism hormone concerned with carbohydrate metabolism. The thyroid hormone (thyroxin) regulates the body's basal metabolic rate. Neither hormone initiates either process.

A third group of hormones have a *morphogenetic* function. These hormones influence the development and growth of body tissues or specific organs. Morphogenetic hormones are represented by growth hormones (secreted by the pituitary) and estrogens, which exert their influence on the uterus and vagina.

The adrenal glands, situated above the kidneys, produce hormones called *steroids.* These steroids are divided into glucocorticoids (sugar hormones) and mineralocorticoids (salt hormones). Glucocorticoids exert their function by regulating glucose metabolism. Mineralocorticoids assure that a balance between various minerals (especially sodium and potassium) is maintained to regulate the body's water content.

The adrenal glands also secrete epinephrine (adrenalin) and norepinephrine (noradrenalin), which increase the heart rate and the beating strength of the heart, and raise blood pressure by constricting blood vessels.

The pancreas is located behind the stomach and is the gland responsible for secreting the insulin hormone and digestive juices. Insulin is produced by the beta cells in the pancreas. Drugs such as tolbutamide and tolazamide are used to stimulate insulin production in failing and defective beta cells.

Refer to Table 7.1 for a summary of endocrine functions.

Associated Disorders

Panhypopituitarism

Hypopituitary cachexia

Diabetes insipidus

Diabetes mellitus

Simple goiter

Hypothyroidism

Hyperthyroidism

Thyroid cancer

Thyroiditis

Hypoparathyroidism

Hyperparathyroidism

Osteomalacia

Osteoporosis

Paget's Disease (osteitis deformans)

Prostatitis

Pancreatitis

Adrenocortical insufficiency

Adrenocortical overactivity (Cushing's Syndrome)

Male hypogonadism and hypergonadism

Female hypogonadism and hypergonadism

Amenorrhea

Drug Classes/Drugs

Steroids: hydrocortisone, prednisone, cortisone, desoxycorticosterone, fludrocortisone

Sex hormones: testosterone, diethylstilbesterol, ethinylestradiol, conjugated estrogens

Fertility drugs: bromocriptine, clomiphene

Hormones: vasopressin, calcitonin, insulin

Diuretics: hydrochlorothiazide, furosemide, ethacrynic acid

Thyroid agents: thyroid extract, levothyroxine, iodine, propylthiouracil (PTU), methimazole, liothyronine, liotrix

Chemotherapeutic agents: doxorubicin

Electrolyte replacement/supplement therapy: calcium gluconate, calcium chloride, calcium carbonate, calcium lactate

TABLE 7.1 Endocrine Glands and Their Functions

Gland	Hormone Secretion	Function	Noteworthy
PITUITARY	growth hormone (GH)	stimulates the rate of cell growth	The pituitary gland is also known as the hypophysis and sometimes referred to as the master gland.
	adrenocorticotropic hormone (ACTH)	stimulates the adrenal gland to produce glucocorticoids	
	thyrotropic hormone (TSH)	stimulates the thyroid to release its hormones called thyroxin	
	follicle-stimulating hormone (FSH)	stimulates the growth of follicle cells surrounding the ovum (female egg cell)	
	germinal-stimulating hormones (GSH)	stimulate cells in the testes to produce sperm	
	leutenizing hormone (LH)	responsible for ovulation in the female (release of a mature egg cell from the ovary)	
	interstitial cell-stimulating hormone (ICSH)	stimulates cells in testes to produce testosterone	
	luteotropic hormone (LTH or prolactin)	responsible for the growth of the breast tissue and milk production in pregnant females	
	melanocyte-stimulating hormone (MSH)	stimulates cells in the skin responsible for pigment production	
	vasopressin (pitressin), antidiuretic hormone (ADH)	responsible for the constriction of coronary arteries, reduction of cardiac output, reduction of urine output	
	oxytocin (pitocin)	acts on the smooth muscle of the uterus during pregnancy by stimulating contractions near the time of child delivery, controls bleeding after delivery, stimulates milk production for nursing	
THYROID	thyroid hormone (thyroxin)	stimulates metabolism of all body cells (increases basal metabolic rate—BMR)	The thyroid promotes the growth and ossification of bones and the development of teeth.
PARATHYROID	parathyroid hormone	regulates calcium and phosphorous metabolism	
PANCREAS	insulin	increases the rate of glucose metabolism, decreases amount of glucose in blood, increases amount of glycogen stored in the tissues (e.g., liver)	
	glucagon	stimulates liver to break down stored glycogen into glucose	
ADRENALS (medulla portion)	epinephrine (adrenalin)	stimulates constriction of skin blood vessels, pupil dilation, piloerection, intestinal muscle relaxation, dilation of skeletal muscle blood vessels, bronchodilation, increase in heart muscle contraction	This gland is also referred to as *suprarenal glands.*

TABLE 7.1 CONTINUED

Gland	Hormone Secretion	Function	Noteworthy
	norepinephrine (noradrenalin)	stimulates constriction of skin blood vessels, pupil dilation, piloerection, intestinal muscle relaxation, increase in heart muscle contraction	
ADRENALS (cortex portion)	cortical hormones glucocorticoids (cortisol, corticosterone)	stimulates gluconeogenesis by the liver, decreases protein stores in body cells, fat storage, and metabolism	As a group, the cortical steroids are called corticosteroids (primarily composed of cortisol, corticosterone, and aldosterone).
	mineralocorticoids (aldosterone)	stimulates the increase reabsorption of sodium by the kidneys, decreases reabsorption of potassium by the kidneys, exchange of sodium transfer into cells while transporting potassium out of cells, and controls water balance in the body	
GONADS	androgens (male hormone) testosterone	responsible for normal growth, development, and functioning of male reproductive organs and sex characteristics (for example, voice, beard growth, muscle tone), stimulates bone growth	In the male, the gonad is called the testes. In the female, the gonad is called the ovaries.
	estrogens (female hormones) estradiol	inhibit FSH stimulation, induces ovulation, stimulation growth of uterus, uterine tubes, and mammary ducts, development of sex characteristics (e.g., voice, fat deposit)	
	progesterone	prepares uterus for implantation of fertilized egg cell, inhibits ovulation during pregnancy	Progesterone is sometimes called the "pregnancy hormone."
THYMUS	"hormone-like" factor	stimulates spleen and lymph nodes to produce lymphocytes	The thymus shrinks with age until it nearly disappears in adulthood. Actual endocrine functions are unknown.

Vitamin therapy: dihydrotachysterol (vitamin D), dihydroxycholecalciferol, calciferol

Antidiabetic agents: tolbutamide, chlorpropamide, tolazamide, glyburide, acetohexamide, glipizide

Terms and Definitions

Adrenocorticotropic hormone (ACTH): secreted by the pituitary, this hormone is responsible for stimulating the adrenal glands to increase the production of glucocorticoids (hormones that affect the metabolism of glucose).

Androgens: male hormones

Antidiuretic hormone (ADH): a pituitary hormone responsible for the reduction of urine by increasing reabsorption of water by the kidney. Also known as vasopressin, pitressin, or pituitrin, this hormone causes the constriction of coronary arteries in the heart, and reduces the cardiac output by lessening the strength of the heart muscle.

Glands: structures in the body that produce secretions such as saliva, pancreatic juice, and hormones

Gluconeogenesis: formation of glucose by the liver from noncarbohydrate sources

Glycogenolysis: breakdown of glycogen from a complex carbohydrate to monosaccharides such as glucose

Goiter: enlargement of the thyroid gland as a result of a gland disorder

Gonads: sex glands

Growth hormone (GH): hormone secreted by the pituitary gland and functions to increase the rate of growth of all body cells

Hormones: chemical substances produced by specific organs; these chemicals have specific regulatory effects on body functions.

Hypophysis: pituitary gland

Insulin: hormone secreted by pancreas and used to decrease the blood sugar level

Ossification: process of hardening into bone

Oxytocin: a hormone secreted by the pituitary, responsible for producing powerful contractions in the uterus

Piloerection: hairs "stand on end"

SYSTEM: MALE REPRODUCTIVE

Branch of Anatomy: Genitourinary

Medical Specialist: Urologist

Components

1. Testes
2. Scrotum
3. Penis
4. Accessory organs
   a. duct of epididymis
      (1) duct of epidiymis
      (2) ductus deferens
      (3) ejaculatory ducts
   b. urethra
5. Glands
   a. seminal vesicles
   b. prostate gland
   c. bulbourethral glands
6. Semen

Function/Responsibility The male reproductive organ is responsible for the perpetuation of the human species through sexual reproduction. In addition, the male reproductive organ produces hormones that assure the development of male characteristics.

Additional Information The male reproductive organ includes two testes. These testes produce spermatozoa and male hormones.

Semen, the reproductive fluid of the male, contains spermatozoa plus fluid from the seminal vesicles, prostate gland, and bulbourethral glands. The penis is the male organ that conveys the reproductive fluid from the male into the female. The ejaculation of fluid from the penis contains from 200 to 400 million sperm cells, maintaining a fertilizing vitality lasting twenty-four to seventy-two hours.

Associated Disorders

Gonorrhea

Syphilis

Urethritis

Balanoposthitis

Balanitis

Lymphogranulomas

Drug Classes/Drugs

Antibiotics: penicillin, ampicillin, amoxicillin, tetracycline, sulfonamides (for example, Gantrisin), streptomycin

Terms and Definitions

Circumcision: surgical removal of a free fold of skin (prepuce) along the base of the end of the penis

Cowper's glands: bulbourethral glands responsible for producing an alkaline fluid that helps to neutralize the acidity of the fluid produced by the prostate gland

Ejaculation: expulsion of semen from the male through the penis

Genitalia: sex organs (male—penis; female—vagina)

Scrotum: sac containing the testes

Semen: reproductive fluid

Spermatic cord: collective term for the ducts, blood vessels, nerves, lymphatics, and tissue coverings ascending from the testes and passing out of the scrotum

Spermatogenesis: production of spermatozoa

Spermatozoa: male sex cells

SYSTEM: FEMALE REPRODUCTIVE

Branch of Anatomy: Gynecology

Medical Specialist: Gynecologist

Components

1. Ovary (gonad)
2. Accessory organs
   a. uterus
   b. uterine tubes (oviducts)
   c. vagina

3. Vulva (genitalia)
4. Mammary glands
5. Menstrual cycle

Function/Responsibility The female reproductive system is responsible for the perpetuation of the human species through sexual reproduction. In addition, the female reproductive organs produce hormones that assure the development of female characteristics.

Additional Information The vagina provides the passageway for the fetus during birth and provides the outlet for the excretion of the menstrual flow. It is also the receptive organ for the penis.

The menstrual cycle is usually completed every twenty-eight days, but may vary in normal healthy women. The blood flow during menses occurs during the last five days of the cycle. Approximately ten days after the menstrual flow stops, an ovum is discharged. This process is known as ovulation.

The areola surrounding the nipple darkens in color during pregnancy.

Spermatozoa are viable in the female reproductive tract for at least forty-eight hours.

Emotional disturbances can cause irregularities in the menstrual cycle.

Menstruation stops during pregnancy.

Menopause usually begins between ages forty-five and fifty. During menopause, reproductive glands have a reduction in secretions, the ovaries atrophy (as do the uterus and other sex organs), and physical and psychological disturbances are usually characterized by hot flushes, headaches, sweating, dizzy spells, worry, fear, and irritability.

Associated Disorders

Gonorrhea

Syphilis

Trichomoniasis

Candidiasis

Urethritis

Lymphogranulomas

Dyspareunia

Infertility

Amenorrhea

Uterine bleeding

Endometriosis

Vulvitis

Salpingitis (pelvic inflammatory disease—PID)

Premenstrual tension

Primary or functional dysmenorrhea

Carcinoma of the breast

Drug Classes/Drugs

Antibiotics: penicillin, ampicillin, amoxicillin, tetracycline, streptomycin, kanamycin

Antiprotozoan: metronidazole

Antifungal: nystatin

Analgesics: aspirin, acetaminophen, codeine, pentazocine

Topical anesthetics: dibucaine, lidocaine

Sedative: phenobarbital

Fertility drugs: clomiphene

Hormones: ethinyl estradio, medroxyprogesterone, conjugated estrogens, estrogen-progestin combinations, testosterone

Antihistamines: diphenhydramine, tripelennamine

Tranquilizers: diazepam

Diuretics: hydrochlorothiazide

Nonsteroidal anti-inflammatory agents (NSAIA): naproxen, ibuprofen

Steroids: prednisone

Nonsteroidal estrogen antagonist: tamoxifen

Cytotoxic chemotherapeutic agents: 5-fluorouracil, cyclophosphamide, methotrexate, chlorambucil, vincristine, doxorubicin, melphalan

Terms and Definitions

Areola: pigmented area around the nipple on the breast

Cervix: the constricted lower end of the uterus

Endometrium: mucous membrane lining the uterus

Fallopian tubes: ovarian tubes, uterine tubes

Fertilization: the union of the male's sperm with the female's egg

Gestation: pregnancy

Hymen: a fold of mucous membrane that partially covers the posterior portion of the entrance to the vagina

Mammary glands: breasts

Menopause: the phase of a woman's life when menstruation ceases

Menstruation: the cyclical discharge of bloody fluid from the uterus that occurs between puberty and menopause

Ovulation: eggs become mature and are shed from the ovary on a specific schedule called a menstrual cycle

Placenta: organ to which the fetus is attached by means of the umbilical cord and which supplies nourishment to the fetus while removing waste products.

PHARMACOKINETIC BASICS

Pharmacology is the study of the actions of drugs on a living system. The study of drug activity includes looking at the properties of the drug, the dose/response relationship (pharmacodynamics), and the effect on living systems. The living human system functions to achieve a state of balance through the basic physiologic processes described.

Adding a drug intended to reestablish a balance to a living system may create a different imbalance. In order to prevent imbalances, the pharmacology of drugs is studied by using the principles of pharmacokinetics.

Pharmacokinetics is the primary tool used to predict drugs in motion. The action of drugs in a living organism follows specific processes that are identified as *absorption, distribution, metabolism,* and *excretion.* You may see other terms or phrases representing the same processes such as localization in tissues (i.e., distribution), biotransformation (i.e., metabolism), and elimination (i.e., excretion). Regardless of the terms, drugs follow the same pathways in pharmacokinetics.

In addition to the established kinetic path, drug action is also influenced by age, gender, race, health condition, and lifestyle. Therefore, the expected action of a drug can vary widely between any two patients.

Let us briefly follow a drug ingested orally. The mouth has enzymes that initially act, however minimally, on the drug. When the drug reaches the stomach, gastric glands, which produce enzymes in addition to hydrochloric acid, contribute to breaking down the chemicals in the medication. Some of the drug may enter systemic circulation at this time. Next, the drug moves to the intestine where the intestinal mucosa produce enzymes to help degrade the drug into a form that enters the circulatory system.

As it circulates throughout the systemic system, the drug composition passes into the liver where it is detoxified and/or metabolized into active and inactive molecules. These molecules find their way into the circulatory system, arrive at their receptor site where they exert their action, or the unusable drug finds its way to the kidney where it is filtered out and eliminated.

Obviously, the pathway and actions on the drug are considerably more complex. Let us look more closely at each stage of the process.

Most drugs are not absorbed in the mouth or stomach. The oral enzymes may begin somewhat of a limited digestive process. In the stomach, the acid environment and gastric enzymes do not favor much drug absorption. However, the tablets, capsules, and so forth begin a significant dissociation and dissolution from the binders and excipients that make up the product.

Absorption continues into the intestinal region where enzymes act on the drug to produce a rapidly absorbable form that passes from the intestine into the blood circulation through capillaries that converge into the portal vein, which leads into the liver.

The liver is a very important organ that contains the enzymes to transform drugs to an active or partially active form from an inactive form of the drug. The liver also reduces that amount of active drug that enters the systemic system. The liver contains a number of metabolizing enzyme systems that transform drugs by chemical reactions such as oxidation, reduction, hydrolysis, dealkylation, and hydroxylation. The most pronounced of the liver enzyme systems is the cytochrome P-450 enzyme system, which is comprised of many families of isoenzymes responsible for specific activities in the metabolism of drugs.

The metabolized form of the original drug entity distributes into the circulatory system and exerts its effect on the specific site for which it is designed. The drugs that have an affinity for water are called hydrophilic drugs. Those drugs that distribute into the fat are referred to as lipophilic drugs. The importance of drug affinity is especially important in persons with excessive fat or obesity. Drugs "locked up" by the fat cells have the potential for unpredictable release from the fat that can eventually create a hyperdose situation.

The final stage of the pharmacokinetics of a drug is elimination or excretion. The kidney is a vital organ for this activity. The body makes every attempt to rid itself of foreign bodies and toxins. The body sees drugs as foreign molecules and toxins. The role of the kidney is to filter out and eliminate waste products (in a liquid form) such as metabolites from food breakdown and drug biotransformations and toxins.

The liver also has a role in eliminating waste and toxins. The liver accomplishes this by secreting the toxins and waste metabolites into bile, which is then removed as solid waste by way of the intestine.

Note the following additional points:

1. A prodrug is an inactive or somewhat active drug that is metabolized in the liver into the active form of the drug.
2. The availability of a drug in the bloodstream depends on the route of administration. Drugs administered intravenously are 100 percent available for use. Drugs administered other than intravenously, such as by oral administration, do not achieve 100 percent availability in the bloodstream because of the metabolic processes that a nonintravenously administered drug must undergo before it ever reaches the bloodstream.
3. Factors that affect the metabolism of a drug include the age, race, health condition, diet, and lifestyle of the patient.
4. Drugs that bind with plasma protein are not free to exert their effect.
5. Drugs that impact on the function of the liver may impact on the metabolism of other drugs taken concurrently.
6. A disease state that affects the liver (e.g., cirrhosis) or kidney (e.g., renal failure) requires the prescriber to implement "close titration." One philosophy to follow is, "start low, and go slow" whereby the prescriber is able to methodically and correctly dose the patient.
7. Foods can affect the metabolism of drugs by binding with the drugs themselves or by affecting the dynamics of the digestive process.
8. Drugs may react with each other chemically to form an entity that can result in a kinetic alteration that affects blood flow (hemodynamics), speed of digestion, the ability of the liver to metabolize drugs through biotransformation, or the kidney's ability to perform its reabsorption and elimination functions.
9. The safety of drug therapy depends on the efficacy of the drug and the ability of the patient to tolerate the drug.
10. Each drug has a dose dependency (i.e., the dose required in a person to elicit a result) and therapeutic dose (ie., the dose determined scientifically needed to elicit a response).

Although pharmacokinetic drug management is beyond the job description for pharmacy technicians, a basic understanding of this tool can assist you in answering many questions. In the ambulatory pharmacy setting, where you are the last link between the ordering of the drug and the consumption of the drug, your importance as a resource is even more evident.

EXERCISES

1. How many systems make up our anatomy?
2. What branch of anatomy deals with cell studies?
3. What is a cell?

4. The process by which the cell membrane selects only certain substances to pass into the cell is called ______________________________.
5. The two major parts of the cell are the ____________ and ____________.
6. Like cells form tissues which form ______________________________.
7. Organs are comprised of any of what five basic tissues?
   a.
   b.
   c.
   d.
   e.
8. What is an anatomic system?
9. The body cannot perform appropriately without a proper balance, called ____________________________.
10. Name three physiologic processes used to transport nutrients and wastes across cell membranes.
    a.
    b.
    c.
11. The chemical name for salt is ____________________________.
12. Equal concentration of particles on either side of the cell membrane is known as ____________________________.
13. What is the difference between ligaments and tendons?
14. Give an example of an involuntary movement of a body organ.
15. Are apnea and dyspnea the same? If not, how are they different?

Complete the following exercise by entering the appropriate information on each quadrant of the following charts labeled with a specific anatomical system.

16. What tool is used in pharmacy to predict the activity of drugs?
17. What are the traditional processes that drugs follow once ingested?
18. Other than the traditional pharmacokinetic processes, list three influences on drug action.
19. What effect does hydrochloric acid in the stomach have on ingested drugs?
20. Where are drugs detoxified in the human organism?
21. What is the function of the kidney in drug activity?
22. How does a drug in the liver get metabolized?
23. What are lipophilic drugs?
24. What happens to drugs bound to plasma protein?
25. How is pharmacokinetics important to the pharmacy technician?

Branch of Anatomy	System Components
System Function/Responsibility	**Representative Disorders**

FIGURE 7.1 Anatomical System: Integumentary

Branch of Anatomy	System Components
System Function/Responsibility	**Representative Disorders**

FIGURE 7.2 Anatomical System: Skeletal

Branch of Anatomy	System Components
System Function/Responsibility	**Representative Disorders**

FIGURE 7.3 Anatomical System: Muscular

Branch of Anatomy	System Components
System Function/Responsibility	**Representative Disorders**

FIGURE 7.4 Anatomical System: Nervous

Branch of Anatomy	System Components
System Function/Responsibility	**Representative Disorders**

FIGURE 7.5 Anatomical System: Cardiovascular/Circulatory

Branch of Anatomy	System Components
System Function/Responsibility	**Representative Disorders**

FIGURE 7.6 Anatomical System: Respiratory/Pulmonary

Branch of Anatomy	System Components
System Function/Responsibility	**Representative Disorders**

FIGURE 7.7 Anatomical System: Digestive

Branch of Anatomy	System Components
System Function/Responsibility	**Representative Disorders**

FIGURE 7.8 Anatomical System: Endocrine

Branch of Anatomy	System Components
System Function/Responsibility	**Representative Disorders**

FIGURE 7.9 Anatomical System: Male Reproductive

Branch of Anatomy	System Components
System Function/Responsibility	**Representative Disorders**

FIGURE 7.10 Anatomical System: Female Reproductive

CHAPTER 8

Common Disease States and Drug Associations

OBJECTIVES

When you have completed this chapter, you will be able to:

1. define a variety of common disease conditions and symptoms by name and characteristics
2. describe the etiology for a variety of common disease states
3. describe the pathophysiology for a variety of common disease states
4. list health-care goals for a variety of common disease states
5. identify treatments for a variety of common disease states

The ambulatory pharmacy setting provides more opportunities for pharmacy technicians to take an active role in a patient's care management, especially when associated with medication therapy (i.e., pharmacotherapy). The hospital pharmacy environment has limited exposure to community-type patient questions. However, once in a while calls about illnesses and medication use come to the pharmacy. Depending on the policy of the individual pharmacy department, a well-prepared pharmacy technician who may provide assistance is very beneficial to both the busy pharmacist and the person calling. A pharmacy technician can be instrumental in patient care and patient communication without actively engaging in patient counseling.

Diseases (or, if you prefer, illnesses, conditions, ailments, sicknesses) or whatever extent of the disease an ambulatory patient has, is probably less threatening than that of the hospitalized patient, who requires around-the-clock skilled care. This section discusses the more common ailments in which you can help the ambulatory patient with self-management of the condition. You are able to assist the patient by knowing about the condition, the pharmacologic remedies (both legend and OTC) prescribed, and the nonpharmacologic remedies available. The scope of this textbook is to present a basic knowledge that you can apply in all areas of pharmacy and many areas of health care, including disease states. Therefore, this text uses a simple format that is intended to help you learn and provide a basic understanding of common illnesses (and symptoms), and the commonly associated remedies used to treat the conditions. These commonly used remedies noted in the "pharmacologic treatment" section of the following formats are enclosed by brackets, and indicated by reference numbers to which you can refer in Chapter 9 of this unit, "Drug Classes and Representative Drugs."

Because the information presented here is basic, your interest may require you to consult any of the medical books listed under *Reference Sources* in Chapter 6, "Special Pharmacy Skills," located in Unit 1. These texts are specifically designed to focus in great detail on disease states and remedies.

This section divides the common conditions alphabetically into disease-type conditions (e.g., arthritis) and symptoms-type conditions (e.g., vomiting). Sometimes there is a lack of clearly identifiable definitions for symptoms or conditions. For instance, "headache" could simply be a symptom. However, migraine headaches are considered to be an ailment. Whereas symptoms may be manifest as a result of any number of conditions (e.g., the "pain" symptom generating from conditions such as cancer, gastroenteritis, sinusitis, etc.), diseases are contained by a relatively strict set of identifying criteria diagnosed through symptoms and tests.

The following formats were developed exclusively for use in this textbook. Each format label is defined. Feel free to embellish the information provided with your own notes and findings. The blank set of formats may be copied for any conditions or drugs you may want to add.

THE CONDITION-FORMAT EXPLANATION

CONDITION

(What is the common name for the illness?)
disease ____ symptom ____ (Is the illness a disease or a symptom?)

Other Names or References

(Are there other names used to refer to the illness?)

Definition

(How is the illness defined in a "textbook" method?)

Etiology

(What is the cause of the ailment?)
internal ____ external ____ (Is the cause of the ailment due to *internal* means such as heredity or immunology? Is the cause precipitated by *external* reasons such as pathogenic organisms?)

Pathophysiology

(What does the ailment cause, or what are its effects?)

Health-Care Goals

(What do we expect to achieve with medical intervention? For example, generally we would expect reduced symptoms, improved organ functions, and/or a reduction in the progression of the condition.)

Treatment

(The treatment focuses on pharmacologic, mediation-oriented treatment that includes prescription or legend drugs, and/or non-pharmacologic treatment dealing with lifestyle modification and nutritional management.)

pharmacologic (legend drugs or OTC drugs)

non-pharmacologic (lifestyle and diet)

Pharmacologic treatments referenced by number are found in Unit 2, Chapter 9, starting on page 252.

Other Worthwhile Notes

(Are there other issues or concerns such as age, gender, organ function, etc. that should be noted?)

Note: This format and the information provided serve as a basic guide only. Refer to a medical textbook or other medical compendium for in-depth information about specific diseases.

CONDITION

disease ____ symptom ____

Other Names or References

Definition

Etiology

internal ____ external ____

Pathophysiology

Health-Care Goals

Treatment

pharmacologic
non-pharmacologic

Other Worthwhile Notes

DRUG-FORMAT EXPLANATION

See Chapter 9 of this unit, "Drug Classes and Representative Drugs," for monographs.

PHARMACOLOGIC TREATMENT

(The pharmacologic treatment can be either a legend/prescription drug or an OTC medication.)
generic: (All generic and brand name drugs will have a generic nomenclature. Few generic drugs have a generic brand name.)
brand/trade name: (The brand name is the property of the patent holder of the drug.)
OTC: (These are the medications sold without requiring a prescription.)

Drug Class (To which general group of drugs does this medication belong? Is it an antibiotic, analgesic, etc.?)

Indications (For what is this drug supposed to be used?)

Action (What is this drug supposed to do?)

Dosage Range (What is the usual lower and upper limits of the dosage?)

Usual Schedule (What is the time interval over which it is usually given?)

Common Side Effects (Are there side effects common to its use?)

Drug/Food Interactions (Does this drug interact with other drugs, including OTC drugs and/or food?)

Other Notable Comments (Is there other notable information such as contraindications, adverse effects, special directions or storage, precautions, auxiliary labels?)

Note: The selected drug information provided in this textbook provides you with a basic introductory knowledge about the drug. This complies with the intended scope of this textbook. Refer to drug compendia for additional information about specific drugs.

Pharmacologic Treatment

generic:

brand/trade name:

OTC:

Drug Class:

Indications:

Action:

Dosage Range:

Usual Schedule:

Common Side Effects:

Drug/Food Interactions:

Other Notable Comments:

CONDITION

Angina Pectoris

disease ____ symptom __x__

Other Names or References

Angina

Definition

Chest pain caused by lack of oxygen and nutrients to the heart. This condition is caused by an insufficient blood flow to the heart due to restricted coronary blood circulation.

Etiology

internal __x__ external __x__

Internally, there are hereditary factors that contribute to angina. Externally, a sedentary lifestyle and inappropriate diet contribute to problems with coronary blood flow.

Pathophysiology

Insufficient blood flow to the heart prevents the necessary oxygen from being supplied to the heart for normal function.

Health-Care Goals

- reduce pain
- decrease the oxygen needs of the heart by decreasing its workload
- improve the blood flow

Treatment

pharmacologic: nitroglycerin, calcium channel blockers [references 6, 25, 66], and beta-blockers (e.g., propranolol, nadolol)

non-pharmacologic: low-fat diet, exercise, smoking cessation, weight management

Other Worthwhile Notes

CONDITION

Arthritis

disease __x__ symptom ____

Other Names or References

osteoarthritis, rheumatoid arthritis, gout, ankylosing spondylitis, degenerative joint disease

Definition

A condition characterized by inflammation of joints, usually accompanied by pain, and frequently changes in joint structure.

Etiology

internal __x__ external ____

Note: The condition is not fully understood, but the aging process is implicated with resulting wear and tear on joints.

Pathophysiology

The condition causes joint pain, inflammation, heat, and redness in the affected region. There is also stiffness and a loss of full range of motion. The disease is chronic and progressive.

Health-Care Goals

- reduce the pain and inflammation
- improve the range of movement
- slow the deterioration of joints

Treatment

pharmacologic: nonsteroidal anti-inflammatory disease drugs (NSAIDs) [references 23, 37, 39, 46, 47], analgesics [references 1, 2, 9, 60], antigout drugs [references 4, 20], antimalarial agents [reference 36], gold compounds [reference 35], chelating agents [reference 54], immunosuppressive agents [reference 10], and antineoplastic agents [reference 22].

non-pharmacologic: Rest. Heating pad to the affected area. Gentle exercises to move joints. Reduce body weight, if necessary, to relieve stress on joints. Home-health devices are available to assist patients with their daily activities.

Other Worthwhile Notes

Osteoarthritis results from deterioration of cartilage. Rheumatoid arthritis is an autoimmune condition. Gout is a metabolic condition that is limited to severe pain and swelling in one joint. Ankylosing spondylitis is ossification (bone formation) localized in the joints that support the spinal column, hips, and shoulders.

CONDITION

Asthma

disease __x__ symptom ____

Other Names or References

Definition

A respiratory condition in which the small breathing passages (bronchioles) narrow or clog with mucus, thereby making difficult the movement of air in and out of the lungs.

Etiology

internal __x__ external __x__

The internal cause is due to hereditary factors. There are external factors such as viral respiratory infection that can precipitate an asthma condition.

Pathophysiology

The development of the condition leads to wheezing, shortness of breath, tightness in the chest, and coughing.

Health-Care Goals

- control the condition acutely and chronically
- abolish symptoms by relaxing the smooth respiratory muscles by means of medications
- restore normal lung function
- minimize the need for relief medication

Treatment

pharmacologic: bronchodilators [reference 3], steroids (e.g., prednisone), and respiratory inhalation products (e.g., cromolyn).

non-pharmacologic: Prepare living quarters to be free of allergens and irritants such as cigarette smoke, pet dander, and dust mites.

Other Worthwhile Notes

Drink plent of clear fluids to assist in loosening mucus.

CONDITION

Atherosclerosis

disease __x__ symptom ____

Other Names or References

"hardening of the arteries"

Definition

A slow, progressive condition in which the large and medium-sized arteries form plaques on the inner walls making the blood vessel narrow and less flexible, thereby reducing blood flow and circulation of blood to organs.

Etiology

internal __x__ external __x__

Internally, hereditary factors and the aging process contribute to the disease. Externally, a sedentary lifestyle and dietary factors contribute to atherosclerosis.

Pathophysiology

Poor blood flow to any organ causes a dysfunctional situation for the specific organ. Therefore, the pathophysiology will reflect a change in the organ's function. For instance, poor blood flow to the kidneys will result in renal failure.

Health-Care Goals

- increase unrestricted blood flow
- reduce strain on the heart
- slow the progression of plaque buildup

Treatment

pharmacologic: anticoagulants [reference 67], antihyperlipidemic agents [references 43, 58, 63]

non-pharmacologic: smoking cessation, low-fat diet, low sodium diet, weight management, exercise program

Other Worthwhile Notes

Three major risk factors contribute to atherosclerosis. They are elevated lipid levels in the blood, hypertension, and smoking.

CONDITION

Chronic Obstructive Pulmonary Disease

disease __x__ symptom ____

Other Names or References

chronic bronchitis, emphysema, chronic obstructive airways disease, chronic obstructive lung disease

Definition

A progressive and irreversible category of respiratory conditions characterized by diminished pulmonary outflow.

Etiology

internal ____ external __x__

Major cause is smoking.

Pathophysiology

Lack of oxygen to tissues may eventually cause a bluing called *cyanosis.* Ultimately, the limited or lack of oxygen to the lungs and heart can cause respiratory arrest or heart failure.

Health-Care Goals

- increase breathing capacity and airflow
- cessation of smoking
- reduce air pollutants
- slow the progression of the condition

Treatment

pharmacologic: bronchodilators [reference 3], antibiotics [references 7, 8, 12, 13, 14, 15, 17, 18, 55], expectorants (e.g, guaifenesin)

non-pharmacologic: no smoking; condition air and living environment through air filters, humidifiers, and air conditioners; drink liberal amounts of water to loosen mucus

Other Worthwhile Notes

CONDITION

Congestive Heart Failure
disease __x__ symptom ____

Other Names or References

CHF, left ventricular failure, heart failure

Definition

An abnormal heart condition characterized by congestion of the circulatory system due to poor blood flow and inadequate movement of water and sodium.

Etiology

internal __x__ external __x__

Internally, hereditary factors and aging factors play a role in this condition. Externally, CHF can be caused by excessive alcohol intake and viral infections.

Pathophysiology

This condition can lead to difficult breathing (dyspnea), high venous blood pressure, prolonged circulation time, fatigue, swelling of the legs and ankles (peripheral edema).

Health-Care Goals

- strengthen the pumping ability of the heart
- prevent irregular heart rhythms
- remove sodium and water from the blood

Treatment

pharmacologic: inotropic drugs [reference 24, isosorbide], diuretics [references 32, 65], ACE inhibitors [references 11, 26, 41], vasodilators (e.g., hydralazine), calcium channel blockers [references 6, 25, 48, 66], beta-blockers (e.g., propranolol, nadolol)

non-pharmacologic: low-fat diet, low sodium diet, exercise program, weight management, smoking cessation, no alcohol, stress management

Other Worthwhile Notes

Daily self-monitoring of blood pressure is important. Keep a record.

CONDITION

Constipation

disease ____ symptom __x__

Other Names or References

Definition

A bowel movement behavior whereby there is difficulty in passing feces (stools).

Etiology

internal ____ external ____

Pathophysiology

Health-Care Goals

- restore normal or usual bowel movements

Treatment

pharmacologic: laxatives (e.g., docusate, senna compound)

non-pharmacologic: Add fiber to the diet. Fruits such as prunes may stimulate bowel movements or apples may add fiber for bulk. Drink fluids liberally.

Other Worthwhile Notes

CONDITION

Depression

disease __x__ symptom __x__

Other Names or References

blues, seasonal affective disorder (SAD)

Definition

An emotional condition that exceeds the realm of reality characterized by feelings of sadness, despair, dejection, worthlessness, and hopelessness.

Etiology

internal __x__ external __x__

Internally, hereditary factors involving an imbalance of neurotransmitters can play a role in depression. Externally, adverse events such as significant loss or dreary days associated with certain seasons of the year can influence the condition.

Pathophysiology

The condition manifests itself in a variety of ways from the lack of motivation to physiological alterations of body functions.

Health-Care Goals

- supportive roles
- educate to deal with adverse events
- chemically, reestablish neurotransmitter imbalance
- prevent worsening of the condition

Treatment

pharmacologic: antidepressants [references 31, 53, 62]

non-pharmacologic: psychotherapy, light therapy for SAD

Other Worthwhile Notes

Antidepressant drugs require 2 to 3 weeks before there is noticeable improvement in the patient.

CONDITION

Diabetes Mellitus

disease __x__ symptom ____

Other Names or References

sugar, diabetes

Definition

A metabolic condition in which the pancreas is unable to produce and/or secrete the hormone, insulin, needed to metabolize carbohydrates (glucose and starches), fats, and proteins.

Etiology

internal __x__ external ____

Hereditary factors are primary.

Pathophysiology

High blood sugar levels can accelerate atherosclerosis, which in turn can contribute to inadequate blood flow to the heart. This situation can potentiate a heart attack, stroke, kidney failure, eye disorders, gangrene, and impotence.

Health-Care Goals

- regular blood and urine sugar testing
- steady blood glucose levels
- assure proper metabolism of carbohydrates
- maintain strict hygiene, especially of the feet
- strict compliance with a diabetic diet and a hypoglycemic drug or insulin

Treatment

pharmacologic: insulin [reference 38], hypoglycemic agents [references 33, 34]

non-pharmacologic: regularly scheduled eye examinations, weight management, limited fat intake, low intake of simple sugars, exercise program, daily monitoring of blood glucose, and smoking cessation

Other Worthwhile Notes

Many OTC liquid preparations contain sugar. However, there are many OTC products available that are sugar-free.

CONDITION

Diarrhea

disease ______ symptom __x__

Other Names or References

"the runs"

Definition

Bowel movements characterized by frequent passing of loose, watery stools.

Etiology

internal ____ external ____

Pathophysiology

Unattended diarrhea can lead to electrolyte depletion.

Health-Care Goals

- restore normal bowel movement activity
- replace electrolytes as needed

Treatment

pharmacologic: antidiarrheals (e.g., loperamide, diphenoxylate/atropine), electrolyte replacement fluids

non-pharmacologic: starchy, binding foods such as rice and potatoes

Other Worthwhile Notes

CONDITION

Epilepsy

disease ______ symptom __x__

Other Names or References

fits, seizures, convulsions

Definition

A neurological condition characterized by seizures.

Etiology

internal __x__ external __x__

Internally, there is an idiopathic-type of condition that has an unknown cause, but tends to run in families. Externally, this condition can be associated with environmental trauma to the head such as infection, tumor, intoxication, or impact.

Pathophysiology

Idiopathic (i.e., no clear identifiable pathway)

Health-Care Goals

- remove the negative stigma attached to epilepsy
- prevent harm or injury to the patient (e.g., during a fall resulting from the seizure)
- reduce or eliminate seizures through medication

Treatment

pharmacologic: antiseizure agents [references 19, 56], tranquilizers (e.g., chlordiazepoxide, diazepam)

non-pharmacologic:

Other Worthwhile Notes

CONDITION

Fever

disease ____ symptom __x__

Other Names or References

temperature

Definition

Fever is an abnormal elevation of the body temperature.

Etiology

internal ____ external ____

Pathophysiology

Unattended, an elevated temperature can lead to seizures.

Health-Care Goals

- reduce temperature to a "normal" body temperature (98.6 degrees Fahrenheit)

Treatment

pharmacologic: antipyretic drugs [references 1, 9, 47]

non-pharmacologic: cool compresses

Other Worthwhile Notes

In children with highly elevated temperatures, phenobarbital may be ordered to prevent the onset of seizures.

CONDITION

Gastroenteritis

disease __x__ symptom ____

Other Names or References

stomach flu

Definition

An acute condition characterized by an inflammation of the stomach and intestines.

Etiology

internal ____ external __x__

The condition has a bacterial, viral, or chemical origin.

Pathophysiology

Diarrhea and vomiting can precipitate substantial water loss, which can lead to dehydration, which, in turn, can result in the loss of electrolytes, which can produce fatigue and weakness.

Health-Care Goals

- supportive treatment until cured

Treatment

pharmacologic: antiemetics (e.g., prochlorperazine, trimethobenzamide), antidiarrheals (e.g., loperamide, diphenoxylate, and atropine)

non-pharmacologic: electrolyte solutions, clear fluids, bland diet

Other Worthwhile Notes

CONDITION

Headache

disease ____ symptom __x__

Other Names or References

Definition

A pain in the head that can vary in location and intensity.

Etiology

internal ____ external ____

Pathophysiology

Health-Care Goals

- eliminate the causative agent of the headache
- relieve the pain

Treatment

pharmacologic: analgesics [references 1, 2, 9, 60], antianxiety agents [reference 5]

non-pharmacologic:

Other Worthwhile Notes

Other treatments, pharmacologic or non-pharmacologic, depend on the nature of the headache. For example, a headache may be caused by seasonal allergy, migraine, sinusitis, stress, or tumor.

CONDITION

Hemorrhoids

disease ____ symptom __x__

Other Names or References

piles

Definition

A condition occurring in the lower rectum or anus characterized by inflamed, swollen, burning, itching veins.

Etiology

internal ____ external __x__

Excessive pressure placed on the affected veins causes bulging.

Pathophysiology

The severity of the hemorrhoids can lead to bleeding.

Health-Care Goals

- reduce the symptoms
- prevent constipation

Treatment

pharmacologic: cortisone-containing ointment or suppositories (e.g., ANUSOL-HC suppositories or ointment, dibucaine ointment), stool softeners (e.g., docusate, senna compound)

non-pharmacologic: apply cold, wet (witch hazel solution) astringent compresses; increase fiber in the diet

Other Worthwhile Notes

CONDITION

Hypertension
disease __x__ symptom ____

Other Names or References

high blood pressure, HBP

Definition

A condition characterized by abnormally high blood pressure in the arteries.

Etiology

internal __x__ external ____

This condition is associated with hereditary factors. The condition can be exacerbated by sedentary lifestyle; poor diet; and unusual, persistent stress.

Pathophysiology

Inadequate blood flow to the heart can lead to heart function complications. Other end-organ complications may involve the kidney, blood vessels in the brain (e.g., stroke), and the eyes.

Health-Care Goals

- achieve and maintain a "normal" blood pressure (*Note:* Blood pressure is age related.)

Treatment

pharmacologic: diuretics [references 32, 65], vasodilators (e.g., hydralazine, terazosin), beta-blockers (e.g., propranolol, nadolol), ACE inhibitors [references 11, 26, 41]

non-pharmacologic: weight management, diet low in sodium and fat, exercise program, stress management, regular schedule for self-monitoring of blood pressure

Other Worthwhile Notes

CONDITION

Insomnia

disease ____ symptom __x__

Other Names or References

Definition

Insomnia is the inability to sleep or remain asleep throughout a sleeping period.

Etiology

internal ____ external ____

Pathophysiology

Health-Care Goals

- determine the cause of the sleeplessness
- enable the patient to sleep

Treatment

pharmacologic: sleeping aids (e.g., zolpidem, triazolam), antianxiety drugs [reference 5]

non-pharmacologic:

Other Worthwhile Notes

It is definitely critical to determine the cause of the insomnia before recommending sleeping aids (i.e., there are OTC sleeping aids available).

CONDITION

Lipid Disorders

disease __x__ symptom ____

Other Names or References

hypercholesterolemia, hyperlipidemia, cholesterol, triglycerides, HDL, and LDL

Definition

A condition characterized by excessive lipids (e.g., cholesterol) in the blood plasma.

Etiology

internal __x__ external __x__

Internally, the condition can be associated with hereditary factors. Externally, a sedentary lifestyle and a diet containing saturated fats can contribute to lipid disorders.

Pathophysiology

Unattended, a lipid disorder can precipitate atherosclerosis (see atherosclerosis in this chapter).

Health-Care Goals

- achieve and maintain "normal" (or near-normal) blood lipid levels

Treatment

pharmacologic: antihyperlipidemic drugs [references 43, 58, 63]

non-pharmacologic: diet free from saturated fats found in foods such as red meats, eggs, and dairy products

Other Worthwhile Notes

Cholesterol is transported through the bloodstream by being attached to lipoproteins. Low-density lipoproteins (LDL) are the "bad" cholesterol, and high-density lipoproteins (HDL) are the "good" cholesterol. HDL prevents the lipids from binding to the inside walls of the blood vessels.

CONDITION

Myocardial Infarction

disease __x__ symptom ____

Other Names or References

MI, infarct, heart attack, coronary thrombosis

Definition

A condition characterized by a number of events that result in the heart being unable to pump enough oxygenated blood to meet the body's metabolic needs.

Etiology

internal __x__ external ____

Atherosclerosis is the primary underlying cause. There are also hereditary factors.

Pathophysiology

Total obstruction of a coronary vessel stops the flow of blood to the heart, thereby depriving the heart of needed oxygen to function.

Health-Care Goals

- reduce pain
- establish support during acute phase
- improve organ function
- slow the progression of the condition

Treatment

pharmacologic: beta-blockers (e.g., propranolol, nadolol), anticoagulants [reference 67, aspirin], calcium channel blocker [references 6, 25, 48, 66], antihyperlipidemics [references 43, 58, 63]

non-pharmacologic: low-fat diet, exercise program, smoking cessation, weight management

Other Worthwhile Notes

CONDITION

Nausea and Vomiting
disease ____ symptom __x__

Other Names or References

"sick to my stomach," throwing up, upchuck, N/V

Definition

Nausea is an unpleasant sensation that can lead to vomiting, which is to orally expel the contents of the stomach.

Etiology

internal ____ external ____

Pathophysiology

Health-Care Goals

- determine the cause of the N/V
- eliminate the feeling of nausea
- stop the vomiting
- replace electrolytes if needed

Treatment

pharmacologic: antiemetic drugs (e.g., prochlorperazine, trimethobenzamide), electrolyte solutions

non-pharmacologic: various alternative medicine approaches

Other Worthwhile Notes

The cause of the N/V is very important. N/V is a symptom of many conditions. In the ambulatory setting, before recommending an OTC product, be assured that you have covered the issue completely with the patient or caregiver.

CONDITION

Pain

disease ____ symptom __x__

Other Names or References

"hurt"

Definition

Pain is an unpleasant sensation characterized by discomfort, stress, or suffering.

Etiology

internal ____ external ____

Pathophysiology

Health-Care Goals

- determine the cause
- relieve the discomfort

Treatment

pharmacologic: analgesics [references 1, 2, 9, 60]

non-pharmacologic: Depending on the type of pain involved, ice packs may aid in the temporary relief of pain.

Other Worthwhile Notes

The determination of the source of the pain is critical before recommending any type of "painkillers." Pain is an indicator that a problem exists.

CONDITION

Ulcer

disease __x__ symptom ____

Other Names or References

peptic ulcer, stomach ulcer, gastric ulcer, duodenal ulcer, esophageal ulcer, peptic ulcer disease, PUD

Definition

A condition characterized by erosion of the lining of any part of the digestive tract exposed to gastric juices that contain acid and pepsin.

Etiology

internal ____ external __x__

The primary causes for ulcerative conditions are smoking, alcohol, drug irritation, or bacterial infection (Helicobacter pylori).

Pathophysiology

The severity of the ulcer can lead to massive blood loss with resulting anemia. The formation of scar tissue can ultimately lead to intestinal obstruction.

Health-Care Goals

- protect the lining of the digestive tract from irritation
- reduce symptoms associated with ulcer disease
- stop the progression of the ulceration

Treatment

pharmacologic: antacids (e.g., calcium carbonate; magnesium or aluminum hydroxides), gastrointestinal agents [references 16, 29, 49, 50, 61], mucosal strengthening drugs (e.g., sucralfate)

non-pharmacologic: diet free from irritating/acidic foods and spicy foods. Avoid alcohol, smoking, coffee, tea, acidic juices, and carbonated drinks.

Other Worthwhile Notes

Oral treatment regimens for ulcer conditions caused by the Helicobactor pylori bacteria include combinations of bismuth subsalicylate, metronidazole, tetracycline, omeprazole, clarithromycin, ranitidine bismuth citrate, and amoxicillin.

Exercises

1. What specific conditions are included in a cardiovascular category?
2. What class of drugs is commonly used when inflammation is involved?
3. What are the causes of asthma?
4. What can you recommend to a patient who asks about non-pharmacologic ways to deal with asthma?

5. Why would the use of antihyperlipidemic agents and a low-fat diet be an important approach to managing atherosclerosis?
6. What three major risk factors contribute to atherosclerosis?
7. Identify the following acronyms:
   CHF
   SAD
   HBP
   LDL
   HDL
   MI
   N/V
   PUD
   NSAID
   ACE
8. Which is the good and the bad cholesterol?
   HDL ______________________________
   LDL ______________________________
9. Why would you explain to an ulcer patient to stay away from irritating, acidic, and spicy foods?
10. What bacteria has been implicated as a cause of ulcer conditions?

CHAPTER 9

Drug Classes and Representative Drugs

OBJECTIVES

When you have completed this chapter, you will be able to:

1. list major drug groupings
2. list representative drug categories within each major grouping
3. name representative drugs within each drug category
4. describe the indications, action, and dosage range for many drugs representing the various drug classes
5. identify common side effects and common interactions for many drugs representing the various drug classes
6. identify drugs by generic and brand names

This section deals with the primary focus of pharmacy—drugs. The FDA estimates the number of drugs for which national codes exist to be around 35,000. How does anyone begin to learn about 35,000 drugs? Fortunately, only 200 drugs comprise approximately 75 percent of the drug market. Even learning about 200 drugs appears to be an enormous task.

We will direct our drug review to drug classes rather than individual drugs. Focusing on major drug classes will enable us to look at characteristics associated with each drug class and, therefore, there is a good possibility that each drug in the class will exhibit those characteristics. An additional advantage of studying drug classes is the large number of drugs with which you will become familiar.

The format of this section is designed to address each major class of drugs, with a brief introductory note followed by a list of categories and generic drugs representing each major class. Where subdivisions of a major class exist, generic drug representatives have been listed for each subdivision. The first class, for instance, defines analgesics as a major class. However, a number of subdivisions occur for analgesics and include salicylates (aspirin is the representative drug), para-aminophenol (acetaminophen is the representative drug), and narcotics (codeine is one of many representative examples listed). The narcotic analgesic subdivision has been further divided into specific groups based on the drug derivatives. Studying drugs to this extreme may not be practical or necessary for the purposes of this text. However, the information is available and provided for your review.

Drugs, as a rule, are not absolute by category. Many drugs exhibit crossover therapeutic activity. Nonsteroidal anti-inflammatory agents (NSAIA) may be classified as analgesics because they reduce pain responses. NSAIAs are also considered to be anti-inflammatory agents and antiarthritic agents. The NSAIAs are also referred to as nonsteroidal anti-inflammatory drugs, or NSAIDS. The terms and acronyms are interchangeable.

There is a lack of absolute consistency in drug classification. Drugs may be classified according to the therapy they elicit (e.g., painkilling), the disorder for which they are intended (e.g., anti-diarrheal), the pharmacologic response (e.g., antihistamine) or the anatomical/physiological effect they have (e.g., anatomic: cardiovascular agents; physiological: diuretic).

The best way to facilitate learning the massive amounts of information about drugs is to review each class. Highlight important features associated with each group. Learn the names of the most commonly used drugs in each group. Interrelate information where possible and, above all, *keep current* by reading drug journals and other drug literature.

Following are 30 major drug classes. Trade names have not been included because it is common for drug patents to expire (patents are valid for 17 years). Once a drug patent has expired, many drug manufacturers ("drug houses") may produce the generic form of the drug using their own coined names for the drug. The generic name, however, does not change.

Identifiers used in the following listings are as follows:

Major drug groupings (e.g., A. antibacterials) are identified by a capital letter.

Subdivisions within a major drug grouping (e.g., 2. cephalosporins) are identified by a number.

Generic drug representatives have no identifiers.

Abbreviated drug profiles follow the discussion about drug classes. These drugs represent many of the most commonly prescribed drugs, especially in the ambulatory pharmacy setting.

The references made to many of these "most commonly" prescribed drugs are found in Chapter 8 of this unit, "Common Disease States and Drug Associations," which contains a selection of illnesses often found in the ambulatory community. I emphasize that the drug monographs that follow contain basic information about the drug. For additional instruction, consult prescribing information in texts written explicitly for the purpose of evaluating drugs in detail.

ANALGESIC

Analgesics are characteristically used to treat pain. Some analgesics are also able to reduce fever (antipyretic properties), reduce inflammation, and/or inhibit blood platelet aggregation. Some narcotic analgesics (e.g., codeine) are used to suppress coughs.

REPRESENTATIVE CATEGORIES AND DRUGS

A. Salicylates
aspirin

B. Para-aminophenol
acetaminophen

C. Narcotic analgesics
1. phenanthrene derivatives
   codeine
   hydrocodone
   hydromorphone
   levorphanol
   morphine
   oxycodone
   butorphanol
   oxymorphone
   nalbuphine
   pentazocine (not considered a narcotic)
2. phenylpiperidine derivatives
   alphaprodine
   anileridine
   fentanyl
   meperidine
   sufentanil

3. diphenylheptane derivatives
   methadone
   propoxyphene (not considered a narcotic)

Nonsteroidal anti-inflammatory drugs (NSAID) possess analgesic properties. As a class of drugs, they will be found under antiarthritic agents.

ANTIDIARRHEAL

Antidiarrheal drugs function to slow intestinal mobility and propulsion. The body interprets diarrhea as a positive response because it may be the only way of eliminating toxins. The problem with diarrhea, however, is the loss of excessive water and electrolytes, which can result in dehydration.

REPRESENTATIVE CATEGORIES AND DRUGS

1. adsorbents
   kaolin and pectin
2. piperidine derivatives
   diphenoxylate
   loperamide
3. bacterial derivatives
   lactobacillus acidophilus
4. opiate derivative
   opium

ANTIHISTAMINE

Drugs of this class neutralize the effects of histamine (i.e., edema, redness, and itching). These effects are allergic responses. The ethyl-enediamine group of antihistamines characteristically produce more adverse gastrointestinal (GI) upset than the other groups. Some antihistamines, especially the ethanolamine group, possess antiemetic properties. This same group also causes a high incidence of drowsiness while showing a low incidence of GI distress. The alkylamine group causes less drowsiness and more central nervous stimulation than the other groups. Although phenothiazine drugs have antihistamine properties, they are used principally for their psychotherapeutic effects. In addition to antihistamine properties, drugs in this and the piperazine class are also used to treat motion sickness (e.g., meclizine), anxiety and pain (e.g., hydroxyzine), restlessness (e.g., diphenhydramine, promethazine), pruritis (e.g., chlorpheniramine), and nausea (e.g., prochlorperazine).

REPRESENTATIVE CATEGORIES AND DRUGS

1. ethylenediamine derivatives
   pyrilamine
   tripelennamine
2. ethanolamine derivatives
   carbinoxamine
   clemastine
   dimenhydrinate
   diphenhydramine
   doxylamine
   phenyltoloxamine

3. alkylamine derivatives
- brompheniramine
- chlorpheniramine
- dexbrompheniramine
- pheniramine
- triprolidine

4. phenothiazine derivatives
- methdilazine
- promethazine
- trimeprazine

5. piperazine derivatives
- buclizine
- cyclizine
- hydroxyzine
- meclizine

6. miscellaneous
- astemizole
- cetirizine
- fexofenadine
- loratadine

ANTI-INFECTIVE

Anti-infective drugs include a large spectrum of agents used to support the body's defense mechanism or directly defend the body against bacterial, fungal, viral, and other biotic invasion. The terms *antibiotic* and *antibacterial* have been used interchangeably. Anti-infectives are comprised of specific classifications based on their primary chemical derivations, such as aminoglycosides, cephalosporins, beta-lactams, and more.

REPRESENTATIVE CATEGORIES AND DRUGS

A. Antibacterial

1. aminoglycosides
   - gentamicin
   - neomycin
   - streptomycin
   - tobramycin
   - kanamycin
   - amikacin
2. cephalosporins

   (Classification by "generation" represents similar activity against bacteria by each drug in the group.)

   (*first generation*)
   - cefadroxil
   - cefazolin
   - cephalexin
   - cephalothin
   - cephapirin
   - cephradine

   (*second generation*)
   - cefaclor
   - cefamandole
   - cefonicid
   - ceforanine
   - cefoxitin
   - cefuroxime

   (*third generation*)
   - cefoperazone
   - cefotaxime
   - ceftizoxime
   - ceftriaxone
3. beta-lactams

   moxalactam (chemically related to third-generations cephalosporins)

   ceftazidime (structurally related to beta-lactams, pharmacologic properties of third-generation cephalosporins)

   penicillins
   - ampicillin
   - methicillin

- amoxicillin
- carbenicillin
- cloxacillin
- dicloxacillin
- hetacillin
- nafcillin
- oxacillin
- penicillin
- ticarcillin

4. tetracyclines
   - demeclocycline
   - doxycycline
   - methacycline
   - minocycline
   - oxytetracycline
   - tetracycline
5. sulfonamides ("sulfas")
   - sulfacytine
   - sulfamethizole
   - sulfamethoxazole
   - sulfasalazine
   - sulfisoxazole
6. sulfones
   - dapsone
   - sulfoxone
7. cephamycin
   - cefoxitin (pharmacologic properties of second-generation cephalosporins)
8. fluoroquinolones
   - ciprofloxacin
   - norfloxacin
   - ofloxacin
9. urinary antiseptics
   - methenamine
   - nalidixic acid
   - nitrofurantoin
   - trimethoprim
10. miscellaneous
   (*bacterial derivatives*)
   - bacitracin
   - colistin
   - chloramphenicol
   - erythromycin
   - novobiocin
   - spectinomycin
   - troleandomycin
   - vancomycin
   - polymixin B
   - polymixin E
   - "lincomycins"
     - clindamycin
     - lincomycin
   - folate-antagonist
     - trimethoprim

B. Antiviral
- acyclovir
- amantadine
- vidarabine
- famciclovir
- stavudine
- zidovudine
- zalcitabine
- foscarnet
- didanosine
- ganciclovir
- rimantadine

C. Antifungal
- clotrimazole
- ketaconazole
- miconazole
- butoconazole
- griseofulvin
- amphotericin B
- nystatin
- fluconazole
- itraconazole

D. Antituberculars
- aminosalicylic acid
- ethambutal
- pyrazinamide
- ethionamide
- isoniazid
- capreomycin
- cycloserine
- rifampin
- streptomycin

E. Antiprotozoans
- chloroquine
- iodoquinol
- hydroxychloroquine
- metronidazole
- pyrimethamine
- sulfadoxine/pyrimethamine
- paromomycin

F. Antiparasitics
- pyrantel
- pyrvinium
- mebendazole
- thiabendazole

ANTINEOPLASTIC

Chemotherapy is a treatment modality using chemical agents. These chemical agents produce a desired and anticipated therapeutic effect. The term has been associated with the treatment of cancer. The treatment of cancer is so complex that new terminology has been added steadily. Terms such as antimetabolite, cytotoxic, immunosuppressive, oncolytic, tumorcidal, and mutagenic are only a few representing the vast approaches that have been taken to treat cancer and the terminology that has resulted from new research. A popular basis for treatment is interference with the cancer cell's life cycle. Therefore, many chemotherapeutic agents exert their effects on the cancer cell's enzyme system used in proliferating cell growth through DNA synthesis.

REPRESENTATIVE CATEGORIES AND DRUGS

A. Antimetabolites
1. folic acid antagonists
   - methotrexate
2. podophyllotoxin derivative
   - etoposide
   - teniposide
3. purine antagonists
   - azathioprine
   - mercaptopurine
   - thioguanine
4. pyrimidine antagonists
   - floxuridine
   - fluorouracil
   - cytarabine
5. vinca alkaloids
   - vinblastine
   - vincristine
6. urea derivative
   - hydroxyurea

B. Alkylating agents
1. nitrogen mustards
   - chlorambucil
   - cyclophosphamide
   - mechlorethamine
   - melphalan
   - uracil mustard
2. ethylenimines
   - thiotepa
3. alkylsulfonates
   - busulfan

4. triazenes
   dacarbazine
5. nitrosoureas
   carmustine
   lomustine
6. piperazines
   pipobroman

C. Antineoplastic antibiotics
dactinomycin
daunorubicin
doxorubicin
mitomycin
bleomycin
plicamycin

D. Hormones
1. adrenals
   prednisone
   prednisolone
2. androgens
   dromostanolone
   testolactone
3. Leuteinizing Hormone-Releasing Factor (LHRF)
   leuprolide
4. estrogens
   diethylstilbestrol (DES)
5. progestogens (progestins)
   medroxyprogesterone
   hydroxyprogesterone
   megestrol

E. Enzymes
asparaginase

F. Miscellaneous
interferon
mitotane
paclitaxel
procarbazine
tamoxifen

ANTIULCER

The drug therapy used for ulcers attempts to promote healing of ulcerations by neutralizing acids, reducing the production of acids, or enhancing a barrier protection against the effects of acids.

REPRESENTATIVE CATEGORIES AND DRUGS

1. anticholinergics
amsotropine
clindinium
glycopyrrolate
hexocyclium
isopropamide
mepenzolate
methantheline
methscopolamine
oxyphencyclimine
oxyphenonium
propantheline
tridihexethyl

2. H_2-receptor antagonists
cimetidine
ranitidine

3. disaccharide
sucralfate

4. proton pump inhibitors
omeprazole

CARDIOVASCULAR

The use of cardiovascular agents depends on the proper diagnosis by a physician. These agents vary widely, from influencing the contractility of the heart muscle to affecting the consistency of blood.

REPRESENTATIVE CATEGORIES AND DRUGS

A. Inotropics (affect heart muscle contraction)
1. cardiac glycosides
   digoxin
   digitoxin
2. beta-adrenergic agonists
   dobutamine
   isoproterenol
3. miscellaneous
   dopamine
   amrinone

B. Antiarrhythmics (stabilize the cardiac beat rhythm)
1. nonspecific adrenergic blocker
   bretyllium
2. beta-adrenergic blocking agents
   propranolol
   nadolol
   acebutolol
3. alkaloid
   quinidine
   papavarine
4. calcium channel blockers
   diltiazem
   nifedipine
   verapamil
5. amides/amines
   lidocaine
   procainamide
   tocainide
   disopyramide
   flecainide
   methoxamine
6. sodium channel blockers
   disopyramide

C. Antianginals (promote adequate blood and oxygen supply to the heart)
1. calcium channel blockers
   (see drugs under *Antiarrhythmics*)
2. nitrates
   erythrityl tetranitrate
   isosorbide dinitrate
   nitroglycerin
   pentaerythritol tetranitrate

3. beta-adrenergic blockers
   (see drugs under *Antiarrhythmics*)
4. miscellaneous
   dipyridamole (non-nitrate)

D. Antihypertensives (reduce elevated blood pressure)
1. alpha-adrenoceptor agonist
   guanfacine
   clonidine
   guanabenz
2. Angiotensin converting enzyme inhibitors
   captopril
   enalapril
   lisinopril
   ramipril

E. Vasodilators (affect dilation of blood vessels)
(see nitrate/nitrite drugs, non-nitrate, and alkaloid drugs under *Antianginals*)

F. Antilipemics (reduce the level of fatty substances in the blood)
cholestyramine
lovastatin
simvastatin
clofibrate
colestipol
dextrothyroxine
pravastatin
gemfibrozil
probucol

DIURETIC

Diuretics are used to eliminate excessive fluid from the body tissues. These drugs are likely to be seen in the treatment of hypertension, edema, congestive heart failure, and glaucoma. Diuretics are categorized by structure (e.g., thiazide diuretics) or action (e.g., carbonic anhydrase inhibitors).

Representative Categories and Drugs

1. thiazide diuretics
   chlorothiazide
   hydrochlorothiazide
   metolazone
   methyclothiazide
   trichlormethiazide

2. loop diuretics
   ethacrynic acid
   furosemide
   bumetanide
   chlorthalidone

3. osmotic diuretics
   mannitol
   urea

4. potassium-sparing diuretics
   amiloride
   spironolactone
   triamterene

5. indolines
   indapamide

6. carbonic anhydrase inhibitors
   acetazolamide

dichlorphenamide
methazolamide

7. sulfonamide diuretics
   acetazolamide
   furosemide
   indapamide

HORMONE

Hormones are very potent chemical substances. Only minute amounts of hormones are required to effect a response. Many hormones are available for many hormone-related disorders. Many hormone drugs exhibit variable mineralocorticoid and glucocorticoid properties.

REPRESENTATIVE CATEGORIES AND DRUGS

A. Adrenocorticosteroids
1. mineralocorticoids
   desoxycorticosterone
   fludrocortisone
2. glucocorticoids
   beclomethasone
   betamethasone
   cortisone
   dexamethasone
   flunisolide
   hydrocortisone
   meprednisone
   methylprednisolone
   paramethasone
   prednisolone
   prednisone
   triamcinolone

(*Note:* Fludrocortisone has properties associated with both mineralocorticoids and glucocorticoids. However, fludrocortisone is used primarily for its mineralocorticoid properties.)

B. Sex hormones
1. androgens (male)
   oxymetholone
   methyltestosterone
   fluoxymesterone
2. estrogens (female)
   ethinyl estradiol
   diethylstibesterol
   estradiol
   quinestrol
   chlorotrianisene
3. progestins (female)
   progesterone
   medroxyprogesterone
   norethindrone

C. Gonadotropins
   chorionic gonadotropin
   leuprolide
   menotropin

D. Pituitary (human growth hormone)
   somatropin
   vasopressin

E. Thyroid
   calcitonin
   liotrix

thyroid extract
levothyroxine
liothyronine
thyroglobulin

F. Antidiabetic agents
insulin
(drugs used to stimulate insulin production)
acarbose
acetohexamide
chlorpropamide
glipizide
glyburide
metformin
tolazamide
tolbutamide

LAXATIVE

Laxatives promote the evacuation of feces from the intestine. Drugs function in a variety of ways to evacuate feces. Drugs have been developed to create "bulk" in the intestine, soften the stools in the intestine, lubricate the intestine, or stimulate the peristaltic action of the intestinal tract.

REPRESENTATIVE CATEGORIES AND DRUGS

1. bulk laxatives
   methylcellulose
   carboxymethylcellulose
   psyllium
2. stool softeners
   docusate
3. saline laxatives
   magnesium citrate
   magnesium sulfate
   sodium phosphate
4. hyperosmotic laxatives
   sorbitol
   lactulose
5. intestinal stimulants
   bisacodyl
   cascara sagrada
   phenolphthalein
   danthron
6. intestinal lubricants
   mineral oil

PSYCHOTHERAPEUTIC

These agents are used for a variety of conditions associated with the mind and brain. They affect the central nervous system (CNS). Drugs are available for depression, anxiety, hyperactivity, and a number of other mental disorders.

REPRESENTATIVE CATEGORIES AND DRUGS

A. Antidepressants
   1. monoamine oxidase (MAO) inhibitors
      isocarboxazid

phenelzine
tranylcypromine

2. tricyclic compounds
   imipramine
   desipramine
   trimipramine
   amitriptyline
   nortriptyline
   protriptyline
   doxepin
   amoxapine
3. tetracyclic compounds
   maprotiline
   trazodone
4. phenothiazines
   promethazine
   ethopropazine
   propriomazine
   chlorpromazine
   methotrimeprazine
   promazine
   triflupromazine
   trimeprazine
   acetophenazine
   fluphenazine
   perphenazine
   prochlorperazine
   thiethylperazine
   trifluoperazine
   thioridazine
   mesoridazine
   methdilazine
   chlorprothixene
   thiothixene
   droperidol
   haloperidol
   loxapine
   molindone

B. Stimulants
amphetamine
benzphetamine
dextroamphetamine
diethylpropion
fenfluramine
phendimetrazine
phenmetrazine
phentermine
mazindol
methamphetamine
methylphenidate
pemoline
caffeine
doxapram

C. Sedatives/hypnotics/anxiolytics

1. barbiturates
   amobarbital
   aprobarbital
   butabarbital
   mephobarbital
   methohexital
   pentobarbital
   phenobarbital
   secobarbital
   talbutal
2. benzodiazepines
   alprazolam
   chlordiazepoxide
   clorazepate
   diazepam
   flurazepam
   halazepam
   lorazepam
   oxazepam
   prazepam
   temazepam
   triazolam
3. miscellaneous
   chloral hydrate
   ethchlorvynol
   chlormezanone
   ethinamate
   meprobamate
   glutethimide
   methyprylon
   hydroxyzine
   methotrimeprazine
   promethazine
   propiomazine

D. Selective serotonin reuptake inhibitors
fluoxetine
sertraline
paroxetine

HYPOTENSIVE

The term *hypotensive agent* denotes the desired results of this class. Drugs used to treat hypertension control high blood pressure. Physicians approach the treatment of high blood pressure (HBP) in steps:

1. oral diuretic (usually a thiazide)
2. sympathetic depressant (e.g., beta-blocker, methyldopa, or reserpine)
3. vasodilator
4. another sympathetic depressant (e.g., clonidine or guanethidine)

REPRESENTATIVE CATEGORIES AND DRUGS

1. beta-adrenergic blockers
   atenolol
   metaprolol
   pindolol
   acebutolol
   timolol
2. Angiotensin-Converting Enzyme (ACE)
   captopril
   enalapril
3. alpha- and beta-adrenergic blocker
   labetalol
4. thiazide derivative
   diazoxide
5. postganglionic adrenergic blockers
   guanadrel
   guanethidine
6. alpha-adrenergic blockers
   prazosin
7. monoamine oxidase (MAO) inhibitors
   pargyline
8. natural derivatives
   reserpine
   deserpidine
9. miscellaneous
   clonidine
   guanabenz
   hydralazine
   methyldopa
   minoxidil
   nitroprusside
   mecamylamine
   trimethaphan

ANTI-INFLAMMATORY

Anti-inflammatory agents are used for a variety of purposes. They may be used by those suffering from menstrual cramps, inflamed joints, or muscular spasms. Nonsteroidal anti-inflammatory agents (NSAIAs) constitute the primary group within this class, because side effects are tolerable or preventable and the benefits are great.

REPRESENTATIVE CATEGORIES AND DRUGS

A. Steroidal
    (see *Hormone* class for drug representatives)
    adrenocorticosteroids

B. Nonsteroidal
1. salicylates
    aspirin
    diflunisal
2. nonsalicylates
    fenoprofen
    ibuprofen
    naproxen
    indomethacin
    meclofenamate
    ketorolac
    mefenamic acid
    phenylbutazone
    piroxicam
    sulindac
    tolmetin
3. cox-2 inhibitor
    celecoxib
    rofecoxib

ANTIGOUT

Gout is a metabolic disorder characterized by inflammation of the joints resulting from uric acid crystals. It follows, therefore, that research would focus on a mechanism to eliminate excessive uric acid from the blood. That path was followed, resulting in a small, but reliable group of drugs.

REPRESENTATIVE CATEGORIES AND DRUGS

1. xanthines
    allopurinol

2. natural derivatives
    colchicine

3. sulfonamide derivatives
    probenecid

4. miscellaneous
    sulfinpyrazone

MUSCLE RELAXANT

Muscle relaxants are prime examples of drugs that experience crossover in identification. There are skeletal muscle relaxants, smooth muscle relaxants, GI tract relaxants, genitourinary (GU) tract relaxants, and respiratory muscle relaxants. Muscle relaxants, for example, may be found under drugs for the gastrointestinal tract or respiratory tract. However, the various classifiers categorize muscle relaxants as agents that ultimately relax skeletal muscle (e.g., voluntary muscle) or smooth muscle (e.g., involuntary muscle).

REPRESENTATIVE CATEGORIES AND DRUGS

1. skeletal muscle relaxants
   - baclofen
   - carisoprodol
   - chlorphenesin
   - chlorzoxazone
   - cyclobenzaprine
   - diazepam
   - metaxalone
   - methocarbamol
2. smooth muscle relaxants
   (*GI tract*)
   - loperamide
   - diphenoxylate

   (*GU tract*)
   - flavoxate
   - oxybutynin

   (*respiratory*)
   - theophylline
3. miscellaneous
   - succinylcholine
   - pancuronium

BRONCHODILATOR

Most bronchodilator drugs are sympathomimetics. These drugs function at the nerve sites, which stimulate the relaxation of smooth muscle. By relaxing these muscles, the passageways in the lung are permitted to expand, thereby enabling a greater airflow. Older compounds stimulated the heart muscle while effecting response in the bronchial smooth muscle. Newer drugs have been developed to reduce or avoid the unwanted effects on the heart muscle.

REPRESENTATIVE CATEGORIES AND DRUGS

1. sympathomimetic drugs (adrenergics)
   - albuterol
   - bitolterol
   - ephedrine
   - isoetharine
   - isoproterenol
   - metaproterenol
   - terbutaline
2. nonsympathomimetics (xanthines)
   - theophylline
   - aminophylline
3. corticosteroids
   - beclomethasone
   - fluticasone
   - budesonide

4. miscellaneous
   - ipratropium
   - cromolyn
   - nedocromil

SUPPLEMENT

Supplements may be classified as nutritional (vitamins), electrolytic (potassium, sodium, calcium, chloride, etc.), and mineral, which in the general sense may refer to electrolytes. In a stricter sense, however, minerals may be construed as those elements that do not possess an electrical charge. Calcium as an electrolyte has an electrical charge of two (Ca++), but as a mineral is referred to as elemental calcium (no electrical charge).

REPRESENTATIVE CATEGORIES AND DRUGS

1. vitamins
   - single vitamin preparations
   - multiple vitamin preparations
   - pediatric vitamins with fluoride
   - pediatric vitamins
   - multiple vitamins with minerals
   - prenatal vitamins
   - geriatric vitamins
   - therapeutic vitamins
2. electrolytes
   - phosphorus
   - phosphate
   - potassium
   - calcium
   - sodium
   - chloride
   - magnesium
   - acetate
   - lactate
3. minerals
   - zinc
   - iron
   - copper
   - iodine
   - calcium
   - magnesium
   - manganese

ANTICONVULSANT

Anticonvulsant drugs function by raising the threshold to stimuli that initiate seizures. The anticonvulsant drugs available are used in the treatment of epilepsy. It should be noted that seizures can occur as a result of conditions other than epilepsy (i.e., drug-induced seizures, tumor, etc.)

REPRESENTATIVE CATEGORIES AND DRUGS

1. barbiturate derivatives
   - phenobarbital
   - primidone
   - mephobarbital
   - metharbital

2. benzodiazepine derivatives
- clonazepam
- clorazepate
- diazepam
- lorazepam

3. hydantoins
- phenytoin
- mephenytoin
- ethotoin
- phenacemide

4. miscellaneous
- trimethadione
- paramethadione
- ethosuximide
- methsuximide
- phensuximide
- carbamazepine
- valproic acid
- divalproex

ANTIARTHRITIC

Drugs found within this class are used to treat disorders of a larger magnitude called *collagen diseases.* These diseases affect the joints, skin, and supporting tissue of various organs. Many of the drugs used for inflammation are found in this class.

REPRESENTATIVE CATEGORIES AND DRUGS

A. Steroids
1. adrenocorticosteroids
   - prednisone
   - cortisone
   - hydrocortisone

B. Nonsteroidal anti-inflammatory drugs (NSAID)
1. salicylates
   - aspirin
   - diflunisal
   - salsalate
2. nonsalicylates
   - fenoprofen
   - ibuprofen
   - naproxen
   - indomethacin
   - ketorolac
   - meclofenamate
   - mefenamic acid
   - phenylbutazone
   - piroxicam
   - sulindac
   - tolmetin

C. Gold derivatives
- auranofin
- aurothioglucose
- gold sodium thiomalate

D. Heavy-metal antagonists
- penicillamine

E. Immunosuppressants
- azathioprine

F. Antimalarial agents
- chloroquine
- hydroxychloroquine

OPHTHALMIC

Sometimes referred to as optic drugs, these agents are used primarily for inflammation, infection, glaucoma, anesthesia, and diagnostics. These drugs should be sterile and free from particulate matter. All products used for the eyes should be in solution. Some drugs are available for both the ear as a suspension and the eye as a solution. These drugs are not interchangeable.

REPRESENTATIVE CATEGORIES AND DRUGS

A. Anti-inflammatory agents
1. steroids
   - dexamethasone
   - fluorometholone
   - hydrocortisone
   - medrysone
   - prednisolone
2. nonsteroids
   - diclofenac
   - epinephrine
   - flurbiprofen
   - ketoralac
   - naphazoline
   - oxymetazoline
   - phenylephrine
   - propylhexedrine
   - suprofen
   - tetrahydrozoline
   - xylometazoline
   - zinc sulfate

B. Anti-infective agents
1. antibacterials
   - bacitracin
   - chloramphenicol
   - erythromycin
   - gentamicin
   - neomycin
   - polymixin B
   - sulfacetamide
   - tetracycline
   - tobramycin
2. antifungal
   - natamycin
3. antiviral
   - idoxuridine
   - trifluridine
   - vidarabine

C. Antiglaucoma
1. carbonic-anhydrase inhibitors
   - acetazolamide
   - dichlorphenamide
   - methazolamide
2. miotics
   - acetylcholine
   - carbachol
   - demecarium
   - echothiophate
   - isoflurophate
   - physostigmine
   - pilocarpine

D. Anesthetic agents
- tetracaine
- proparacaine

E. Diagnostic agents
- demecarium bromide
- echothiophate iodide
- tropicamide
- homatropine

fluorescein
isoflurophate
cyclopentolate
phenylephrine
hydroxyamphetamine

F. Lubricants/artificial tears
hydroxypropyl cellulose
methylcellulose

G. Miscellaneous agents
timolol
epinephrine
glycerine

HYPOGLYCEMIC

Hypoglycemic agents are used to treat hyperglycemic (diabetic) conditions. In many diabetics, the insulin-producing portion of the pancreas does not function properly. Hypoglycemic agents stimulate these cells (beta cells) to produce adequate insulin needed for the metabolism of carbohydrates.

REPRESENTATIVE CATEGORIES AND DRUGS

1. sulfonylureas
   acetohexamide
   chlorpropamide
   glipizide
   glyburide
   tolazamide
   tolbutamide
2. biguanides
   metformin
3. hormones
   insulin
4. alpha-glucosidase inhibitor
   acarbose
5. meglitinides
   repaglinide
6. glitazones
   pioglitazone
   rosiglitazone

ANTINAUSEANT/ANTIEMETIC

Drugs in this class include those which are used for motion sickness and vertigo. There are numerous causes of vertigo, nausea, and vomiting. Pregnancy, toxins, microbial infections, and radiation are only a few of the causes. In each situation, the approach to treatment is symptomatic. The drugs used alleviate the symptoms and not the cause. The purpose for these drugs is to provide comfort for the patient until other treatment dealing with the cause takes effect, resulting in the elimination of nausea, vomiting, or vertigo.

REPRESENTATIVE CATEGORIES AND DRUGS

A. Antihistamine derivatives
- diphenhydramine
- meclizine
- cyclizine
- dimenhydrinate
- hydroxyzine
- promethazine
- trimethobenzamide

B. Antidopaminergic derivatives
1. phenothiazines
   - chlorpromazine
   - promazine
   - triflupromazine
   - fluphenazine
   - perphenazine
   - prochlorperazine
   - thiethylperazine
2. miscellaneous
   - haloperidol
   - metoclopramide

C. Marijuana derivatives
- nabilone
- dronabinol

D. Miscellaneous
- ondansetron
- granisetron

BLOOD MODIFIER

Blood-modifying drugs represent a multitude of agents used for almost anything involving the blood. If the problem is anemia, there are iron preparations. If the blood is too thick, anticoagulants are available to remedy the situation. There is even a drug to treat calf muscle pain due to an inadequate blood supply.

REPRESENTATIVE CATEGORIES AND DRUGS

A. Antianemic agents
- iron preparations
- cyanocobalamine
- folic acid

B. Anticoagulant agents
1. coumarin derivatives
   - dicumarol
   - phenprocoumon
   - warfarin
2. miscellaneous
   - anisindione
   - heparin

C. Hemostatic agents
- aminocaproic acid
- antihemophilic factor
- factor IX complex
- thrombin

D. Hemorrheologic agent
- pentoxifylline

E. Thrombolytic agents
- streptokinase
- urokinase

ANTISPASMODIC

Spasms are sudden, involuntary muscle contractions. The drugs in this group focus primarily on gastrointestinal spasms and urinary spasms. Muscle relaxants focus on spasms occurring in the skeletal muscles.

REPRESENTATIVE CATEGORIES AND DRUGS

A. Gastrointestinal
1. natural alkaloids
   - atropine
   - belladonna
   - hyoscyamine
2. semisynthetic derivatives
   - homatropine
   - methscopolamine
3. synthetic
   - anisotropine
   - clidinium
   - glycopyrrolate
   - hexocyclium
   - isopropamide
   - mepenzolate
   - methantheline
   - oxyphenonium
   - propantheline
   - tridihexethyl dicyclomine
   - oxyphencyclimine

B. Urinary
1. natural alkaloids
   - atropine
   - hyoscyamine
2. synthetic compounds
   - flavoxate
   - oxybutinin

ANTIPARKINSON

Parkinson's Disease is characterized by a progressive central nervous system involvement. Shaking is perhaps the most characteristic symptom. The disease occurs in the middle-aged and elderly, and eventually may become incapacitating. Drug treatment provides only symptomatic relief.

REPRESENTATIVE CATEGORIES AND DRUGS

1. anticholinergic agents
- benztropine
- biperiden
- cycrimine
- hyoscyamine
- procyclidine
- trihexyphenidyl

2. antihistamine agents
   chlorphenoxamine
   diphenhydramine
   orphenadrine
3. phenothaizine derivative
   ethopropazine
4. dopamine-releasing drug
   amantadine
5. dopamine-elevating drugs
   levodopa
   levodopa/carbidopa

ANTITUSSIVE

Antitussive compounds are used to treat coughing. Coughing can be due to many factors, but the symptomatic treatment is the same. Most drugs are effective at the central nervous system site (i.e., the "cough center"). Some drugs may work at the site of irritation causing the cough.

REPRESENTATIVE CATEGORIES AND DRUGS

A. Centrally acting agents
   1. narcotic derivatives
      codeine
      hydrocodone
   2. non-narcotic derivatives
      dextromethorphan
      diphenhydramine
B. Peripherally acting agents
   benzonatate (non-narcotic)
   noscapine (non-narcotic)

OTIC

Otic agents are drugs intended specifically for the ear. Preparations are available to treat inflammation, infection, pain, and accumulated cerumen (wax).

REPRESENTATIVE CATEGORIES AND DRUGS

1. anti-inflammatory agents
   hydrocortisone
   dexamethasone
   prednisolone
   desonide
2. analgesic agents
   benzocaine
   pramozine
   antipyrine
3. anti-infective agents
   chloramphenicol
   colistin
   acetic acid
   domiphen

neomycin
polymixin B
parachlormetaxylenol

4. cerumenolytic
   triethanolamine polypeptide
   carbamide peroxide

5. decongestant
   phenylephrine

DERMATOLOGIC

Dermatology has one of the most elusive groups of diagnoses. However, there are many drugs available to combat the wide variety of disorders associated with the skin and hair.

REPRESENTATIVE CATEGORIES AND DRUGS

A. Anti-inflammatory agents
   fluocinonide
   fluocinolone
   amcinonide
   dexamethasone
   diflorasone
   hydrocortisone
   betamethasone
   triamcinolone
   desoximetasone
   desonide
   clocortolone
   flurandrenolide
   halcinonide
   methylprednisolone

B. Antihistamine agents
   diphenhydramine
   chlorcyclizine
   tripelennamine

C. Anti-infective agents
   1. antibacterial
      clindamycin
      tetracycline
      chloramphenicol
      erythromycin
      nitrofurazone
      gentamicin
      neomycin
      gramicidin
      polymixin B
      bacitracin
      mafenide
      povidone-iodine
      silver sulfadiazine
      iodoquinol
      iodochlorhydroxyquin
   2. antifungal
      nystatin
      iodochlorhydroxyquin (clioquinol)
      iodoquinol
      griseofulvin
      triacetin
      amphotericin B
      haloprogin
      ciclopirox olamine
      clotrimazole
      miconazole
      econazole
      thiosulfate
      tolfanate
      zinc undecylanate
   3. antiviral/antiherpes agents
      acyclovir
   4. scabicide agents
      crotamiton
      lindane

5. pediculicide agents
   - lindane
   - pyrethrins/piperonyl butoxide

D. Antiacne agents
- benzoyl peroxide
- isotretinoin
- sulfur

E. Antiseborrhea agents
- chloroxine
- coal tar
- sulfur
- salicyclic acid
- selenium
- zinc pyrithione

F. Antipsoriasis agents
- coal tar
- anthralin

G. Miscellaneous
1. depigmenting agents
   - monobenzone
   - hydroquinone
2. repigmenting agents
   - methoxsalen
   - trioxsalen
3. keratolytic agent
   - salicyclic acid
4. sunscreen
   - para-aminobenzoic acid (PABA)
5. topical analgesic/anesthetic agents
   - benzocaine
   - pramoxine
   - dibucaine
   - dyclonine
6. cell-stimulating agent
   - tretinoin
7. debridement agents
   - collagenase
   - dextranomer
   - sutlains
   - fibrinolysin/desoxyribonuclease

VAGINAL

Most gynecologic disorders involve the vagina. Inflammation, discharge, and bleeding are a few common symptoms that require the physician to choose from an assortment of vaginal preparations. Perhaps the most common problem associated with the vagina is the fungal infection.

REPRESENTATIVE CATEGORIES AND DRUGS

1. antifungal agents
- clotrimazole
- nystatin
- miconazole

2. antitrichomonal agent
- metronidazole

3. antibacterial agents
   "sulfonamides"
   triple sulfa
4. hormone agents
   dienestrol
   estropipate
   conjugated estrogens

ANTIOBESITY

Obesity is characterized by the accumulation of excessive body fat. Obesity is not considered a disease in the sense of how we traditionally view diseases. The cause of obesity is the consumption of more calories than are expended. Therefore, drug therapy (anorectic drugs) attempts to convince the individual that he or she is not hungry and can consume less food.

REPRESENTATIVE CATEGORIES AND DRUGS

1. amphetamine agents
   benzphetamine
   dextroamphetamine
   methamphetamine
2. nonamphetamine agents
   diethylpropion
   fenfluramine
   phendimetrazine
   phenmetrazine
   phentermine
   mazindol
   phenylpropanolamine
   dexfenfluramine
3. satient agents
   cholecystokinin
   carboxymethylcellulose
   guar gum
   vegetable bran

COMMONLY USED PHARMACOTHERAPIES

Most of the following drugs are commonly prescribed to patients who are ambulatory. The abbreviated information presents a basic guideline and provides the type of detail that you will most likely need at your immediate disposal to respond to an inquiry.

The "side effects" represent reported observable occurrences in more than 10 percent of the patients taking the drug. Therefore, there is significant chance that the patient taking a particular drug will not experience any of the side effects. However, you and the patient should be aware of the potential for these side effects. Remember, that you are a resource to the patient, especially in the outpatient setting.

The dosing and scheduling listed present the most usual dosing for children and adults for the oral form of the drug. In those cases where the dosing is available for adults only, the dose and schedule will be reflected as such. Dosing depends greatly on age, weight, the condition being treated, and the condition of the patient. Therefore, in actual practice you can expect to see variations from the "usual" dose.

The food and drug interactions do not indicate the significance of the interaction. Listing a drug or food merely notes that there is a possibility based on experience, studies, or pharmacokinetic modeling.

The notable comments provide you with probable needs for auxiliary labeling. This is highlighted by the use of capital letters. This part of the drug profile also gives you some useful hints that you can pass on to the patient.

There are a number of acronyms used within each drug profile. Use the following list of acronyms to help you in reviewing the drug information.

ACE inhibitor—Angiotensin Converting Enzyme inhibitor

CHF—congestive heart failure

CNS—central nervous system

COPD—chronic obstructive pulmonary disease

DNA—deoxyribonucleic acid

/d—per day

FU—fluorouracil, as in 5-FU or 5-fluorouracil

GERD—gastroesophageal reflux disease

GI—gastrointestinal

g/d—grams per day

IM—intramuscular

IV—intravenously

mg/d—milligrams per day

mg/kg/dose—milligrams per kilogram of body weight per dose

NSAIDs—nonsteroidal anti-inflammatory drugs

OCT—over-the-counter

PCN—penicillin

PUD—peptic ulcer disease

RA—rheumatoid arthritis

RNA—ribonucleic acid

SOB—shortness of breath

SSRI—selective serotonin reuptake inhibitor

TCAs—tricyclic antidepressants

TCN—tetracycline

UTI—urinary tract infection

PHARMACOLOGIC TREATMENT 1

generic: acetaminophen

brand/trade name: Tylenol (one of many)

over-the-counter (OTC): yes

Drug Class

analgesic, antipyretic

Indications

fever and moderate pain

Action

relieves pain, lowers elevated body temperature

Dosage Range

children: up to 480 mg/d (age-dependent)
adult: up to 4 g/d

Usual Schedule

children: q 4–6 h (no more than 5 doses in 24 h)
adult: q 4–6 h (up to 650 mg/dose)
3–4 times/d (1,000 mg/dose)

Common Side Effects

rare

Drug/Food Interactions

rifampin, barbiturates, carbamazepine, hydantoins, sulfinpyrazone

Other Notable Comments

toxicity affects liver

PHARMACOLOGIC TREATMENT 2

generic: acetaminophen with codeine
brand/trade name: Tylenol with codeine
over-the-counter (OTC):

Drug Class

analgesic

Indications

moderate pain

Action

relieves pain

Dosage Range

children: up to 1 mg/kg/dose of codeine portion
adults: up to 60 mg/dose of codeine portion

Usual Schedule

children: q 4–6 h
adults: q 4–6 h

Common Side Effects

lightheadedness, dizziness, sedation, constipation

Drug/Food Interactions

CNS depressants, phenothiazines, TCAs, guanabenz, MAO inhibitors

Other Notable Comments

C-III schedule

Tablets and capsules—
#2 contains codeine 15 mg.
#3 contains codeine 30 mg.
#4 contains codeine 60 mg.

MAY CAUSE DROWSINESS

limit to 10-day use unless otherwise advised by physician

PHARMACOLOGIC TREATMENT 3

generic: albuterol

brand/trade name: Proventil, Ventolin

over-the-counter (OTC):

Drug Class

bronchodilator

Indications

reversible restricted airway flow due to respiratory airway disease such as asthma and COPD

Action

relax bronchial smooth muscle to permit less resisted pulmonary ariflow

Dosage Range

children: up to 24 mg/d (divided doses)

adults: up to 32 mg/d (divided doses)

Usual Schedule

children: TID

adults: 3–4 times/d

Common Side Effects

tachycardia, nervousness, tremor

Drug/Food Interactions

beta-adrenergic blockers, ipratropium (enhanced therapy), MAO inhibitors, TCAs, sympathomimetics

Other Notable Comments

availabe in oral and inhalation forms

DO NOT exceed the recommended dosage

PHARMACOLOGIC TREATMENT 4

generic: allopurinol

brand/trade name: Zyloprim

over-the-counter (OTC):

Drug Class

antigout agent

Indications

gouty arthritis

Action

prevents formation of uric acid crystals in joints

Dosage Range

children: 10 mg/kg/d, maximum 600 mg/24 h

adults: maximum 800 mg/d

Usual Schedule

children: 2–3 divided doses

adults: divided doses for doses greater than 300 mg.

Common Side Effects

itching rash, diarrhea, nausea, vomiting, drowsiness

Drug/Food Interactions

alcohol, azathioprine, mercaptopurine, ampicillin, amoxicillin, theophylline

Other Notable Comments

TAKE AFTER MEALS

TAKE WITH LIBERAL FLUIDS

MAY CAUSE DROWSINESS

PHARMACOLOGIC TREATMENT 5

generic: alprazolam

brand/trade name: Xanax

over-the-counter (OTC):

Drug Class

antianxiety agent (benzodiazepine)

Indications

anxiety disorders

Action

affects the body's neurotransmission chemicals

Dosage Range

adults (at least 18 years old): maximum 4 mg/d

Usual Schedule

adults: BID or TID

Common Side Effects

drowsiness, fatigue, lightheadedness, insomnia, decreased libido, headache, constipation, decreased salivation (dry mouth), nausea, vomiting, tachycardia, chest pain, impact on appetite

Drug/Food Interactions

carbamazepine, disulfiram, oral contraceptives, CNS depressants, cimetidine, lithium

Other Notable Comments

AVOID ALCOHOL

MAY CAUSE DROWSINESS

avoid CNS depressants

may cause drug dependence

Schedule C-IV

discontinue gradually after prolonged use

avoid activities that require alertness

PHARMACOLOGIC TREATMENT 6

generic: amlodipine

brand/trade name: Norvasc

over-the-counter (OTC):

Drug Class

cardiovascular agent (calcium channel blocker)

Indications

hypertension, angina

Action

dilates coronary vessels by relaxing the smooth muscles of the coronary vessels

Dosage Range

adults: up to 10 mg/d

Usual Schedule

once daily

Common Side Effects

peripheral edema, headache, fatigue, dizziness, flushing, palpitations

Drug/Food Interactions

fentanyl

Other Notable Comments

report dizziness, SOB, palpitations, edema

PHARMACOLOGIC TREATMENT 7

generic: amoxicillin

brand/trade name: Amoxil, Larotid, Polymox, Trimox

over-the-counter (OTC):

Drug Class

anti-infective

Indications

bacterial infection

Action

bactericidal

Dosage Range

children: up to 100 mg/kg/d (in divided doses)

adults: maximum 3 g/d

Usual Schedule

children: q 8 h

adults: q 8 h

Common Side Effects

rash, diarrhea

Drug/Food Interactions

oral contraceptives, tetracycline

Other Notable Comments

hypersensitivity crossover between amoxicillin and penicillin

complete full course of therapy (10 d–14 d)

take in equal intervals around the clock

report symptoms of vaginal fungus infections

PHARMACOLOGIC TREATMENT 8

generic: amoxicillin/clavulanic acid

brand/trade name: Augmentin

over-the-counter (OTC):

Drug Class

anti-infective

Indications

bacterial infection

Action

bactericidal

Dosage Range

children: up to 40 mg/kg/d (in divided doses)

adults: maximum 2 g/d

Usual Schedule

children: q 8 h

adults: q 8 h

Common Side Effects

rare, if the patient has no hypersensitivity

Drug/Food Interactions

oral contraceptives, probenecid, allopurinol

Other Notable Comments

complete full course of therapy (10 d–14 d)

take in equal intervals around the clock

report symptoms of vaginal fungus infection

hypersensitivity crossover between amoxicillin and penicillin

PHARMACOLOGIC TREATMENT 9

generic: aspirin, acetylsalicylic acid

brand/trade name: various

over-the-counter (OTC): yes

Drug Class

analgesic, anti-inflammatory, antipyretic (salicylate)

Indications

mild to moderate pain, inflammation, fever

Action

relieves pain, reduces inflammation, lowers body temperature

Dosage Range

children: analgesic/antipyretic, up to 15 mg/kg/dose
anti-inflammatory, up to 100 mg/kg/day (maximum 3.6 g/d)

adults: analgesic/antipyretic, maximum 4 g/d
anti-inflammatory, maximum 5.4 g/d

Usual Schedule

children: analgesic/antipyretic, q 4–6 h
anti-inflammatory, q 6–8 h

adults: analgesic/antipyretic, q 4–6 h
anti-inflammatory, divided doses

Common Side Effects

heartburn, nausea, stomach pains, indigestion

Drug/Food Interactions

probenecid, NSAIDs, methotrexate, valproic acid, warfarin

Other Notable Comments

use with caution in patients with PUD

DO NOT use in children under 16 years old who have chicken pox or flu

watch for bleeding gums

TAKE WITH FOOD OR MILK

report tinnitus (ringing in the ears) or continual GI pain

PHARMACOLOGIC TREATMENT 10

generic: azathioprine

brand/trade name: Imuran

over-the-counter (OTC):

Drug Class

immunosuppressive agent

Indications

kidney transplant, RA

Action

prevents rejection of a kidney transplant

affects immune system in the treatment of RA (used in lieu of unresponsiveness of traditional RA drug therapy)

Dosage Range

transplant, up to 3 mg/kg/d

RA, titration up to 2.5 mg/kg/d

Usual Schedule

once daily

Common Side Effects

nausea, vomiting, anorexia (loss of appetite), fever, chills

Drug/Food Interactions

allopurinol

Other Notable Comments

RA response may take up to 3 months

report sore throat, bleeding, bruising, fatigue

PHARMACOLOGIC TREATMENT 11

generic: captopril

brand/trade name: Capoten

over-the-counter (OTC):

Drug Class

cardiovascular (ACE inhibitor)

Indications

hypertension, CHF

Action

produces vasodilation, enabling blood to flow without resistance

Dosage Range

children: titrate to maximum 6 mg/kg/d (2–4 divided doses)

adults: titrate to maximum 450 mg/d

Usual Schedule

children: q 12–24 h

adults: q 8–12 h

Common Side Effects

dysgeusia (impairment of the taste senses), oliguria (reduced urine formation), tachycardia, palpitations, insomnia, headache, dizziness, fatigue, nausea, transient cough

Drug/Food Interactions

indomethacin, NSAIDs, potassium-sparing diuretics

Other Notable Comments

report swelling of face, lips, or tongue

report development of persistent cough

PHARMACOLOGIC TREATMENT 12

generic: cefaclor

brand/trade name: Ceclor

over-the-counter (OTC):

Drug Class

anti-infective

Indications

bacterial infection

Action

bactericidal

Dosage Range

children: maximum 1 g/d

adults: maximum 1.5 g/d

Usual Schedule

children: q 8–12 h

adults: q 8 h or BID (divided doses)

Common Side Effects

pseudomembranous colitis, diarrhea

Drug/Food Interactions

probenecid, oral contraceptives

Other Notable Comments

DO NOT FREEZE
report persistent diarrhea
complete full course of therapy (10 d–14 d)
take in equal intervals around the clock
report symptoms of vaginal fungus infections

PHARMACOLOGIC TREATMENT 13

generic: cefprozil
brand/trade name: Cefzil
over-the-counter (OTC):

Drug Class

anti-infective

Indications

bacterial infection

Action

bactericidal

Dosage Range

children: up to 30 mg/kg/d
adults: up to 1 g/d

Usual Schedule

children: q 12 h (10 d)
adults: q 12–24 h (10 d–14 d)

Common Side Effects

diarrhea, nausea, vomiting

Drug/Food Interactions

probenecid, oral contraceptives

Other Notable Comments

DO NOT FREEZE
report continuous diarrhea
complete full course of therapy
take in equal intervals around the clock
report symptoms of vaginal fungus infections

PHARMACOLOGIC TREATMENT 14

generic: cefuroxime
brand/trade name: Ceftin, Kefurox, Zinacef
over-the-counter (OTC):

Drug Class

anti-infective (cephalosporin)

Indications

bacterial infection

Action

bactericidal

Dosage Range

children: up to 500 mg/d
adults: up to 1 g/d

Usual Schedule

children: BID
adults: BID

Common Side Effects

nausea, vomiting, diarrhea, stomach cramps

Drug/Food Interactions

probenecid, oral contraceptives

Other Notable Comments

complete full course of therapy (10 d–14 d)
take in equal intervals around the clock
report symptoms of vaginal fungus infections

PHARMACOLOGIC TREATMENT 15

generic: cephalexin
brand/trade name: Keflex, Keftab
over-the-counter (OTC):

Drug Class

anti-infective (cephalosporin)

Indications

bacterial infection

Action

bactericidal

Dosage Range

children: maximum 3 g/d
adults: maximum 4 g/d

Usual Schedule

children: q 6 h
adults: q 6 h

Common Side Effects

diarrhea

Drug/Food Interactions

probenecid, oral contraceptives

Other Notable Comments

refrigerate suspension and give it a 14-day expiration date
complete full course of therapy (10 d–14 d)
take in equal intervals around the clock
report symptoms of vaginal fungus infections

PHARMACOLOGIC TREATMENT 16

generic: cimetidine
brand/trade name: Tagamet
over-the-counter (OTC): available

Drug Class

GI agent (histamine H_2 blocker)

Indications

PUD

Action

reduces gastric acid secretion

Dosage Range

children: up to 40 mg/kg/d (in divided doses)
adults: maximum 2.4 g/d (depending on condition being treated)

Usual Schedule

children: q 4 h
adults: QID, HS, BID, q 6 h (depends on condition being treated and the convenience of the schedule)

Common Side Effects

headache, diarrhea, dizzines, drowsiness, vomiting

Drug/Food Interactions

ciprofloxacin, theophylline, phenytoin, metronidaxole, triamterene, procainamide, quinidine, propranolol, warfarin, TCAs, diazepam, cyclosporine

Other Notable Comments

short term ulcer treatment, up to 8 weeks

TAKE WITH MEALS

TAKE 1 HOUR BEFORE OR 2 HOURS AFTER ANTACIDS

MAY CAUSE DROWSINESS

avoid excessive alcohol

PHARMACOLOGIC TREATMENT 17

generic: ciprofloxacin

brand/trade name: Cipro

over-the-counter (OTC):

Drug Class

anti-infective (fluoroquinolone)

Indications

bacterial infection

Action

bactericidal

Dosage Range

adults: up to 1.5 g/d

Usual Schedule

adults: q 12 h

Common Side Effects

nausea, diarrhea, vomiting, abdominal pain, headache, rash

Drug/Food Interactions

antacids (containing aluminum, magnesium, or calcium), caffeine, warfarin, cyclosporine, theophylline, azlocillin, cimetidine, probenecid

Other Notable Comments

NOT recommended for use by children under 18 years old

may take with food

AVOID ANTACIDS CONTAINING ALUMINUM, MAGNESIUM, OR CALCIUM

avoid products containing ZINC or IRON

MAY CAUSE DROWSINESS

DRINK FLUIDS LIBERALLY

PHARMACOLOGIC TREATMENT 18

generic: clarithromycin

brand/trade name: Biaxin

over-the-counter (OTC):

Drug Class

anti-infective (macrolide)

Indications

bacterial infection

Action

bactericidal

Dosage Range

adults: up to 1 g/d

Usual Schedule

adults q 12 h (7 d–14 d)

Common Side Effects

diarrhea, nausea, abnormal taste, indigestion, abdominal pain, headache

Drug/Food Interactions

theophylline, carbamazepine

Other Notable Comments

may take with food

complete full course of therapy (7 d–14 d)

DO NOT USE with terfenidine or astemizole (non-sedating antihistamines)

PHARMACOLOGIC TREATMENT 19

generic: clonazepam

brand/trade name: Klonopin

over-the-counter (OTC):

Drug Class

antiseizure (benzodiazepine)

Indications

seizures

Action

suppresses the neurotransmission causes that precipitate seizures

Dosage Range

children: maximum 0.2 mg/kg/d

adults: maximum 20 mg/d

Usual Schedule

children: TID

adults: 3 divided doses

Common Side Effects

drowsiness, fatigue, impaired coordination, lightheadedness, insomnia, anxiety, decreased libido, depression, headache, dry mouth, nausea, vomiting, chest pain, blurred vision, change in appetite

Drug/Food Interactions

phenytoin, barbiturates, valproic acid

Other Notable Comments

AVOID ALCOHOL

avoid CNS depressants

may cause drug dependence

Schedule C-IV

avoid abrupt stop after prolonged use

avoid using machinery

PHARMACOLOGIC TREATMENT 20

generic: colchicine

brand/trade name:

over-the-counter (OTC):

Drug Class

antigout agent

Indications

gouty arthritis

Action

reduces the deposit of uric acid crystals in joints

Dosage Range

adults: maximum 8 mg/3 d (0.5 mg and 0.6 mg tablets)

Usual Schedule

adults: [acute attacks] q 1–2 h until relief occurs or GI side effects (nausea, vomiting, diarrhea) occur

[prevent recurrence of attacks] 0.5 mg or 0.6 mg q.o.d.

Common Side Effects

nausea, vomiting, diarrhea, abdominal pain

Drug/Food Interactions

sympathomimetic amines, vitamin B-12, CNS depressants

Other Notable Comments

AVOID ALCOHOL

STOP if GI symptoms noted under *Usual Schedule* occur

PHARMACOLOGIC TREATMENT 21

generic: conjugated estrogens

brand/trade name: Premarin

over-the-counter (OTC):

Drug Class

hormones

Indications

various conditions attributed to hormone imbalance or used to *treat* some conditions not associated with hormone balance

Action

replaces insufficient levels of estrogen

effects the synthesis of DNA and RNA

Dosage Range

consult prescribing information for dosage and schedule for specific conditions

Usual Schedule

consult prescribing information for dosage and schedule for specific conditions

Common Side Effects

nausea, peripheral edema, breast enlargement and tenderness, bloating, loss of appetite

Drug/Food Interactions

rifampin, corticosteroids, anticoagulants

Other Notable Comments

report severe headache, vomiting, vision or speech disturbance, numbness, chest pain, depression, unusual bleeding

DO NOT take if pregnant or planning to become pregnant

PHARMACOLOGIC TREATMENT 22

generic: cyclophosphamide

brand/trade name: Cytoxan, Neosar

over-the-counter (OTC):

Drug Class

antineoplastic agent

Indications

specific carcinomas

Action

interferes with DNA function to reduce or retard neoplastic condition

Dosage Range

consult prescribing information for individual dosing protocols

Usual Schedule

consult prescribing information for individual dosing protocols

Common Side Effects

loss of hair, CHF, nausea, vomiting, loss of appetite, diarrhea, stomatitis, bladder irritation, sterility

Drug/Food Interactions

digoxin, phenobarbital, phenytoin, allopurinol, chloramphenicol, cimetidine, doxorubicin, thiazide diuretics

Other Notable Comments

drink fluids liberally before and after each dose

void frequently

DO NOT take drug at nighttime

report blood in the urine

PHARMACOLOGIC TREATMENT 23

generic: diclofenac sodium
brand/trade name: Voltaren
over-the-counter (OTC):

Drug Class

NSAID

Indications

pain and inflammation associated with RA, ankylosing spondylitis, osteoarthritis

Action

relieves pain and reduces inflammation

Dosage Range

adults: maximum 200 mg/d

Usual Schedule

adults: TID, two to five divided doses depending on condition

Common Side Effects

skin rash, abdominal cramps, heartburn, indigestion, nausea

Drug/Food Interactions

thiazides, furosemide, aspirin, digoxin, methotrexate, cyclosporine, lithium, insulin, sulfonylureas, potassium-sparing diuretics

Other Notable Comments

DO NOT crush tablets
TAKE WITH FOOD OR MILK
report signs of blood in the stools

PHARMACOLOGIC TREATMENT 24

generic: digoxin
brand/trade name: Lanoxin
over-the-counter (OTC):

Drug Class

cardiovascular agent (ionotropic)

Indications

CHF, irregular heartbeat

Action

strengthens the heartbeat (and, therefore, the blood flow) by potentiating the activity of the contractile heart muscle and regulates the beat rhythm

Dosage Range

children: consult prescribing information

adults: initially up to 1.5 mg (loading dose)

maintenance, up to 0.5 mg/d

Usual Schedule

Adults: initial dose, once (digitalization)

maintenance dosing, once daily

Common Side Effects

loss of appetite, nausea, vomiting

Drug/Food Interactions

antacids containing aluminum or magnesium, cholestyramine, colestipol, kaolin/pectin, aminoglutethimide, barbiturates, hydantoins, rifampin, amiodarone, nifedipine, quinidine, quinine, verapamil, thiazide diuretics

Other Notable Comments

report loss of appetite or visual disturbances

PHARMACOLOGIC TREATMENT 25

generic: diltiazem

brand/trade name: Cardizem, Dilacor

over-the-counter (OTC):

Drug Class

cardiovascular (calcium channel blocker)

Indications

hypertension, angina

Action

dilates coronary vessels by relaxing the smooth muscles of the coronary vessels

Dosage Range

adults: [capsules] up to 300 mg/d

[tablets] up to 480 mg/d

Usual Schedule

adults: [capsules] QD, BID

[tablets] three to four times/d

Common Side Effects

headache

Drug/Food Interactions

histamine H_2-antagonists, carbamazepine, cyclosporine, digitalis glycosides, fentanyl

Other Notable Comments

discontinue gradually

report dizziness, SOB, heart palpitations, edema

take with a full 8 oz. of water

PHARMACOLOGIC TREATMENT 26

generic: enalapril
brand/trade name: Vasotec
over-the-counter (OTC):

Drug Class

cardiovascular agent (ACE inhibitor)

Indications

hypertension, CHF

Action

produces vasodilation, enabling blood to flow without resistance

Dosage Range

adults: up to 20 mg/d

Usual Schedule

adults: [hypertension] once daily or two divided doses

[CHF] once daily

Common Side Effects

chest pains, palpitations, tachycardia, insomnia, headache, dizziness, fatigue, malaise, impairment of taste senses, abdominal pain, nausea, vomiting, loss of appetite, changes in bowel movement habits, cough

Drug/Food Interactions

NSAIDs, lithium

Other Notable Comments

report vomiting, excessive sweating, swelling of the lips or tongue

report difficulty breathing

report persistent cough

PHARMACOLOGIC TREATMENT 27

generic: ethinyl estradiol/levonorgestrel

brand/trade name: Triphasil 28, Nordette

over-the-counter (OTC):

Drug Class

hormones (oral contraceptives)

Indications

prevent pregnancy, hypermenorrhea, endometriosis, hypogonadism

Action

alters hormone levels to inhibit ovulation or to replace imbalanced levels of hormones

Dosage Range

memory-minder manufacturer's packaging

Usual Schedule

memory-minder manufacturer's packaging

Common Side Effects

peripheral edema, breast enlargement and tenderness, bloating, nausea, loss of appetite

Drug/Food Interactions

barbiturates, hydantoins, rifampin, antibiotics (PCNs, TCNs, griseofulvin), acetaminophen, anticoagulants, benzodiazepines, caffeine, corticosteroids, metoprolol, theophylline, TCAs

Other Notable Comments

report severe headache, vomiting, vision or speech disturbance, numbness or weakness in the extremities, chest pain, calf pain, SOB, abdominal pain, depression, or unusual bleeding

discontinue if you are pregnant or intend to become pregnant

PHARMACOLOGIC TREATMENT 28

generic: ethinyl estradiol/norethindrone

brand/trade name: Ortho-Novum 7/7/7 28

over-the-counter (OTC):

Drug Class

hormones (oral contraceptives)

Indications

prevent pregnancy, hypermemorrhea, endometriosis, hypognadism

Action

alters hormone levels to inhibit ovulation or to replace imbalanced levels of hormones

Dosage Range

memory-minder manufacturer's packaging

Usual Schedule

memory-minder manufacturer's packaging

Common Side Effects

peripheral edema, breast enlargement and tenderness, bloating, nausea, loss of appetite

Drug/Food Interactions

barbiturates, hydantoins, rifampin, antibiotics (PCNs, TCN, griseofulvin), acetaminophen anticoagulants, benzodiazepines, caffeine, corticosteroids, metoprolol, theophylline, TCAs

Other Notable Comments

report severe headache, vomiting, vision or speech disturbance, numbness or weakness in the extremities, chest pain, calf pain, SOB, abdominal pain, depression, or unusual bleeding

discontinue if you are pregnant or intend to become pregnant

PHARMACOLOGIC TREATMENT 29

generic: famotidine

brand/trade name: Pepcid

over-the-counter (OTC): available

Drug Class

GI agent (histamine H_2 blocker)

Indications

PUD

Action

reduces gastric acid secretion

Dosage Range

children: 1–2 mg/kg/d

adults: initially, up to 640 mg.

maintenance, up to 40 mg/d

Usual Schedule

children: single daily dose

adults: initially, single dose

maintenance, BID or hs (depending on the condition)

Common Side Effects

dizziness, headache, change in bowel movements

Drug/Food Interactions

ketaconazole, itraconazole

Other Notable Comments

once daily dosing, take at bedtime

twice daily dosing, take in the morning and at bedtime

PHARMACOLOGIC TREATMENT 30

generic: fluconazole

brand/trade name: Diflucan

over-the-counter (OTC):

Drug Class

anti-infective (antifungal)

Indications

candida infections

Action

fungicidal

Dosage Range

consult prescribing information for dose and scheduling for specific infections

Usual Schedule

consult prescribing information for dose and scheduling for specific infections

Common Side Effects

headache, skin rash, nausea, vomiting, abdominal pain, diarrhea

Drug/Food Interactions

rifampin, cyclosporine, phenytoin, warfarin

Other Notable Comments

may take with food

report any of the side effects

complete full course of therapy

PHARMACOLOGIC TREATMENT 31

generic: fluoxetine

brand/trade name: Prozac

over-the-counter (OTC):

Drug Class

antidepressant (bicyclic antidepressant)

Indications

major depression

Action

effects neurotransmission of neurotransmitter by inhibiting serotonin (the neurotransmitter) uptake

Dosage Range

children: dose and safety has not been established for children under 18 years old

adults: maximum 80 mg/d

Usual Schedule

adults: [20 mg or less] once in the A.M.

[greater than 20 mg] BID (A.M. and NOON)

Common Side Effects

headache, nervousness, insomnia, drowsiness, nausea, diarrhea, dry mouth

Drug/Food Interactions

TCAs, lithium, diazepam, trazadone, MAO inhibitors, alcohol

Other Notable Comments

AVOID ALCOHOL and alcoholic beverages

MAY CAUSE DROWSINESS

an observable response may take several weeks

PHARMACOLOGIC TREATMENT 32

generic: furosemide

brand/trade name: Lasix

over-the-counter (OTC):

Drug Class

diuretic (loop-type)

Indications

edema

Action

increases the excretion of water, sodium, chloride, magnesium, and calcium

Dosage Range

children: minimum 6 mg/kg/*dose*

adults: consult prescribing information for specific condition and titration

Usual Schedule

children: no more often than q 6 h

adults: qd, BID

Common Side Effects

orthostatic hypotension, dizziness

Drug/Food Interactions

hypoglycemic agents, indomethacin, antihypertensive agents, lithium, aminoglycoside antibiotics, and other ototoxic drugs

Other Notable Comments

may take with food or milk

rise slowly from a lying or sitting position

take early enough to prevent nocturia

PHARMACOLOGIC TREATMENT 33

generic: glipizide

brand/trade name: Glucotrol

over-the-counter (OTC):

Drug Class

hypoglycemic agent

Indications

manage noninsulin-dependent diabetes mellitus (NIDDM)

Action

stimulation of the beta cells in the pancreas releases insulin

Dosage Range

adults: up to 40 mg/d

Usual Schedule

adults: [under 15 mg] once daily

[greater than 15 mg] BID in divided doses

Common Side Effects

headache, loss of appetite, nausea, vomiting, epigastric bloating, heartburn, change in bowel movements

Drug/Food Interactions

beta-blockers, cholestyramine, hydantoins, rifampin, thiazide diuretics, urinary alkalizers and acidifiers, histamine H_2-blockers, anticoagulants, fluconazole, salicylates, gemfibrozil, sulfonamides, TCAs, probenecid, MAO inhibitors, methyldopa, digitalis glycosides

Other Notable Comments

DO NOT skip meals

carry source of sugar if needed

take a missed dose as soon as possible, except if it is close to your next dose, in which case, skip the missed dose

DO NOT take double doses

avoid OTC cough/cold preparations, appetite control preparations, hay fever and asthma preparations

possible photosensitivity

PHARMACOLOGIC TREATMENT 34

generic: glyburide

brand/trade name: Diabeta, Glynase, Micronase

over-the-counter (OTC):

Drug Class

hypoglycemic agent

Indications

manage noninsulin-dependent diabetes mellitus (NIDDM)

Action

stimulation of the beta cells in the pancreas releases insulin

Dosage Range

adults: up to 20 mg/d (consult prescribing information for GLYNASE *Prestab)*

Usual Schedule

adults: once daily or BID in divided doses (consult prescribing information for GLYNASE Prestab)

Common Side Effects

headache, loss of appetite, nausea, vomiting, epigastric bloating, heartburn, change in bowel movements

Drug/Food Interactions

thiazides, beta-blockers, oral anticoagulants, hydantoins, salicylates, NSAIDs, sulfonamides, alcohol, phenylbutazone

Other Notable Comments

DO NOT skip meals

carry source of sugar if needed

take a missed dose as soon as possible, except if it is close to your next dose, in which case, skip the missed dose

DO NOT take double doses

avoid OTC cough/cold preparations, appetite control preparations, hay fever and asthma preparations

possible photosensitivity

PHARMACOLOGIC TREATMENT 35

generic: gold sodium thiomalate

brand/trade name: Myochrysine

over-the-counter (OTC):

Drug Class

gold salts

Indications

progressive RA

Action

lessens the symptoms and slows the progression of RA

Dosage Range

consult prescribing information

Usual Schedule

consult prescribing information

Common Side Effects

tongue irritation or soreness, metallic taste, skin rash, itching, bleeding gums, ulcers or sores in mouth region (i.e., mouth, throat, lips), inflammation of the eyes

Drug/Food Interactions

penicillamine

Other Notable Comments

administered by deep IM injection

auranofin (Ridaura brand) is an oral form of a gold preparation

PHOTOSENSITIVITY

benefits of gold therapy may not be seen for 3 months

report rash and oral problems

PHARMACOLOGIC TREATMENT 36

generic: hydroxychloroquine

brand/trade name: Plaquenil

over-the-counter (OTC):

Drug Class

antimalarial

Indications

malaria, RA

Action

destroys malarial parasites

impairs antigen-antibody reactions, thereby reducing symptoms associated with RA

Dosage Range

consult prescribing information for various indications

Usual Schedule

consult prescribing information for various indications

Common Side Effects

headache, itching, diarrhea, loss of appetite, nausea, vomiting, stomach cramps, visual disturbances

Drug/Food Interactions

none of significance

Other Notable Comments

TAKE WITH FOOD OR MILK

complete full course of therapy

protect eyes from sunlight

report blurring vision, tinnitus

PHARMACOLOGIC TREATMENT 37

generic: ibuprofen

brand/trade name: Motrin

over-the-counter (OTC): available

Drug Class

NSAID

Indications

mild to moderate pain and inflammation associated with RA, osteoarthritis, and other inflammatory diseases

Action

relieves stiffness, redness, and swelling (anti-inflammatory activity) and relieves pain (analgesic effects) in treating the pain and inflammation associated with inflammatory diseases

Dosage Range

children: maximum 40 mg/kg/d

adults: maximum 3.2 g/d

Usual Schedule

children: q 6–8 h

adults: [analgesic] q 4–6 h

[anti-inflammatory] TID or QID

Common Side Effects

dizziness, fatigue, rash, itching, heartburn, indigestion, nausea, abdominal cramps

Drug/Food Interactions

aspirin, digoxin, methotrexate, lithium, furosemide, histamine H_2-blockers, warfarin

Other Notable Comments

TAKE WITH FOOD

MAY CAUSE DROWSINESS

report prolonged heartburn and abdominal pain

PHARMACOLOGIC TREATMENT 38

generic: insulin

brand/trade name: Humulin, Novolin

over-the-counter (OTC): "insulins" are OTC

Drug Class

hypoglycemic agent (hormone)

Indications

insulin-dependent diabetes mellitus (IDDM)

Action

replaces the hormone "insulin" in sufficient amount to metabolize carbohydrates (sugars and starches)

Dosage Range

consult the prescribing information for determining dosages and schedules

Usual Schedule

consult the prescribing information for determining dosages and schedules

Common Side Effects

sweating, palpitations, tachycardia, fatigue, tingling in the fingers, headache, itching, hypothermia, hunger, pallor, nausea, muscle weakness, visual disturbances

Drug/Food Interactions

oral contraceptives, corticosteroids, diltiazem, epinephrine, smoking, thiazide diuretics, thyroid hormones, niacin, alcohol, alpha blockers, anabolic steroids, beta-blockers, clofibrate, MAO inhibitors, pentamidine, salicylates, sulfinpyrazone, TCN, fenfluramine, guanethidine

Other Notable Comments

keep injection site aseptic

alcohol and tobacco affect insulin dosing

respond to symptoms of low blood sugar, which include: cold sweats, confusion, difficulty in concentration, drowsiness, excessive hunger, headache, nausea, nervousness, rapid pulse, shakes, and visual disturbances

PHARMACOLOGIC TREATMENT 39

generic: ketorolac

brand/trade name: Toradol

over-the-counter (OTC):

Drug Class

NSAID

Indications

short-term management of pain

Action

relief of pain

Dosage Range

adult: maximum 40 mg/d (oral dosage form)

Usual Schedule

adult: q 4–6 h

Common Side Effects

edema, drowsiness, dizziness, headache, GI pain, indigestion, diarrhea, increased sweating

Drug/Food Interactions

diuretics, lithium, methotrexate, salicylates, probenecid

Other Notable Comments

limit use to a maximum of 5 days

PHARMACOLOGIC TREATMENT 40

generic: levothyroxin

brand/trade name: Synthroid, Levothroid

over-the-counter (OTC):

Drug Class

hormone (thyroid)

Indications

underactive thyroid

Action

replaces or supplements insufficient amount of thyroid hormone, thereby enabling the thyroid gland to function appropriately

Dosage Range

children: up to 150 mcg (0.150 mg)/d

adults: up to 200 mcg (0.200 mg)/d

Usual Schedule

children: qd

adults: qd

Common Side Effects

palpitations, heart arrhythmias, tachycardia, chest pain, nervousness, sweating, headache, insomnia, hair loss, changes in menstrual cycle, changes in appetite, changes in bowel movements, tremors, SOB, sensitivity to heat

Drug/Food Interactions

phenytoin, cholestyramine, oral anticoagulants, TCAs

Other Notable Comments

report chest pain, increased pulse, heart palpitations, excessive sweating

stay with the same brand of medicine

noticeable effects may take a few weeks

PHARMACOLOGIC TREATMENT 41

generic: lisinopril

brand/trade name: Zestril, Prinvil

over-the-counter (OTC):

Drug Class

cardiovascular agent (ACE inhibitor)

Indications

hypertension, CHF

Action

produces vasodilation, enabling blood to flow without resistance

Dosage Range

adults: up to 40 mg/d

Usual Schedule

adults: qd

Common Side Effects

dizziness, headache, fatigue, cough, diarrhea

Drug/Food Interactions

NSAIDs, lithium

Other Notable Comments

report vomiting, diarrhea, excessive sweating

report swelling of the face, lips, or tongue

report persistent cough and difficult breathing

PHARMACOLOGIC TREATMENT 42

generic: loratidine

brand/trade name: Claritin

over-the-counter (OTC):

Drug Class

antihistamine

Indications

symptoms of seasonal allergy

Action

relieves the "runny" nose and other symptoms of seasonal allergy

Dosage Range

adults: 10 mg/d

Usual Schedule

adults: qd

Common Side Effects

headache, somnolence (sleepiness), fatigue, dry mouth

Drug/Food Interactions

caution with triazole antifungals (e.g., ketoconazole), cimetidine, ranitidine, theophylline, macrolide antibiotics (e.g., erythromycin)

Other Notable Comments

TAKE ON AN EMPTY STOMACH

drink fluids liberally

can impair coordination

PHARMACOLOGIC TREATMENT 43

generic: lovastatin

brand/trade name: Mevacor

over-the-counter (OTC):

Drug Class

antihyperlipidemic agent

Indications

hypercholesterolemia

Action

decreases elevated serum cholesterol levels

Dosage Range

adults: maximum 80 mg/d

Usual Schedule

adults: qd

Common Side Effects

headache, flatus (intestinal gas), abdominal cramps, rash, changes in bowel movements, indigestion, heartburn, dizziness, muscle pain

Drug/Food Interactions

levothyroxine, gemfibrozil, clofibrate, niacin, erythromycin, cyclosporine, oral anticoagulants

Other Notable Comments

use in conjunction with dietary therapy

PHARMACOLOGIC TREATMENT 44

generic: medroxyprogesterone acetate

brand/trade name: Provera, Depo-Provera (injection)

over-the-counter (OTC):

Drug Class

hormones

Indications

endometrial carcinoma, renal carcinoma, uterine bleeding caused by hormone imbalance

Action

palliative treatment that lessens the intensity of the symptoms caused by the carcinoma

hormone replacement to treat uterine bleeding

Dosage Range

consult prescribing information for dosing and scheduling for specific condition and route of administration

Usual Schedule

consult prescribing information for dosing and scheduling for specific condition and route of administration

Common Side Effects

bleeding, spotting, changes in menstrual flow, amenorrhea, loss of appetite, edema, weakness

Drug/Food Interactions

aminoglutethimide

Other Notable Comments

take exactly as directed

report visual problems or migraine headaches

may cause photosensitivity

PHARMACOLOGIC TREATMENT 45

generic: methotrexate

brand/trade name: Folex, Rheumatrex

over-the-counter (OTC):

Drug Class

antirheumatic agent, antipsoriatic agent, antineoplastic agent

Indications

carcinomas, leukemias, psoriasis, RA

Action

inhibits reproduction of cancer cells

may affect immune system, thereby intervening with RA immunopathway and symptomatically controlling the symptoms of psoriasis

Dosage Range

consult prescribing information for the specific condition

Usual Schedule

consult prescribing information for the specific condition

Common Side Effects

observable side effects include ulceration and inflammation of the mouth, throat, tongue, and gums; skin reddening; nausea

Drug/Food Interactions

corticosteroids, phenytoin, 5-FU, NSAIDs, live virus vaccines, cyclosporine, vincristine, salicylates, sulfonamides, probenecid, penicillins (in high doses)

Other Notable Comments

report infections, bruising, bleeding, SOB, burning urination

TAKE ON AN EMPTY STOMACH

AVOID ALCOHOL

PHOTOSENSITIVITY

PHARMACOLOGIC TREATMENT 46

generic: nabumetone

brand/trade name: Relafen

over-the-counter (OTC):

Drug Class

NSAIDs

Indications

management of pain and inflammation associated with osteoarthritis and RA

Action

relieves pain and reduces inflammation

Dosage Range

adults: up to 2 g/d

Usual Schedule

adults: qd or BID

Common Side Effects

heartburn, abdominal cramps, indigestion, nausea, skin rash, dizziness

Drug/Food Interactions

warfarin

Other Notable Comments

report stomach disturbances, visual disturbances, rash, weight gain, edema, blackened stools

AVOID ALCOHOL

AVOID ASPIRIN

PHARMACOLOGIC TREATMENT 47

generic: naproxen

brand/trade name: Naprosyn, Anaprox

over-the-counter (OTC): available

Drug Class

NSAIDs

Indications

RA, acute gout, dysmenorrhea, fever, inflammatory disease

Action

relieves pain and reduces inflammation

reduces elevated body temperature

Dosage Range

children: maximum 10 mg/kg/d (over 2 years old)

adults: 1.5 g/d (limited time)

Usual Schedule

children: two divided doses

adults: two divided doses, q 6–8 h (depending on condition)

Common Side Effects

skin rash, dizziness, abdominal cramps, heartburn, indigestion, nausea

Drug/Food Interactions

furosemide, methotrexate, aspirin, probenecid

Other Notable Comments

TAKE WITH FOOD OR MILK

MAY CAUSE DROWSINESS

PHARMACOLOGIC TREATMENT 48

generic: nifedipine

brand/trade name: Procardia, Adalat

over-the-counter (OTC):

Drug Class

cardiovascular agent (calcium channel blocker)

Indications

angina, hypertension

Action

dilates coronary vessels by relaxing the smooth muscles of the coronary vessels

Dosage Range

children: up to 0.9 mg/kg/24 h

adults: maximum 180 mg/24 h (capsules), 120 mg/d (sustained release form)

Usual Schedule

children: three to four divided doses

adults: once daily, TID, QID (depending on drug form)

Common Side Effects

dizziness, lightheadedness, giddiness, flushing, headache, weakness, nausea, heartburn

Drug/Food Interactions

warfarin, fentanyl, cimetidine phenytoin

Other Notable Comments

DO NOT CHEW, CRUSH, OR BREAK (sustained release form of the drug)

rise slowly from a lying or sitting position

PHARMACOLOGIC TREATMENT 49

generic: nizatidine

brand/trade name: Axid

over-the-counter (OTC): available

Drug Class

GI drug (histamine H_2-blocker)

Indications

duodenal ulcer, GERD

Action

suppresses gastric acid secretion

Dosage Range

adults: up to 300 mg/d

Usual Schedule

adults: qd, BID, hs (depending on treatment and convenience)

Common Side Effects

constipation, diarrhea, dizziness, headache

Drug/Food Interactions

salicylates

Other Notable Comments

avoid aspirin, cough and cold preparations

avoid black pepper, caffeine, alcohol, harsh spices

MAY CAUSE DROWSINESS

PHARMACOLOGIC TREATMENT 50

generic: omeprazole

brand/trade name: Prilosec

over-the-counter (OTC):

Drug Class

GI agent (proton pump inhibitor)

Indications

erosive esophagitis, GERD, PUD

Action

suppresses gastric acid secretions

Dosage Range

adults: maximum 360 mg/d (depending on the condition and if "initial" or "maintenance" dosing)

Usual Schedule

adults: qd, TID (divided doses for doses greater than 80 mg.)

Common Side Effects

headache, changes in bowel movements, nausea, vomiting, abdominal pain, dizziness, rash, cough, back pain, UTI

Drug/Food Interactions

ketaconazole, itraconazole, diazepam, phenytoin, warfarin

Other Notable Comments

TAKE BEFORE EATING

SWALLOW CAPSULE WHOLE

DO NOT CHEW, CRUSH OR BREAK

PHARMACOLOGIC TREATMENT 51

generic: ondansetron

brand/trade name: Zofran

over-the-counter (OTC):

Drug Class

antiemetic

Indications

emesis associated with emetogenic chemotherapeutic agents

Action

blocks the serotonin that affects the chemoreceptor trigger zone for emesis

Dosage Range

consult prescribing information for special dosing requirements

Usual Schedule

consult prescribing information for special dosing requirements

Common Side Effects

constipation, diarrhea, headache, fever

Drug/Food Interactions

barbiturates, carbamazepine, rifampin, phenytoin, phenylbutazone, cimetidine, allopurinol, disulfiram

Other Notable Comments

maximum daily dose of 8 mg. in patients with liver disease

give dose 30 minutes before chemotherapy dosing

PHARMACOLOGIC TREATMENT 52

generic: paclitaxel

brand/trade name: Taxol

over-the-counter (OTC):

Drug Class

antineoplastic agent

Indications

ovarian carcinoma, breast carcinoma

Action

antitumor activity

Dosage Range

consult prescribing information for specific regimen requirements

Usual Schedule

consult prescribing information for specific regimen requirements

Common Side Effects

myalgia, loss of hair, numbness in lower extremities

Drug/Food Interactions

ketaconazole

Other Notable Comments

parenteral administration only

premedicate with dexamethasone, diphenhydramine, and cimetidine or ranitidine

use special IV tubing that does not react with the drug

PHARMACOLOGIC TREATMENT 53

generic: paroxetine

brand/trade name: Paxil

over-the-counter (OTC):

Drug Class

antidepressant

Indications

depression

Action

effects neurotransmission of neurotransmitter by inhibiting serotonin (the neurotransmitter) uptake

Dosage Range

adults: maximum 50mg/d

Usual Schedule

adults: once daily

Common Side Effects

headache, asthenia (loss of strength), nausea, changes in bowel movements, dry mouth, dizziness, changes in sleeping behavior, sweating, ejaculatory disturbance

Drug/Food Interactions

phenobarbital, phenytoin, alcohol, cimetidine, MAO inhibitors, TCAs, fluoxetine, sertraline, phenothiazines, warfarin, IC antiarrhythmics (flecainide, propafenone)

Other Notable Comments

adjust doses at 7-day intervals

AVOID ALCOHOL and beverages containing alcohol

MAY CAUSE DROWSINESS

observable response may take several weeks

PHARMACOLOGIC TREATMENT 54

generic: penicillamine

brand/trade name: Cuprimine, Depen

over-the-counter (OTC):

Drug Class

chelating agent

Indications

heavy metal (lead, mercury, iron) poisoning, RA

Action

binds with heavy metal to make them soluble and excreted in the urine

depresses rheumatoid factor in the immune system, thereby being useful as adjunctive therapy in RA

Dosage Range

consult prescribing information for specific condition

Usual Schedule

consult prescribing information for specific condition

Common Side Effects

fever, joint pain, skin rash, hives, itching, lessened ability to taste

Drug/Food Interactions

iron and zinc salts, antacids (containing calcium or magnesium), digoxin, gold, antimalarials, immunosuppressive agents, phenylbutazone

Other Notable Comments

TAKE AT LEAST 1 HOUR BEFORE MEALS

DRINK FLUIDS LIBERALLY

report bruising, unusual bleeding, persistent fever, sore throat, fatigue, unusual coughing, SOB, or rash

may lose taste sensation

PHARMACOLOGIC TREATMENT 55

generic: penicillin VK

brand/trade name: Veetids, Pen Vee K, V-Cillin K

over-the-counter (OTC):

Drug Class

anti-infective

Indications

bacterial infection

Action

bactericidal

Dosage Range

consult prescribing information for specific determinations made according to the sensitivity and severity of the causative pathogen

children (under 12 years old): up to 50 mg/kg/d (in divided doses)

adults: up to 2/g/d

Usual Schedule

children: q 6–8 h (acute infections), BID (prophylaxis)

adults: q 6–8 h (acute infections), BID (prophylaxis)

Common Side Effects

diarrhea, vomiting, nausea

Drug/Food Interactions

probenecid, oral contraceptives, TCN

Other Notable Comments

complete full course of therapy (minimum 10 days)

report rash, SOB, wheezing, black tongue, bruising, swollen joints

take around the clock

PHARMACOLOGIC TREATMENT 56

generic: phenytoin

brand/trade name: Dilantin

over-the-counter (OTC):

Drug Class

antiseizure agent

Indications

grand mal seizures, ventricular arrhythmias

Action

decreases seizure activity

shortens the action potential in the heart

Dosage Range

consult prescribing information for specific condition and medication regimen

Usual Schedule

consult prescribing information for specific condition and medication regimen

Common Side Effects

psychiatric changes, slurred speech, trembling, constipation, nausea, vomiting, dizziness, drowsiness

Drug/Food Interactions

rifampin, cisplatin, vinblastine, bleomycin, folic acid, cimetidine, chloramphenicol, isoniazid, trimethoprim, sulfonamides, valproic acid, ethosuximide, primidone, warfarin, oral contraceptives, corticosteroids, cyclosporine, theophylline, doxycycline, quinidine, mexiletine, disopyramide

Other Notable Comments

use the same manufacturer brand of drug

MAY CAUSE DROWSINESS

TAKE WITH FOOD

PHARMACOLOGIC TREATMENT 57

generic: potassium chloride

brand/trade name: Kay Ciel, Kaochlor, K-Tab, K-Lyte/CL

over-the-counter (OTC):

Drug Class

electrolyte

Indications

hypokalemia (low blood potassium)

Action

potassium replacement elevates blood potassium level

Dosage Range

consult prescribing information for dosing requirements and routes of administration

Usual Schedule

consult prescribing information for dosing requirements and routes of administration

Common Side Effects

diarrhea, nausea, vomiting, stomach pain, flatulance (excessive amount of gas in the stomach and intestine causes distention)

Drug/Food Interactions

potassium-sparing diuretics, salt substitutes, ACE inhibitors

Other Notable Comments

SWALLOW TABLETS WHOLE

DILUTE BEFORE USING oral liquid potassium supplements with water or fruit juice

PHARMACOLOGIC TREATMENT 58

generic: pravastatin

brand/trade name: Pravachol

over-the-counter (OTC):

Drug Class

antihyperlipidemic agent

Indications

hypercholesterolemia

Action

decreases elevated serum cholesterol levels

Dosage Range

adult: up to 40 mg/d

Usual Schedule

adults: qdhs

Common Side Effects

headache, flatus (intestinal gas), abdominal cramps, rash, changes in bowel movements, indigestion, heartburn, dizziness, muscle pain

Drug/Food Interactions

gemfibrozil, clofibrate, oral anticoagulants, cholestyramine

Other Notable Comments

use in conjunction with dietary therapy

report muscle pain, weakness, malaise, fever

PHARMACOLOGIC TREATMENT 59

generic: prazosin

brand/trade name: Minipress

over-the-counter (OTC):

Drug Class

cardiovascular (alpha adrenergic blocker)

Indications

hypertension, severe CHF

Action

vasodilation of veins and arterioles resulting in decreased peripheral resistance to blood flow

Dosage Range

children: maximum 0.025 mg/kg/dose

adults: maximum 20 mg/d

Usual Schedule

children: q 6 h

adults: two to four times/d in divided doses

Common Side Effects

orthostatic hypotension, dizziness, lightheadedness, drowsiness, headache, malaise

Drug/Food Interactions

NSAIDs, diuretics, beta-blockers

Other Notable Comments

rise slowly from a sitting or lying position

report persistent, painful erection

PHARMACOLOGIC TREATMENT 60

generic: propoxyphene napsylate/acetaminophen

brand/trade name: Darvocet-N

over-the-counter (OTC):

Drug Class

analgesic

Indications

mild to moderate pain

Action

relieves pain

Dosage Range

adults: maximum up to 600 mg/d

Usual Schedule

adults: q 4 h

Common Side Effects

weakness, fatigue, nausea, vomiting, drowsiness, dizziness, constipation

Drug/Food Interactions

CNS depressants, carbamazepine, phenobarbital, TCAs, warfarin, MAO inhibitors, rifampin, hydantoins, sulfinpyrazone

Other Notable Comments

Schedule C-IV

cigarette smoking decreases the effect of the drug

MAY CAUSE DROWSINESS

AVOID ALCOHOL and sedatives

report visual disturbances

PHARMACOLOGIC TREATMENT 61

generic: ranitidine

brand/trade name: Zantac

over-the-counter (OTC): available

Drug Class

GI agent (histamine H_2-blocker)

Indications

PUD, GERD

Action

reduces gastric acid secretion

Dosage Range

children: up to 2.5 mg/kg/dose

adults: up to 6 g/d

Usual Schedule

children: q 12 h

adults: BID or hs

Common Side Effects

skin rash, nausea, vomiting, headache, drowsiness, dizziness, changes in bowel movements

Drug/Food Interactions

itraconazole, ketaconazole, cynaocobalamin, diazepam, cyclosporine, gentamicin, glyburide, glipizide, midazolam, metoprolol, pentoxifylline, phenytoin, quinidine, atropine

Other Notable Comments

MAY CAUSE DROWSINESS

a 6 P.M. dose may be more beneficial than a bedtime dose because a chronobiologic elevated acid secretion begins around 7 P.M.

PHARMACOLOGIC TREATMENT 62

generic: sertraline

brand/trade name: Zoloft

over-the-counter (OTC):

Drug Class

antidepressant

Indications

major depression

Action

affects neurotransmission of neurotransmitter by inhibiting serotonin (the neurotransmitter) uptake

Dosage Range

adults: maximum 200 mg/d

Usual Schedule

adults: qd

Common Side Effects

nausea, vomiting, diarrhea, dry mouth, CNS stimulation, male sexual dysfunction

Drug/Food Interactions

warfarin, MAO inhibitors, CNS drugs, diazepam, tolbutamide

Other Notable Comments

dose changes may be made at 1-week intervals

AVOID ALCOHOL and alcoholic beverages

MAY CAUSE DROWSINESS

observable response may take several weeks

PHARMACOLOGIC TREATMENT 63

generic: simvastatin

brand/trade name: Zocor

over-the-counter (OTC):

Drug Class

antihyperlipidemic agent

Indications

hypercholesterolemia

Action

decreases elevated serum cholesterol levels

Dosage Range

adults: up to 40 mg

Usual Schedule

adults: once daily

Common Side Effects

headache, flatus (intestinal gas), abdominal cramps, rash, changes in bowel movements, indigestion, heartburn, dizziness, muscle pain

Drug/Food Interactions

gemfibrozil, cyclosporine, oral anticoagulants

Other Notable Comments

use in conjunction with dietary therapy

report muscle pain, malaise, weakness, fever

PHARMACOLOGIC TREATMENT 64

generic: cetirizine

brand/trade name: Zyrtec

over-the-counter (OTC):

Drug Class

antihistamine

Indications

symptoms of seasonal allergy

Action

relieves the "runny" nose and other symptoms of seasonal allergy

Dosage Range

children: up to 10 mg

adults: up to 10 mg

Usual Schedule

children: once daily

adults: once daily

Common Side Effects

headache, fatigue, increased appetite, nervousness, dizziness, nausea, diarrhea, abdominal pain, dry mouth, joint pain

Drug/Food Interactions

CNS depressants, theophylline, alcohol

Other Notable Comments

do not use if sensitive to hydoxyzine

MAY CAUSE DROWSINESS

not recommended for women who are breastfeeding

PHARMACOLOGIC TREATMENT 65

generic: triamterene/hydrochlorothiazide

brand/trade name: Dyazide, Maxzide

over-the-counter (OTC):

Drug Class

diuretic

Indications

mild to moderate hypertension, edema in CHF

Action

body water elimination

Dosage Range

adults: up to four capsules or tablets/d

Usual Schedule

adults: BID

Common Side Effects

loss of appetite, nausea, vomiting, stomach cramps

Drug/Food Interactions

oral hypoglycemic drugs, cholestyramine, colestipol, loop diuretics (e.g., furosemide), lithium, amiloride, spironolactone, ACE inhibitors

Other Notable Comments

TAKE AFTER MEALS

take early during day to avoid nocturia

possible PHOTOSENSITIVITY

report headache, weakness, persistent nausea

PHARMACOLOGIC TREATMENT 66

generic: verapamil

brand/trade name: Calan, Isoptin, Verelan

over-the-counter (OTC):

Drug Class

cardiovascular (calcium channel blocker)

Indications

angina, hypertension

Action

dilates coronary vessels by relaxing the smooth muscles of the coronary vessels

Dosage Range

children: not well established

adults: up to 480 mg/d (depending on condition)

Usual Schedule

adults: three to four divided doses, qd, TID (depending on the condition being treated)

Common Side Effects

skin rash, peripheral edema, dizziness, lightheadedness, nausea, tiredness, weakness, constipation

Drug/Food Interactions

phenobarbital, phenytoin, sulfinpyrazone, rifampin, digoxin, quinidine, carbamazapine, cyclosporine, cimetidine, ranitidine

Other Notable Comments

TAKE WITH FOOD (sustained-release products)

DO NOT CRUSH (sustained-release products)

limit caffeine intake

report SOB

PHARMACOLOGIC TREATMENT 67

generic: warfarin

brand/trade name: Coumadin

over-the-counter (OTC):

Drug Class

cardiovascular (anticoagulant)

Indications

thromboembolic disorders (blood clots)

Action

thins blood

Dosage Range

children: up to 0.34 mg/kg/d

adults: usual maintenance is up to 10 mg/d

Usual Schedule

children: qd

adults: qd

Drug/Food Interactions

barbiturates, carbamazepine, cholestyramine, glutethimide, griseofulvin, phenytoin, rifampin, sucralfate, anabolic steroids, chloral hydrate, allopurinol, chloramphenicol, cimetidine, ciprofloxacin, clofibrate, alcohol, danazol, disulfiram, erythromycin, fluconazole, gemfibrozil, thyroid, ketaconazole, metronidazole, NSAIDs, miconazole, quinidine, cotrimoxazole, sulfonamides

Common Side Effects

Other Notable Comments

DO NOT TAKE WITH FOOD

report bleeding or black stools

possible CHANGE IN URINE COLOR

ADDITIONAL DRUG MONOGRAPHS

DRUG atenolol (Tenormin)

Drug Class

cardiovascular (beta-adrenergic blocker)

Indications

hypertenion, angina pectoris

Action

decreases cardiac output, peripheral vascular resistance, and oxygen consumption

Dosage Range

maximum oral dose: 100 mg (hypertension), 200 mg (angina pectoris)

Usual Schedule

single daily dose

Common Side Effects

fatigue, dizziness, bronchospasm (life-threatening)

Drug/Food Interactions

antihypertensives, cardiac glycosides, cardizem, verapamil, insulin, oral antidiabetic agents, reserpine

Other Notable Comments

dosage adjustments in hemodialysis patients

DRUG acyclovir (Zovirax)

Drug Class

anti-infective

Indications

antiviral (herpes simplex, varicella zoster)

Action

inhibits viral DNA synthesis

Dosage Range

maximum oral daily dose: 1,200 mg. (genital herpes)
1,000 mg. (recurrent genital herpes)
3,200 mg. (varicella infection in immunocompetent patients)
4,800 mg. (acute herpes zoster infection in immunocompetent patients)

Usual Schedule

every 4 hours while awake or every 8 hours for 7–10 days (initial genital herpes)

every 4 hours while awake for 5 days (recurrent genital herpes)

BID up to 12 months (chronic recurrent genital herpes)

QID for 5 days (varicella infection in immunocompetent patients)

every 4 hours five times daily for 7–10 days (acute herpes zoster infection in immunocompetent patients)

Common Side Effects

malaise, headache, lethargy, tremor, confusion, hallucinations, agitation, seizures (life-threatening), nausea, vomiting

Drug/Food Interactions

interferon, probenecid, zidovudine

Other Notable Comments

adjust dose in renal-compromised patients

DRUG amitriptyline (Elavil)

Drug Class

CNS (tricyclic antidepressant [TCA])

Indications

depression

Action

tricyclic compound that blocks reuptake of norepinephrine, serotonin

Dosage Range

maximum oral dose: 300 mg

Usual Schedule

daily (at bedtime)

Common Side Effects

coma (life-threatening), seizures (life-threatening), orthostatic hypotension, tachycardia, dry mouth

Drug/Food Interactions

barbiturates, CNS depressants, cimetidine, fluoxetine, fluvoxamine, oral contraceptives, paroxetine, sertraline, clonidine, epinephrine, norepinephrine, MAO inhibitors, alcohol

Other Notable Comments

smoking may affect drug concentration

increased risk of photosensitivity

cautioned-use in glaucoma patients

parenteral form of drug for intramuscular use ONLY (i.e., not intravenous)

strong anticholinergic effects

very sedating

drug withdrawn gradually

DRUG carisoprodol (Soma)

Drug Class

muscle relaxant

Indications

muscle pain

Action

CNS (modifies perception of pain)

Dosage Range

up to 1,400 mg orally

Usual Schedule

350 mg TID and hs

Common Side Effects

drowsiness, dizziness, orthostatic hypotension, skin reaction

Drug/Food Interactions

CNS depressants, alcohol

Other Notable Comments

avoid activities that require alertness

avoid sudden changes in posture

take with food or milk if GI upset occurs

DRUG cefadroxil (Duricef)

Drug Class
anti-infective

Indications
infections caused by susceptible organisms

Action
bactericidal

Dosage Range
maximum daily oral adult dosage: 2 Gm.

Usual Schedule
once daily or BID

Common Side Effects
seizures (life-threatening), diarrhea, skin rash, anaphylaxis (life-threatening)

Drug/Food Interactions
probenecid

Other Notable Comments
potential cross allergenicity to penicillin

dosage adjustments in patients with impaired renal function

take with food or milk to lessen GI discomfort

take entire amount of drug prescribed for the drug regimen

DRUG clindamycin (Cleocin)

Drug Class
anti-infective

Indications
infections caused by susceptible organisms

Action
bactericidal

Dosage Range
maximum oral daily dose: 1,800 mg (1.8 Gm.)

Usual Schedule

orally, every 6 hours

Common Side Effects

nausea, anaphylaxis (life-threatening)

Drug/Food Interactions

erythromycin, kaolin, neuromuscular blocking agents, diet foods containing sodium cyclamate

Other Notable Comments

take with a full glass of water

do not treat diarrhea with opioid antidiarrheals

DRUG clonidine (Catapres-TTS [patches], Catapres [oral])

Drug Class

cardiovascular (alpha adrenergic-receptor)

Indications

essential hypertension, renal hypertension

Action

decreased peripheral vascular resistance, decreased systolic and diastolic blood pressure, decreased heart rate

Dosage Range

maximum daily oral adult dosage: 0.6 mg

Usual Schedule

daily in divided doses

Common Side Effects

drowsiness, dizziness, sedation, weakness, rebound hypertension (life-threatening), constipation, dry mouth, pruritus, skin responses (resulting from patches)

Drug/Food Interactions

CNS depressants, diuretics, antihypertensive agents, levodopa, MAO inhibitors, prazosin, tricyclic antidepressants, propranolol (and other beta-blockers), verapamil, capsicum (herb)

Other Notable Comments

do not discontinue prior to surgery

do not discontinue drug abruptly

take last dose of day immediately before going to sleep

DRUG clorazepate (Traxene)

Drug Class
CNS (benzodiazepine)

Indications
anxiety, seizure disorders, acute alcohol withdrawal

Action
anxiolytic

Dosage Range
maximum oral dose: 90 mg (acute alcohol withdrawal)
60 mg (anxiety)
90 mg (seizure disorder)

Usual Schedule
reducing dosage schedule (acute alcohol withdrawal)

daily (anxiety)

TID (seizure disorder)

Common Side Effects
drowsiness

Drug/Food Interactions
cimetidine, CNS depressants, digoxin, alcohol

Other Notable Comments
smoking decreases effectiveness of drug

avoid drug use during prenancy

controlled substance schedule IV

avoid activities that require alertness

DRUG cyclobenzaprine (Flexeril)

Drug Class
muscle relaxant

Indications
muscle spasm

Action
relieves skeletal muscle spasm at point of origin

Dosage Range

maximum oral daily dose: 60 mg

Usual Schedule

TID (maximum duration of treatment is 3 weeks)

Common Side Effects

drowsiness, dizziness, seizures (life-threatening), dry mouth

Drug/Food Interactions

anticholinergics, CNS depressants, MAO inhibitors, alcohol

Other Notable Comments

avoid activities that require alertness

DRUG diazepam (Valium)

Drug Class

CNS (benzodiazepine)

Indications

anxiety, alcohol withdrawal, muscle spasm, preoperative sedation, cardioversion, adjunct in seizure disorders

Action

potentiates the effects of GABA (an inhibitory neurotransmitter)

Dosage Range

maximum oral adult daily dose: 40 mg

Usual Schedule

BID, TID, QID depending on the indication

Common Side Effects

drowsiness, bradycardia (life-threatening), respiratory depression (life-threatening)

Drug/Food Interactions

cimetidine, CNS depressants, digoxin, phenobarbital, alcohol

Other Notable Comments

avoid during pregnancy

caution in patients with open-angle glaucoma

controlled substance Schedule IV drug

avoid activities requiring alertness

smoking may decrease effectiveness of drug

do not stop drug abruptly

DRUG doxycycline (Vibramycin)

Drug Class

anti-infective

Indications

infections caused by susceptible organisms

Action

bacteriostatic

Dosage Range

maximum oral dose: 300 mg

Usual Schedule

daily in one or two divided doses (7 days for gonorrhea, 10 days epididymitis, 10 days for primary or secondary syphilis, 14 days for pelvic inflammatory disease)

Common Side Effects

epigastric distress, nausea, diarrhea, skin events, photosensitivity, urticaria

Drug/Food Interactions

antacids and laxatives containing aluminum, calcium, or magnesium, carbamazepine, phenobarbital, ferrous sulfate (products containing ferrous sulfate), zinc products, methoxyflurane, oral anticoagulants, oral contraceptives, penicillins, alcohol

Other Notable Comments

photosensitivity reactions

discoloration of tooth enamel (children under age 9)

DRUG etodolac (Lodine)

Drug Class

NSAID

Indications

osteoarthritis, rheumatoid arthritis, pain

Action

inhibition of prostaglandins

Dosage Range

maximum adult oral daily dose: 1200 mg

Usual Schedule

every 6 to 8 hours as needed

Common Side Effects

heart failure (life-threatening), dyspepsia, GI bleeding (life-threatening)

Drug/Food Interactions

antacids, aspirin, beta blockers, diuretics, cyclosporine, digoxin, lithium, methotrexate, phenytoin, warfarin, alcohol

Other Notable Comments

avoid sun exposure

fewer GI problems than with other NSAIDs

avoid use during last trimester of pregnancy

DRUG gemfibrozil (Lopid)

Drug Class

cardiovascular

Indications

antihyperlipidemic

Action

lower serum triglyceride levels, increase HDL cholesterol level

Dosage Range

maximum oral dose: 1,200 mg

Usual Schedule

daily in two divided doses 30 minutes before morning and evening meals

Common Side Effects

abdominal and epigastric pain, dyspepsia

Drug/Food Interactions

lovastatin, simvastatin, oral anticoagulants

Other Notable Comments

nondrug management includes weight control, exercise, and smoking cessation

DRUG hydrochlorothiazide (Esidrix, Hydrodiuril)

Drug Class

cardiovascular (fluid and electrolyte balance)

Indications

edema, hypertension

Action

increases water excretion

Dosage Range

maximum oral dose: 100 mg, but 200 mg (limited)

Usual Schedule

daily (for edema)

daily or BID (for hypertension)

Common Side Effects

dizziness, vertigo, headache, weakness, orthostatic hypotension, polyuria, urinary frequency

Drug/Food Interactions

amphotericin B, corticosteroids, antidiabetic agents, antihypertensive agents, barbiturates, opiates, cardiac glycosides, cholestryramine, colestipol, diazoxide, lithium, NSAIDs, alcohol

Other Notable Comments

take with food to minimize gastrointestinal upset

take last dose of drug well before bedtime to avoid nocturia

potential for photosensitivity reactions

DRUG ipratroprium (Atrovent)

Drug Class

respiratory tract

Indications

bronchodilator

Action

antagonize acetylcholine at receptors on bronchial smooth muscle

Dosage Range

no more than 12 inhalations in 24 hours

Usual Schedule

QID

Common Side Effects

bronchitis, upper respiratory tract infections, bronchospasm (life-threatening)

Drug/Food Interactions

anticholinergics

Other Notable Comments

not for acute episodes of bronchospasm

wait more than 2 minutes between sprays

use at least 5 minutes before using a steroid inhaler

DRUG isosorbide dinitrate (Isordil)

Drug Class

cardiovascular

Indications

acute anginal attacks

Action

reduces cardiac oxygen demand

Dosage Range

maximum oral dose: 120 mg daily (for prophylaxis)

Usual Schedule

TID or QID (oral tablet for prophylaxis)

every 5 to 10 minutes (three doses for each 30 minute period, sublingual tablet relief of anginal pain)

Common Side Effects

headache, dizziness, orthostatic hypotension, tachycardia, palpitations, ankle edema, flushing

Drug/Food Interactions

antihypertensives, alcohol

Other Notable Comments

discontinue over a 1- to 2-week period

DRUG lorazepam (Ativan)

Drug Class

anxiolytic

Indications

anxiety, insomnia

Action

CNS

Dosage Range

maximum dose: 10 mg per day orally, 4 mg parenterally

Usual Schedule

daily divided doses

Common Side Effects

drowsiness, sedation

Drug/Food Interactions

CNS depressants, alcohol, digoxin

Other Notable Comments

contraindicated in patients with acute angle-closure glaucoma

DRUG methyphenidate (Ritalin)

Drug Class

CNS

Indications

attention deficit disorder with hyperactivity (children), narcolepsy (adults)

Action

CNS calming effect in children
CNS stimulation effect in adults

Dosage Range

maximum oral dose: 60 mg (children)
30 mg (adults)

Usual Schedule

once daily (children)

BID or TID (adults)

Common Side Effects

nervousness, insomnia, seizures (could be life threatening), palpitations, tachycardia, skin changes

Drug/Food Interactions

centrally acting hypertensive drugs, MAO inhibitors, tricyclic antidepressants, caffeinated beverages

Other Notable Comments

controlled substance (Schedule II)

DRUG methylprednisolone (Medrol [oral], Solu-Medrol [injectable])

Drug Class

hormone (corticosteroid)

Indications

inflammation, immunosuppression

Action

decreases inflammation, immunosuppression

Dosage Range

maximum oral dose: 48 mg

Usual Schedule

daily or in divided doses

Common Side Effects

euphoria, insomnia, seizures (life threatening), arrhythmias (life threatening), peptic ulcers

Drug/Food Interactions

aspirin, NSAIDs, indomethacin, barbiturates, rifampin, phenytoin, oral anticoagulants, potassium-depleting drugs, salicylates, skin test antigens, toxoids, vaccines

Other Notable Comments

avoid use in patients with systemic fungal infections

alternate-day therapy is acceptable

best results from once daily morning dosing

drug may mask infections

monitor blood glucose levels closely in diabetic patients

do not discontinue drug abruptly

take with food or milk

DRUG metoprolol (Lopressor [tartrate salt], Toprol XL [succinate salt])

Drug Class

cardiovascular (beta blocker)

Indications

hypertension, angina pectoris

Action

decreases myocardial contractility, heart rate, cardiac output, oxygen consumption

Dosage Range

maximum oral dose: 400 mg per day

Usual Schedule

once daily or in 2 or 3 divided doses (hypertension)

once daily or in 2 equally divided doses (angina pectoris)

Common Side Effects

fatigue, dizziness, hypotension, bronchospasm (life threatening)

Drug/Food Interactions

barbiturates, rifampin, cardiac glycosides, cardizem, verapamil, reserpine, H_2 antagonists, MAO inhibitors, chlorpromazine, cimetidine, indomethacin, insulin, oral antidiabetic agents, propafenone, terbutaline, any foods may enhance absorption

Other Notable Comments

gradually withdraw drug over a 1- to 2-week period

DRUG minocycline (Minocin)

Drug Class

anti-infective

Indications

infections caused by susceptible organisms

Action

bacteristatic action

Dosage Range

maximum oral dose: 200 mg per day

Usual Schedule

orally

- initially 200 mg, then 100 mg every 12 hours for at least 4 days (gonorrhea in penicillin-resistent patients)
- initially 200 mg, then 100 mg every 12 hours for 10 to 15 days (syphillis in penicillin-resistent patients)

100 mg every 12 hours for 5 days (meningococcal state)

100 mg BID for at least 7 days (uncomplicated infection caused by Chlamydia tranchomatis or Ureaplasma urealyticum)

100 mg BID for 5 days (uncomplicated gonococcal urethritis)

Common Side Effects

anorexia, nausea, diarrhea, skin changes, photosensitivity, urticaria, permanent teeth discoloration

Drug/Food Interactions

antacids and laxatives containing aluminum, calcium, or magnesium, antidiarrheals, iron products, zinc products, oral anticoagulants, oral contraceptives, penicillins

Other Notable Comments

avoid exposure to sun

DRUG nitroglycerin (Nitrostat, Nitro-Bid, Nitro-Dur)

Drug Class

cardiovascular (nitrate, inotropic)

Indications

anginal attacks (angina pectoris), heart failure associated with myocardial infarction

Action

reduces cardiac oxygen demand, increases blood flow through coronary vessels

Dosage Range

depends on titration and form of drug

Usual Schedule

sustained release is every 8 to 12 hours titrated to BID to QID, ointment or transdermal disc is daily, sublingual is every 5 minutes as needed for 15 minutes, intravenously is every 3 to 5 minutes until response

Common Side Effects

headache, dizziness, orthostatic hypotension, tachycardia, flushing, palpitations

Drug/Food Interactions

antihypertensives, heparin (IV)

Other Notable Comments

avoid alcohol

do not use drug in patients with severe anemia, angle-closure glaucoma, orthostatic hypotension, allergy to adhesives (transdermal form)

avoid abrupt discontinuation of drug

take oral tablets on an empty stomach

do not inhale spray (aerosol form)

do not chew sublingual form

store drug in tightly closed container in cool, dark place

store sublingual form in original container

DRUG nortriptyline (Aventyl, Pamelor)

Drug Class

CNS (tricyclic antidepressant [TCA])

Indications

depression

Action

blocks reuptake of norepinephrine and serotinin thereby making them more available

Dosage Range

maximum oral dose: 150 mg

Usual Schedule

TID, QID, or at bedtime

Common Side Effects

drowsiness, dizziness, seizures (life threatening), tachycardia, blurred vision, constipation, urinary retention

Drug/Food Interactions

barbiturates, CNS depressants, cimetidine, fluoxetine, sertraline, clonidine, epinephrine, norepinephrine, MAO inhibitors, alcohol

Other Notable Comments

smoking may lower drug concentration

avoid exposure to sunlight

avoid activities that require alertness

do not stop drug abruptly

DRUG pentoxifylline (Trental)

Drug Class
cardiovascular

Indications
intermitten claudication due to occlusive vascular disease

Action
improves capillary blood flow

Dosage Range
maximum oral dose: 1,200 mg

Usual Schedule
TID (BID if there are central nervous system or gastrointestinal adverse effects)

Common Side Effects
headache, nausea

Drug/Food Interactions
anticoagulants, antihypertensives, theophylline

Other Notable Comments
avoid smoking

take with meals

do not break or crush drug

DRUG prednisone (Deltasone)

Drug Class
hormone (corticosteroid)

Indications
inflammation, immunosuppression

Action
anti-inflammatory, immunosuppressant

Dosage Range
maximum oral dose: individualized up to 200 mg

Usual Schedule
daily in a single dose or two to four divided doses

Common Side Effects

euphoria, insomnia, seizures (life threatening), heart failure (life threatening), peptic ulcers

Drug/Food Interactions

aspirin, indomethacin, NSAIDs, barbiturates, phenytoin, rifampin, oral anticoagulants, potassium-depleting drugs, salicylates, toxoids, vaccines

Other Notable Comments

adverse reactions are dose or duration dependent

abrupt withdrawal can be fatal

contraindicated in patients with systemic fungal infections

take drug with food or milk

early signs of adrenal insufficiency are fatigue, muscular weakness, joint pain, fever, anorexia, nausea, dyspnea, dizziness, fainting

long-term therapy subjects patient to potential for weight gain, swelling, infections

DRUG propranolol (Inderal)

Drug Class

cardiovascular

Indications

angina pectoris, arrythmias, tachyarrythmias, hypertension, migraine or vascular headache

Action

reduces cardiac oxygen demand, prevents cerebral vasodilation

Dosage Range

maximum oral daily doses:
320 mg (angina pectoris)
120 mg (arrhythmia and tachyarrhythmia)
480 mg (hypertension)
240 mg (migraine and vascular headache)

Usual Schedule

BID, TID, or QID (angina pectoris)

TID or QID (maintenance for arrythmia and tachyarrhythmia)

daily in two to four divided doses (hypertension)

TID or QID (maintenance dose for migraine or vascular headache)

Common Side Effects

fatigue, lethargy, bradycardia, hypotension, heart failure (life threatening), blood disorders (life threatening)

Drug/Food Interactions

aminophylline, cardiac glycosides, ditiazem, verapamil, cimetidine, epinephrine, glucagon, isoproterenol, haloperidol, insulin, oral antidiabetic drugs, phenothiazines, reserpine, betel palm (herbal product)

Other Notable Comments

take with food

discontinuation of drug should be gradual

DRUG tamoxifen (Nolvadex)

Drug Class

antineoplastic

Indications

advanced breast cancer

Action

estrogen antagonist

Dosage Range

maximum oral dosage: up to 20 mg BID

Usual Schedule

BID

Common Side Effects

nausea, vomiting, diarrhea, vaginal discharge, irregular menses, skin changes, hot flashes, weight gain/loss, fluid retension

Drug/Food Interactions

antacids, bromocriptine, warfarin-type anticoagulants

Other Notable Comments

monitor for hypercalcemia

DRUG temazepam (Restoril)

Drug Class

CNS (benzodiazepine)

Indications

insomnia

Action

acts on CNS to produce hypnotic effects

Dosage Range

maximum oral adult dosage: 30 mg

Usual Schedule

at bedtime

Common Side Effects

lethargy, daytime sedation

Drug/Food Interactions

CNS depressants, alcohol

Other Notable Comments

controlled drug under Schedule IV

elderly are especially sensitive to the drug's effects

do not discontinue drug abruptly if take for more than a month

onset of drug effects may take up to 2 1/2 hours

DRUG trazodone (Desyrel)

Drug Class

CNS

Indications

antidepressant

Action

inhibits serotonin uptake in the brain

Dosage Range

maximum oral daily dose: 400 mg

Usual Schedule

daily in divided doses

Common Side Effects

dizziness, drowsiness

Drug/Food Interactions

antihypertensives, clonidine, CNS depressants, digoxin, phenytoin, MAO inhibitors, St. John's Wort (herbal product), alcohol

Other Notable Comments

priapism is potential problem for male patients

avoid activities that require alertness

DRUG trimethoprim/sulfa [co-trimoxazole] (Bactrim, Septra)

Drug Class

anti-infective

Indications

infections caused by susceptible organisms

Action

bactericidal

Dosage Range

maximum oral daily dose: 960 mg (trimethoprim portion)—urinary tract infections

Usual Schedule

every 12 hours (10 to 14 days for urinary tract infections and chronic bronchitis/ upper respiratory infections, 5 days for shigellosis)

BID for 3 to 5 days (traveler's diarrhea)

BID for 3 to 6 days (urinary tract infections in men with prostatitis)

daily or three times a week for 3 to 6 months (prophylaxis for chronic urinary tract infections)

daily (prophylaxis for Pneumocystis carinii pneumonia)

Common Side Effects

nausea, vomiting, diarrhea, seizures (life threatening), generalized skin eruptions

Drug/Food Interactions

cyclosporine, methotrexate, oral anticoagulants, oral antidiabetic agents, oral contraceptives, phenytoin

Other Notable Comments

photosensitivity may occur when exposed to sun

adjust dose in renal-compromised patients

EXERCISES

1. Complete the following chart by entering the appropriate answer under "DRUG CLASS" or "USE."
2. Other than reducing pain, what other characteristics do some analgesics have?

Drug Class	Use
analgesic agents	reduce pain level
antipyretic agents	
	stop diarrhea
	neutralize effects of antihistamines
anti-infective agents	
antineoplastic agents	
antiulcer agents	
cardiovascular agents	
	remove excessive fluid from body tissues
hormones	
	stimulate evacuation of feces
psychotherapeutic agents	
	control hypertension
anti-inflammatory agents	
antigout agents	
muscle relaxants	
	enable breathing passageways to expand, thereby enabling greater airflow
supplements	
anticonvulsant agents	
antiarthritic agents	
ophthalmic agents	
	treat diabetes
	symptomatic relief of nausea and vomiting
	control muscle spasms in the gastrointestinal tract and the urinary system
antiparkinson agents	
	drug compounds used to treat coughing
otic agents	
dermatologic agents	
vaginal agents	
antiobesity agents	

3. Why are physicians concerned about patients with diarrhea?
4. What are the characteristic effects of a histamine response?
5. Many chemotherapeutic agents exert their effectiveness by _________with the cancer cell's life cycle.
6. What is the primary cause of gastric ulcers?
7. Why does the choice of cardiovascular agent used vary?
8. How do inotropic agents work?
9. What do antiarrhythmic agents do?
10. What do antianginal agents do?

11. What do antihypertensive agents do?
12. What is another term for antihypertensive agent?
13. What does a vasodilator do?
14. What do antilipidemic agents do?
15. What is the function of diuretics?
16. What conditions commonly require the use of a diuretic?
17. What is the collective term for male sex hormones?
18. What are the collective terms for female sex hormones?
19. What are the different means laxatives use to evacuate feces?
20. What is peristaltic action?
21. What does the term *anxiolytic* mean?
22. What does the acronym HBP represent?
23. What type of agents are used to lower HBP?
24. What makes up the stepwise approach to controlling HBP?
25. What does the acronym ACE mean?
26. Inflammation is a condition resulting from histamine response. What are the characteristics of inflammation?
27. What type of crystals form in skeletal joints that characterize a metabolic disorder known as gout?
28. What is the primary intended effect of a muscle relaxant?
29. Into which class do most bronchodilators fall?
30. By what mechanism do bronchodilators effect their response?
31. By what mechanism do anticonvulsant drugs effect their response?
32. What is a collective term for all diseases that affect joints, skin, and supporting tissue?
33. What should a pharmacy technician check for prior to dispensing an ophthalmic solution?
34. Are ear suspensions and eye solutions of the same drug interchangeable?
35. What is a miotic ophthalmic preparation?
36. What happens in the diabetic to cause excessive levels of glucose in the blood?
37. What is insulin?
38. What is the difference between nausea and emesis?
39. What is a commonly used acronym for nausea and vomiting?
40. What is the role of anticoagulant drugs?
41. What is the primary indication for iron use?
42. What is a spasm?
43. What is the primary observable symptom that characterizes the condition known as Parkinsonism?

44. How are most coughs controlled?

45. What commonly used narcotic analgesic is also used as an antitussive?

46. What is a cerumenolytic?

47. What is PABA?

48. What is the primary use for PABA?

49. What are anorectic drugs?

50. Review each of the following representative drugs from the drug classes discussed in the text. Complete the charts by filling in the drug use, class, function, or some other identifying feature, and the trade name(s), if appropriate. You may find it necessary to consult additional texts or references for trade names.

Drug Representative	Identifying Feature	Trade Name(s)
nifedipine	calcium channel blocker	Procardia, Adalate
procainamide		
disopyramide		
nitroglycerin		
clonidine		
quinidine		
probucol		
gemfibrozil		
hydrochlorothiazide		
furosemide		
mannitol		
spironolactone		
indapamide		
acetazolamide		
fludrocortisone		
cortisone		
methyltestosterone		
estradiol		
progesterone		
chorionic gonadotropin		
vasopressin		
levothyroxine		
insulin		
carboxymethylcellulose		
docusate		
magnesium citrate		
lactulose		
bisacodyl		
mineral oil		
phenelzine		
doxepin		
trazodone		
promethazine		
chlorpromazine		

TABLE 9.1

ANSWER SHEET

Drug Representative	Identifying Feature	Trade Name(s)

TABLE 9.2

Drug Representative	Identifying Feature	Trade Name(s)
methylphenidate		
phenobarbital		
triazolam		
atenolol		
captopril		
labetolol		
diazoxide		
guanadrel		
prazosin		
pargyline		
reserpine		
diflunisal		
indomethacin		
allopurinol		
colchicine		
probenecid		
diazepam		
loperamide		
oxybutinin		
theophylline		
ephedrine		
terbutaline		
primidone		
clorazepate		
prednisone		
aspirin		
piroxicam		
auranofin		
penicillamine		
azathioprine		
chloroquine		
physostigmine		
pilocarpine		
chlorpropamide		
prochlorperazine		
dimenhydrinate		
belladonna		
propantheline		

TABLE 9.3

ANSWER SHEET

Drug Representative	Identifying Feature	Trade Name(s)

TABLE 9.4

Drug Representative	Identifying Feature	Trade Name(s)
oxybutinin		
benztropin		
levodopa		
dextromethorphan		
carbamide peroxide		
clotrimazole		
metronidazole		
phentermine		
acetaminophen		
codeine		
morphine		
pentazocine		
meperidine		
propoxyphene		
loperamide		
clemastine		
gentamicin		
amikacin		
cephalexin		
cefaclor		
cefamandole		
cefoxitin		
penicillin		
ampicillin		
amoxicillin		
tetracycline		
sulfamethoxazole		
sulfasalazine		
sulfisoxazole		
erythromycin		
clindamycin		
acyclovir		
amantadine		
clotrimazole		
miconazole		
isoniazid		
metronidazol		
methotrexate		

TABLE 9.5

ANSWER SHEET

Drug Representative	Identifying Feature	Trade Name(s)

TABLE 9.6

Drug Representative	Identifying Feature	Trade Name(s)
mercaptopurine		
fluorouracil		
vinblastine		
cyclophosphamide		
bleomycin		
dromostanolone		
leuprolide		
diethylstilbesterol		
megestrol		
asparginase		
propantheline		
cimetidine		
ranitidine		
sucralfate		
digoxin		
dobutamine		
propranolol		

TABLE 9.7

ANSWER SHEET

Drug Representative	Identifying Feature	Trade Name(s)

TABLE 9.8

Additional Assignment

The following pages contain samples of patient profiles. Review each profile. Identify the one drug interaction contained in each profile and discuss the potential unwanted drug effect.

PATIENT NAME: Harraway, Seth
ADDRESS: 456 Elm St.
Parkville
PHONE: 543-5678

AGE: 22
SEX: M
ALLERGIES: none

DOCTOR:
#1 Lucra #2 Tu
#3 #4
#5 #6

	DATE FILLED	Rx No.	DRUG	QUANTITY	DIRECTIONS	Dr. I.D.	No. of REFILLS	DATE REFILLED 1	2	3	4	5	6	PRN
1	2/12/01	127-224	Multiple Vitamins with Iron (Generic) Tablets	100	i q d p̄ breakfast	2								X
2	3/7/01	128-974	Amoxicillin 250mg Caps	30	i TID	2	1	3/18						
3	3/29/01	130-514	TCN 250 mg Caps	40	i QID	1	∅							
4	5.5.01	133-179	Haloprogin Cream	30 Gm	apply between toes AM and HS	2	4							
5	5.5.01	OTC	Benzoyl Peroxide Gel 5%	1 tube	Pkg. instructions	2								

FIGURE 9.1

PATIENT NAME: Jane Doe
ADDRESS: 123 Main St.
Balto.
PHONE: 321-7890

AGE: 43
SEX: F
ALLERGIES: PCN

DOCTOR:
#1 Smith
#2 Hyde
#3 Pardo
#4 Conners
#5
#6

	DATE FILLED	Rx No.	DRUG	QUAN-TITY	DIRECTIONS	Dr. I.D.	No. of RE FILLS	DATE REFILLED 1	2	3	4	5	6	PRN
1	1/17/01	125-614	chloramphenicol otic drops	1X 7.5ml	2-3 gtt Ⓛ ear TID	3	∅							
2	2/15/01	127-574	Warfarin 5mg tablets	30	i tab d	1	2							
3	3/1/01	128-694	clotrimazole vag. cr. 1%	45 G.	i applicator vaginally q hs	4	∅							
4	3/10/01	129-324	Propoxyphene c̄ aspirin	20	i q 4°	2	∅							
5	6/8/01	135-484	HC 1% Cr.	30 Gm.	Apply to rash QID	3								X

FIGURE 9.2

PATIENT NAME: Patent, Constance
ADDRESS: 75 Oak Leaf Lane, Balto.
PHONE: 321-0040

AGE: 67
SEX: F
ALLERGIES: none

DOCTOR:
#1 Hart
#2 Conners
#3 Foster
#4
#5
#6

	DATE FILLED	Rx No.	DRUG	QUANTITY	DIRECTIONS	Dr. I.D.	No. of REFILLS	DATE REFILLED 1	2	3	4	5	6	PRN
1	7/11/01	137-794	Digox 0.25mg tabs	30	i d	1								X
2	7/15/01	OTC	Bisacodyl Suppos	8	per package									
3	7/30/01	OTC	guaifenesin expectorant	120ml	per package									
4	8/9/01	139-754	Kaolin-Pectin Susp.	60 ml	2-4 TBSP p̄ each loose BM	3	Ø							
5	10/22/01	141-869	triazolam 0.25mg tabs	15	ss-i hs prn	2	1							

FIGURE 9.3

PATIENT NAME: Walter Pyle
ADDRESS: 1247 Water Way
Annapolis
PHONE: 771-1357

AGE: 71
SEX: Male
ALLERGIES: nuts, choc., TCN

DOCTOR:
#1 Cardi
#2 Mann
#3
#4
#5
#6

	DATE FILLED	Rx No.	DRUG	QUANTITY	DIRECTIONS	Dr. I.D.	No. of REFILLS	DATE REFILLED 1	2	3	4	5	6	PRN
1	1/17/01	125-614	digoxin 0.25mg tabs	100	i̇ qd	1		4/5	7-12					X
2	1/17/01	125-615	HCTZ 50mg tabs	100	i̇ qd	1		4/5						X
3	3/23/01	130-234	acyclovir 5% oint.	1 tube	Apply to lip lesion as dir	2	∅							
4	5/2/01	132-964	flurazepam 15mg caps	20	i̇ hs prn sleep	2	3	5-25						
5	8/12/01	139-964	Digox. 0.125mg. tablets	30	i̇ daily	1	∅							

FIGURE 9.4

PATIENT NAME: Nui, Irsay
ADDRESS: 6801 Ledem Apt. B
Balto.
PHONE: 321-9753

AGE: 27
SEX: F
ALLERGIES: fish

DOCTOR:
#1 Peale **#2** Cunningham
#3 O'Wheel **#4**
#5 **#6**

	DATE FILLED	Rx No.	DRUG	QUANTITY	DIRECTIONS	Dr. I.D.	No. of REFILLS	DATE REFILLED 1	2	3	4	5	6	PRN
1	9/3/01	141-434	Ortho-Novum (ortho) 435	21	Per pkg instructions	3	6							
2	9/15/01	142-274	betamethasone 0.05% Cream	1x 30Gm	Apply to rash AM and PM	2	2							
3	9/19/01	142-275	DPH 50mg Caps	20	i TID	2	∅							
4	10/12/01	144-029	Propranolol 40mg tabs	60	i BID Migraine	1	∅							
5	11/1/01	145-494	Ampicillin 250mg Caps	40	i QID	2	∅							

FIGURE 9.5

PATIENT NAME: Gaulston, Ursula
AGE: 37
SEX: F
DOCTOR:
#1 Conners
#2 O'Dell
#3 Farmer
#4
#5
#6

ADDRESS: 1111 Eleven Way
Hampden
ALLERGIES: Hayfever

PHONE: 742-1234 (Unlisted)

	DATE FILLED	Rx No.	DRUG	QUANTITY	DIRECTIONS	Dr. I.D.	No. of REFILLS	DATE REFILLED 1	2	3	4	5	6	PRN
1	4/7/01	134-214	propranolol 40mg	120	$\dot{\text{T}}$ QID (BP)	2								X
2	4/30/01	135-824	Sulfacetamide 10% Eye Soln	Small bottle	$\dot{\text{T}}$-$\ddot{\text{TT}}$ gtts q 2-3° during the day	3	∅							
3	5·14·01	143-524	Ortho Novum 1/35-28 (ortho)	1 Pkg.	Pkg. Insert	1	6							
4	6·6·01	145-060	Clotrimazole 1% Soln	1 bottle	Apply to affected area TID	3	∅							
5														

FIGURE 9.6

PATIENT NAME: Childer, Ernest
ADDRESS: 905 Littleway Pl
Severna Park
PHONE: 377-0767

AGE: 11
SEX: M
ALLERGIES: none

DOCTOR:
#1 Kidd #2 Young
#3 Small #4
#5 #6

	DATE FILLED	Rx No.	DRUG	QUANTITY	DIRECTIONS	Dr. I.D.	No. of REFILLS	DATE REFILLED 1	2	3	4	5	6	PRN
1	1/5/01	124-475	phenytoin 50 mg chew. Tabs	100	ii TID	3								X
2	2/9/01	126-870	BACTRIM SUSP (Roche)	480 ml	℥iv q12° x 10d	1	ø							
3	5-6-01	133-169	prochlorperazine 5mg Suppos	6	i or ii q6° pr nausea and vomiting	2	ø							
4	6-4-01	OTC	pseudoephedrine LIQ	1	Pkg. instruct.									
5	6-4-01	OTC	Xylometazoline nose drops	1	pkg. instruct.									

FIGURE 9.7

PATIENT NAME: Maher, Richard W.
ADDRESS: 55 Ageway Circle
Balto.
PHONE: 321-9991

AGE: 65
SEX: M
ALLERGIES: 0

DOCTOR:
#1 Hart **#2** Vassal
#3 Pedo **#4** Sykes
#5 **#6**

	DATE FILLED	Rx No.	DRUG	QUANTITY	DIRECTIONS	Dr. I.D.	No. of REFILLS	DATE REFILLED 1	2	3	4	5	6	PRN
1	10/4/01	143-601	Geriatric Multiple V.t.	100	T QD	2								X
2	11/9/01	146-050	Quinidine SO4 200mg Caps	100	T QID	1								X
3	12/7/01	(replaces OLD Rx #106,210) 148-014	Digoxin 0.25mg. tabs	100	T qd	1								X
4	12/14/01	148-555	phenobarbital 30mg.	30	T TID	4	1							
5														

FIGURE 9.8

PATIENT NAME: Cybill Naughton
ADDRESS: The Towers Apt. E
Balto.
PHONE: 321-2468

AGE: 53
SEX: F
ALLERGIES: none

DOCTOR:
#1 Tufolk #2 Bonner
#3 Hart #4 Sykes
#5 Moody #6 L.E. Waters

	DATE FILLED	Rx No.	DRUG	QUANTITY	DIRECTIONS	Dr. I.D.	No. of REFILLS	DATE REFILLED 1	2	3	4	5	6	PRN
1	4/27/01	132-610	Chlorpropamide 250 mg tabs	30	i daily	5								X
2	5/1/01	132-894	triethanolamine polypeptide	1 bottle	use as dir for earwax removal	2	∅							
3	5/18/01	OTC	dextromethorphan cough med	1 bottle	per pkg instruct									
4	5/20/01	134-225	phenylbutazone 100mg tab	28	i QID c̄ meals or snack X7d	1	∅							
5	6/2/01	OTC	oxymetazoline nasal spray	1	Pkg instruct									

FIGURE 9.9

PATIENT NAME: John Doe
ADDRESS: 123 Main St.
Balto.
PHONE: 321-7890

AGE: 45
SEX: M
ALLERGIES: nkda
sensitive to perfume
and cologne

DOCTOR:
#1 Smith **#2** Hyde
#3 Pardo **#4**
#5 **#6**

	DATE FILLED	Rx No.	DRUG	QUANTITY	DIRECTIONS	Dr. I.D.	No. of REFILLS	DATE REFILLED 1	2	3	4	5	6	PRN
1	2/17/01	129-811	erythomycin 250 mg. tablets	42	Ṫ TID	2	∅							
2	5·8·01	133-381	theophylline 300 mg	60	Ṫ q 12H	1	3							
3	6·1·01	134-994	pseudoephedrine 30 mg.	20	Ṫ prn for stuffy nose - DO NOT exceed 4/d	1	∅							
4	6·4·01	135-201	Cimetidine 300mg. tabs	90	Ṫ in the Am and ṪṪ hs	3	2							
5	6·11·01	135-694	albuteral inhaler	1	ṪṪ puffs as dir	1	2							

FIGURE 9.10

Over-the-Counter Drugs

Nonprescription medications are commonly used by people as another part of their health-care self-involvement for managing their personal wellness status. As a pharmacy technician in the community pharmacy environment, there are numerous opportunities to share information and offer recommendations about nonprescription medications known also as over-the-counter (OTC) drugs. In busy settings where phones are ringing, calls being made to doctors and insurance companies, people waiting for new and refill prescriptions to be filled, and patrons looking for information about their new prescriptions, your value is enhanced as a significant knowledge source for OTC preparations for those individuals looking for an OTC recommendation for such conditions as a cough, runny nose, chapped lips, and itchy eyes.

OTC preparations are labeled with directions for use. The dosing is individually specific for children and adults. The labeling also contains warnings to alert individuals with certain ailments such as hypertension, diabetes, or glaucoma to check with their physician before taking the medication.

As a pharmacy technician who upholds the position as a professional, become knowledgeable about the common ailments for which people are seeking OTC advice. Learn about the nonpharmacologic alternatives as well as the pharmacologic therapies available for common ailments. Learning and listening should be the cornerstone of your position as a pharmacy technician. As a health-care person you will be asked for advice. You have a duty to inquire to be assured that the products you recommend are appropriate for the ailment and the individual.

What follows is a compilation of common ailments and popular OTC products used to treat them. The active ingredient, identified by lower case letters, is followed by a sample of trade-name products that begin in capital letters. The following compilation provides only a sampling of drugs. There are many brandname OTC medications that contain a variety of active ingredients. Refer to a comprehensive nonprescription drug reference for the many choices that are available.

Acne

benzoyl peroxide (Oxy 10 Wash, Fostex 10% Wash, Benoxyl 5)—antiseptic agents

Allergy

chlorpheniramine—antihistamine

clemastine (Tavist)—antihistamine

diphenhydramine—antihistamine

Analgesics

acetaminophen—analgesic

ibuprofen—nonsteroidal anti-inflammatory drug (NSAID)

Calcium Supplements

calcium carbonate (Oscal, Tums)

Canker Sores

benzocaine (Orabase gel, Anbesol)—topical anesthetic

lidocaine (Zilactin-L liquid)—topical anesthetic

carbamide peroxide (Cankaid, Gly-Oxide)—topical antiseptic

Chapped Lips

white petrolatum (Lip Treatment, Chapstick, Blistex)—emollient

Cold

acetaminophen—analgesic, antipyretic

chlorpheniramine—antihistamine

dextromethorphan—cough suppressant

guaifenesin—expectorant

pseudoephedrine—nasal decongestant

Constipation

bisacodyl (Dulcolax)—stimulant laxative

casanthranol—stimulant

cascara sagrada—stimulant laxative

docusate sodium (Colace)—lubricant laxative

magnesium citrate—saline laxative

phenolphthalein—stimulant laxative

psyllium hydrophilic fiber (Metamucil, Konsyl, Modane)—bulk laxative

SAMPLING OF COLD PRODUCTS

Product	Acetaminophen	Chlorpheniramine	Dextromethorphan	Guaifenesin	Pseudoephedrine
Tylenol	X				
Chlor-Trimeton		X			
Benylin			X		
Robitussin				X	
Sudafed					X
Alka-Seltzer Plus Cold Medicine	X	X	X		X
Allerest[1]	X	X			X
Ambenyl-D			X	X	X
Coricidin[2]	X	X			

[1] *There are multiple variations containing different combinations of active ingredients.*
[2] *There are multiple variations containing different combinations of active ingredients.*

Cuts

bacitracin (Baciguent)—topical antibiotic

bacitracin-polymyxin (Polysporin)—topical antibiotic

bacitracin-neomycin-polymyxin (Neosporin)—topical antibiotic

Diarrhea

attapulgite (Donnagel, Kaopectate)

loperamide (Imodium A-D)

Dry Skin

glycerin—humectant

petrolatum—skin softener

urea—skin softener

Eye Irritation

naphazoline (Naphcon-A, Opcon-A, Vaso Clear)—vasoconstrictor

phenylephrine (Isopto-Frin, Prefrin)—vasoconstrictor

oxymetazoline (Ocu Clear, Visine L.R.)—vasoconstrictor

tetrahydrolozine (Collyrium, Murine, Visine)—vasoconstrictor

Flatulence

simethicone (Phazyme, Mylanta Gas)—antiflatulant

Fungus

clotrimazole (Lotrimin, Mycelex)—antifungal

miconazole (Micatin)—antifungal

tolfanate (Tinactin, Ting, Tritin)—antifungal

turbinafine (Lamisil AT)—antifungal

undecylanate (Desenex, Cruex)—antifungal

Headache

acetaminophen (Tylenol)—analgesic

aspirin (Anacin, Ascriptin, Bayer)—analgesic

ibuprofen (Advil, Excedrin IB, Motrin IB, Nuprin)—nonsteroidal anti-inflammatory drug (NSAID)

naproxen sodium (Aleve)—nonsteroidal anti-inflammatory drug (NSAID)

Heartburn

aluminum hydroxide (Mylanta, Maalox)—aluminum salts

calcium carbonate (Alka-Mints, Titralac, Tums)—calcium salts

cimetidine (Tagamet HB)—histamine H_2-receptor antagonist

famotidine (Pepcid AC)—histamine H_2-receptor antagonist

magnesium hydroxide (Mylanta, Phillips' Milk of Magnesia)—magnesium salts

magnesium carbonate (Maalox)—magnesium salts

magnesium oxide (Mag-Ox)—magnesium salts

magnesium trisilicate (Gaviscon)—magnesium salts

nizatidine (Axid AR)—histamine H_2-receptor antagonist

ranitidine (Zantac 75)—histamine H_2-receptor antagonist

sodium bicarbonate (Alka-Seltzer Gold)—systemic antacid

Hemorrhoids

benzocaine (Americaine, Lanacane)—topical anesthetic

dibucaine (Nupercainal)—topical anesthetic

lanolin (Nupercainal, Pazo)—protectant

petrolatum (Nupercainal, Preparation H)—protectant

pramoxine (Anusol)—topical anesthetic

witch hazel (Tucks)—astringent

zinc oxide (Anusol, Nupercainal)—astringent

Insomnia

diphenhydramine (Benadryl, Sleepinal, Sominex, Tylenol PM, Unisom)—antihistamine

doxylamine (Nytol, Unisom)—antihistamine

Lice

permethrin (Nix)—pediculicide

piperonyl butoxide (RID, A-200)—pediculicide

Menstrual Pain

acetaminophen (Pamprin, Premsyn PMS)—analgesic

ibuprofen (Advil, Midol, Motrin IB, Nuprin)—nonsteroidal anti-inflammatory drug (NSAID)

naproxen sodium (Aleve)—nonsteroidal anti-inflammatory drug (NSAID)

pamabron (Pamprin, Premsyn PMS)—diuretic

Motion Sickness

cyclizine (Marezine)—antihistamine

dimenhydrinate (Dramamine)—antihistamine

diphenhydramine (Benadryl)—antihistamine

meclizine (Bonine)—antihistamine

Nasal Congestion

naphazoline (4-Way)—sympathomimetic vasoconstrictor

oxymetazoline (Afrin, Benzedrex, Vicks)—sympathomimetic vasoconstrictor

phenylephrine (Dristan, 4-Way, Neo-Synephrine)—sympathomimetic vasoconstrictor

xylometazoline (Otrivin)—sympathomimetic vasoconstrictor

Sore Throat

benzocaine (Cepastat, Chloraseptic)—topical anesthetic

cetylpyridinum (Cepacol)—antibacterial agent

hexylresorcinols (Sucrets)—antibacterial agent

menthol (Cepacol)—topical anesthetic, antipruritic agent

phenol (Cepastat)—antimicrobial agent

Unit 3

Pharmacy Environments

OBJECTIVES

Upon completion of this unit, the student will be able to distinguish between pharmacy practices in different health-care settings.

GENERAL OVERVIEW

Pharmacy practices are found in many settings. Although most practices are found in community retail settings and hospitals, pharmacies are also found in nursing homes, residential care and boarding homes, mental institutions, home health agencies, correctional institutions, rehabilitation centers, health maintenance organizations, adult day-care settings, surgical care centers, and mail-order facilities. As laws change to accommodate the health needs of people, we will see additional practice settings.

As a pharmacy technician, you possess the skills and talents necessary to competently practice pharmacy in any setting. Your choice of practice depends on a number of factors that this unit outlines in order to assist your selection.

Why did you become a pharmacy technician? You probably recognized the growing need for pharmacy technicians. Health care is a complex field full of challenges. Your accomplishments reap the rewards associated with the proper delivery of high-quality pharmaceutical care. You are an important part of a health-care team, and you exercise your knowledge, skills, and abilities in any pharmacy location.

What practice setting is best for you? The distributive pharmacy process is generally constant regardless of the pharmacy environment. There are differences, which will be discussed, that may present one pharmacy setting over another as more suited to your liking.

What knowledge, skills, and abilities (KSAs) are relevant to the different practice environments? The basic KSAs attributable to competent pharmacy practice include the ability to:

- Read and understand medical terminology and pharmacy jargon (including abbreviations)
- Read and interpret prescriptions and hospital orders
- Select the correct drug, especially under a formulary system
- Accurately perform pharmaceutical calculations
- Dispense medications within the limits of the law
- Identify potential drug problems
- Prepare a final product containing the correct medication, in the appropriate container, with the necessary labeling and auxiliary labeling

A grasp of these basic dispensing KSAs prepares you for any pharmacy environment.

And, finally, what are the tasks associated with each type of pharmacy practice? We have established that the basic distributive drug flow, the tenets supporting proper handling of drugs, and how you process these needs are fairly standard. Some tasks are prominent to retail pharmacy practice and unnecessary in the hospital setting, and vice versa. Some tasks are expanded more in certain pharmacies than in others. For instance, in the community pharmacy we would expect a greater role for the pharmacy technician in patient communication and OTC drug-product merchandising. In hospitals, you would expect to have more tasks involving intravenous admixtures, emergency cart refills, stocking the floor's medicine cabinets, and unit dose repackaging.

RETAIL PHARMACY

The primary distinction between retail pharmacy (also referred to as community, ambulatory, or outpatient pharmacy) and hospital pharmacy (also known as institutional or inpatient pharmacy) is the contact with the patient. In retail pharmacy the customer, who is usually also a patient (i.e., ill) or the patient's caregiver, is the focal point. The patient enters a pharmacy looking for support, reliance, assurance, and competence. This direct contact with the patient does not occur in the inpatient setting.

Responsibility is an integral part of direct patient contact. The pharmacy technician easily becomes a resource to the patient and a product adviser, without interfering with the counseling role of the pharmacist. The technician's services include assistance with OTC pharmaceutical products and nonpharmaceutical products such as medical equipment, answering general questions about illness and drugs, and other miscellaneous patient-oriented tasks.

As patients become more knowledgeable about health and illness, they insist on a more pronounced involvement in their own health care. The self-care movement focuses on preventative medicine and self-treatment options. Many people are committed to use the local pharmacy as a resource for assistance in self-care.

The first line of inquiry and treatment is often about OTC medications. As the knowledgeable intermediary, you are able to participate in nonprescription drug selection. First, you must be aware of the available pharmaceutical and nonpharmaceutical categories of products. These categories include:

Pharmaceutical Products

- Analgesics
- Antipyretics
- Menstrual products
- Cough, cold, and allergy products
- Decongestants
- Sore throat products
- Asthma products (*Note:* Asthma can be a dangerous condition that should be treated by a physician.)
- Sleeping aids
- Antacids
- Antiemetics
- Antidiarrheals
- Laxatives
- Vitamins (multiple or individual vitamins and minerals, such as vitamin A, vitamin E, and iron)
- Appetite suppressants

- Ophthalmic products
- Otic products
- Dental products (including mouth and gums)
- Birth control products
- Hemorrhoidal products
- Topical anti-infectives (including antifungals)
- Acne products
- Skin products
- Burn products
- Seasonal products (e.g., for poison ivy, poison oak, insect stings, etc.)

Nonpharmaceutical Products

- Blood pressure monitors
- Fecal occult blood test kits
- Ovulation test kits
- Pregnancy test kits
- Testing kits for some diseases
- Air purifiers
- Humidifiers
- Insulin supplies
- Blood sugar testing machines
- Denture products
- Sunscreens and blocks

Become familiar with products within each category. Be prepared to answer questions and assist customers with product selection. Read product literature to familiarize yourself with specific products. Consult references such as the *Physicians' Desk Reference for Nonprescription Drugs* and The American Pharmaceutical Association publication, *Handbook of Nonprescription Drugs.*

Nonprescription medications can be harmful to patients taking prescribed medications. If a patient is a routine customer who has his or her prescriptions filled at the pharmacy, check the patient profile for potential interactions between the prescribed drugs and the OTC products being considered. Your surveillance and intervention in these situations is very important.

Patients are interested in information about illnesses. You may be a significant resource by providing general information about usual drug therapy and changes in lifestyle. Review Unit 2, Chapter 8, "Common Disease States and Drug Associations," for specific illness guidelines. Try to generalize some common aspects for illnesses and drugs. For instance, the diet and activity in a person's lifestyle is critical if the person has cardiovascular disease (e.g., angina, hypertension). Explain the importance of a low-sodium, low-fat diet, moderate exercise, and compliance in taking medication. You may provide information on the type of diet that is restrictive for certain drugs. For instance, a diet free from milk, cheese, ice cream, yogurt, and other milk products is in order for a patient taking tetracycline.

Being in direct contact with patients makes the use of both verbal and nonverbal communication skills important. The expertise you develop in communications is needed to explain clearly the instructions to a patient, to demonstrate the use of a medical device, to convince a patient not to take an OTC medication, and to verbalize over the telephone. You are the last link between the customer and the medication.

Some nonpharmaceutical tasks are more prevalent in the community pharmacy than the institutionalized pharmacy setting. These include drug ordering, inventory, and drug merchandising.

Every pharmacy works within a budget. There is a budget for supplies, utilities, insurance, labor, and so forth. Within the overall budget there is usually one for drugs. The profit in a retail pharmacy is influenced by what you spend on drugs. You want the source of your drugs to be reputable, reliable, service-oriented, and approachable. The supplier should provide quality at a fair price. Ordering and inventory may be part of your job description.

The elements of business and management are beyond the scope of this book. However, there are many texts that you can consult for instruction on business practices, formulas, management, and merchandising.

The following sample of pharmacy technician job tasks have been extracted from various job descriptions and conversations with pharmacy managers:

- Accurately interpret and enter prescription information into the computer
- Fill prescriptions; select correct drug from inventory; count the appropriate amount
- Compound drugs under the pharmacist's supervision
- Complete all records and paperwork accurately and in a timely way (i.e., patient profiles and drug/merchandise "short" list)
- Assist customers courteously
- Provide courteous telephone service
- Operate the cash register accurately
- Process third-party payer billings (e.g., insurance companies, unions, government agencies)
- Order and process inventory and supplies; placing orders to appropriate vendors, checking received orders for accuracy, following up on back orders
- Process returns (i.e., outdated and incorrect merchandise)
- Maintain stock levels; bottles and vials, bags and supplies, and drugs (e.g., unit-of-use packaging)
- Prepare accurate prescription labels

HOSPITAL PHARMACY

In contrast to the retail setting, there is no patient contact between the patient and the pharmacy technician in the hospital setting. The inpatient patient is a much sicker individual requiring more services provided by the pharmacy department. The pharmaceutical care delivered includes intravenous administration of drugs, maintenance of emergency care carts, intravenous nutrition, and stocking of floor medicine cabinets.

The technician in the hospital pharmacy has additional tasks that are not applicable in the outpatient pharmacy practice. Drugs that are not available in unit dose packaging are repackaged to unit dose from bulk stock. Customized specific single dose preparations are often ordered by physicians for newborn (neonates) or children (peds). These are made by pharmacy technicians and checked by supervising pharmacists.

We have seen that the distributive pharmacy process is the same for all pharmacy practices. The changes are common in calculations, dosage sizes, and quantities. Most hospitals fill drug requirements for patients on a daily basis. Most drugs are in unit dose or are repackaged to be a single dose. The inventory selection is based on a hospital formulary system that limits the drugs used in that specific hospital to the drugs evaluated by the Pharmacy and Therapeutics (PT) Committee and determined to be safe, effective, and economical.

The following is a compilation of pharmacy technician job tasks in an institutional setting. These job elements were collected from a variety of position descriptions and vary by institution.

- Select and retrieve drug from stock
- Fill patient dose charts
- Prepare, package, and label unit dose tablets and liquids
- Reconstitute drugs as needed
- Prepare intravenous admixtures
- Deliver controlled drug substances to the floors
- Check inventory levels
- Prepare large-volume solutions
- Maintain floor stock medications (replacing outdated medications and drugs used from stock)
- Package and label unit dose injectables
- Perform mathematical calculations for compounding
- Enter orders into the computer
- Prepare IV chemotherapy
- Compound topical preparations
- Inspect and maintain emergency medication carts
- Conduct counts of controlled substances
- Provide drug information as needed and appropriate

Your choice for a practice setting is a decision you make based on what you like. In helping you make your decision, answer these questions:

- Do I like to have direct contact with patients? (community)
- Do I like the challenge of a more clinical pharmacy setting? (institutional)
- Do I like the potential for career ladders? (institutional)
- Do I require more standardized training? (institutional)
- Do I prefer more levels of review to safeguard patient drug therapy? (institutional)
- Do I like business? (community)
- Do I like merchandising? (community)

Visit various facilities. Observe the operations in progress. Speak with pharmacists. Be sure to speak with other pharmacy technicians.

Unit 4

The Pharmacy Technician Coach

INTRODUCTION

The Pharmacy Technician COACH is designed with a very special feature. Every pharmacy order used in the *"COACH"* is real. Each exhibit is excerpted directly from a pharmacy order that was faxed to the pharmacy, pneumatically tubed to the pharmacy, or brought by hand to the pharmacy. These excerpted orders represent the knowledge, background, and penmanship of physicians, physician assistants, residents, and interns. What better way is there to learn pharmacy than from an on-the-job experience? The *"COACH"* provides the next best way to experience real pharmacy on the job, and that is by means of real pharmacy orders.

The orders contain each and every aspect unchanged as presented to the pharmacist and the pharmacy technician. If the order is illegible when received in the pharmacy, you have it reproduced exactly as is, without any doctoring or enhancements. *What you see is what we got.*

Each excerpt, defined as an "Exhibit" in *The Pharmacy Technician COACH,* presents unique challenges that test your skills as a pharmacy technician. There is ample opportunity to exercise your interpretations of drugs and their directions for use. You will be tested on your ability to identify omissions, incorrect routes of administration, strange dosages, and dosage forms. You will be put to the challenge of multiple issues such as allergies, unique abbreviations, interactions, and drug combinations.

The *"COACH"* also introduces brand name and generic name recognition, drug class, drug cohorts, and calculations. The real orders present examples of polypharmacy, special drug and condition associations, and the need to take action with illegible pharmacy orders. Strange spellings, questionable strengths, and unique scheduling of drugs present you with a forum to think about and discuss what you need to do to assure that the patient receives the right drug and right strength, in the right form, and at the right time.

Until you are practicing in the actual pharmacy setting, the *"COACH"* is the next best thing to prepare you for the real thing. Learning is a lifetime journey. Every era, every new set of practitioners, each new class of drugs that enters the market brings with it new challenges for pharmacy practitioners. New challenges bring new opportunities to exercise your importance to health care delivery.

WELCOME TO THE REAL WORLD OF PHARMACY PRACTICE.

PATIENT:
AGE:
SEX:
RACE:
CHART NO.

MEMORIAL HOSPITAL
BALTIMORE, MARYLAND
PHYSICIAN'S ORDER RECORD

BEAR DOWN ON HARD SURFACE WITH BALL POINT PEN

GENERIC EQUIVALENT IS AUTHORIZED UNLESS CHECKED IN THIS COLUMN

ALLERGY OR SENSITIVITY	DIAGNOSIS		COMPLETED OR DISCONTINUED
TO			
NONE KNOWN ☐ SIGNED:			

DATE	TIME	ORDERS	PHYSICIAN'S SIG.		NAME	DATE	TIME
		Admit ō Med C					
		Dx Pancreatitis					
		EtOH Withdrawal					
		Stable					
		Vitals q6°					
		NKDA					
		OOB – Bathroom					
		NHO T >101, HR >120 <60					
		SBP >180 <90 DBP >110 <60					
		RR >28 <8					
		Strict I/O, Daily Wts					
		NPO x meds					
		IVF NS at 150cc/hr x 2L					

PHARMACY COPY

Exhibit 1

EXHIBIT 1 QUESTIONS

1. What is the actual meaning of ETOH?
2. What is meant by NKDA?
3. What are the meanings of:
   NHO
   SBP
   DBP
   NPO
   IVF

PATIENT:
AGE:
SEX:
RACE:
CHART NO.

MEMORIAL HOSPITAL
BALTIMORE, MARYLAND
PHYSICIAN'S ORDER RECORD

BEAR DOWN ON HARD SURFACE WITH BALL POINT PEN

GENERIC EQUIVALENT IS AUTHORIZED UNLESS CHECKED IN THIS COLUMN

ALLERGY OR SENSITIVITY TO____ NONE KNOWN ☐ SIGNED:____	DIAGNOSIS		COMPLETED OR DISCONTINUED

DATE	TIME	ORDERS	PHYSICIAN'S SIG.		NAME	DATE	TIME
		d/c Unasyn; ↑ Dopamine to 3 mcg/kg					
		Zofran 8 → IV q8 prn N/V					
		BMP, Ca, Mg, phos, LOH @ 6PM					
		Senokot † PO BID					

PHARMACY COPY

Exhibit 2

EXHIBIT 2 QUESTIONS

1. How would you interpret the drugs and directions listed in Exhibit 2?
2. What is the drug class or use for each drug listed?
3. List the trade name and generic name for each drug.

PATIENT:
AGE:
SEX:
RACE:
CHART NO.

MEMORIAL HOSPITAL
BALTIMORE, MARYLAND
PHYSICIAN'S ORDER RECORD

BEAR DOWN ON HARD SURFACE WITH BALL POINT PEN

GENERIC EQUIVALENT IS AUTHORIZED UNLESS CHECKED IN THIS COLUMN

ALLERGY OR SENSITIVITY	DIAGNOSIS		COMPLETED OR DISCONTINUED
TO______			
NONE KNOWN ☐ SIGNED:______			

DATE	TIME	ORDERS	PHYSICIAN'S SIG.		NAME	DATE	TIME
		Act OOB as tolerated					
		V. tals routine, telemetry					
		Diet cooked foods only					
		Allergies: sulfa + codeine					
		Meds toprol XL 50 mg po q d					
		IVF D_5 ½ NS with 40 mEq KCl,					
		2 gm $MgSO_4$ 1 amp HCO_3 per					
		liter × total 2L at 100 cc/hr					
		premarin 0.5 mg po q d					
		Vit B_6 50 mg po bid					
		coumadin 1 mg po q d					
		MVI 1 po q d					
		neupogen 480 mcg SQ q d					
		procrit 10 000 u SQ q M/W/F					
		Oscal 500 mg po tid					
		Compazine 25 mg PR q 8° prn					
		Ativan 0.5 mg IV or po q 6° prn					
		LABS 4 PM 7/10 basic metabolic profile					
		AM 7/11 CBC, CPT, Ca, Mg, PO_4					
		Call HO T > 101.5 SBP < 90 > 180					

PHARMACY COPY

Exhibit 3

EXHIBIT 3 QUESTIONS

1. What brand names are listed on the order sheet?
2. What are the indications for each of the drugs listed?
3. List the generic name for each brand name drug.
4. What allergies should concern you?
5. List the various routes of administration applicable to these medications noted on the orders.
6. What is another name for Vit B_6?
7. What is meant by MVI?
8. How does the physician want Procrit to be given?
9. What is the dosage for Neupogen?

PATIENT:
AGE:
SEX:
RACE:
CHART NO.

MEMORIAL HOSPITAL
BALTIMORE, MARYLAND
PHYSICIAN'S ORDER RECORD

BEAR DOWN ON HARD SURFACE WITH BALL POINT PEN

GENERIC EQUIVALENT IS AUTHORIZED UNLESS CHECKED IN THIS COLUMN

ALLERGY OR SENSITIVITY TO ____ NONE KNOWN ☐ SIGNED: ____

DIAGNOSIS

COMPLETED OR DISCONTINUED

DATE	TIME	ORDERS	PHYSICIAN'S SIG.	NAME	DATE	TIME
		Pamelor 25 mg po 1 hr. before sleep				
		Nerve conduction studies – lower ext.				
		~~B12, folic acid tests~~ error.				
		glycosylated HS.				
		KCl - 90 meq po x 1				
		TUMS - 500 mg po x 1				

PHARMACY COPY

Exhibit 4

EXHIBIT 4 QUESTIONS

1. What drugs are you able to identify in this order?
2. Which drug is being used for sleep?
3. What drug class does Pamelor belong to?
4. What are the directions for using Tums?
5. What is the generic name for Pamelor?
6. What is the generic name for Tums?
7. What dosage forms does Pamelor come in?
8. What are the directions for using Pamelor?
9. What strength of potassium chloride is being requested?
10. What are the directions for using potassium chloride?
11. What are the primary uses for Tums?

PATIENT: AGE: SEX: RACE: CHART NO.	**MEMORIAL HOSPITAL** BALTIMORE, MARYLAND **PHYSICIAN'S ORDER RECORD** BEAR DOWN ON HARD SURFACE WITH BALL POINT PEN

GENERIC EQUIVALENT IS AUTHORIZED UNLESS CHECKED IN THIS COLUMN

ALLERGY OR SENSITIVITY TO NONE KNOWN ☐ SIGNED:	DIAGNOSIS		COMPLETED OR DISCONTINUED		

DATE	TIME	ORDERS	PHYSICIAN'S SIG.		NAME	DATE	TIME
		① CBC Daily ×3					
		② SMA 7 ē AM					
		③ Viscous lidocaine 5cc					
		ē 15cc Maalox					
		P.O. q6h PRN sore throat					

PHARMACY COPY

Exhibit 5

EXHIBIT 5 QUESTIONS

1. What does CBC stand for?
2. What drugs do you find in this order?
3. Will this preparation require compounding?
4. What total volume of drug will be needed for 3 days?
5. How much of each drug is required to make enough for 3 days?
6. What is the indication for viscous lidocaine?
7. What are the directions for using the viscous lidocaine and Maalox preparation?
8. What is the brand name for lidocaine?

PATIENT:
AGE:
SEX:
RACE:
CHART NO.

MEMORIAL HOSPITAL
BALTIMORE, MARYLAND
PHYSICIAN'S ORDER RECORD

BEAR DOWN ON HARD SURFACE WITH BALL POINT PEN

GENERIC EQUIVALENT IS AUTHORIZED UNLESS CHECKED IN THIS COLUMN

ALLERGY OR SENSITIVITY	DIAGNOSIS		COMPLETED OR DISCONTINUED
TO			
NONE KNOWN ☐ SIGNED:			

	DATE	TIME	ORDERS	PHYSICIAN'S SIG.		NAME	DATE	TIME
			Vancomycin 14.1 mg IV q18					
			Trough & hold Serial					
			to 2nd dose.					
			Cefotaxime 47 mg IV q12°					
			Amphotericin B 5 mg in 50cc D5W					
			to run @ 0.9cc/hr x 5 hours (Total 4.7)					
			WT = .940 Kg (0.5 u/Kg/day)					

PHARMACY COPY

Exhibit 6

EXHIBIT 6 QUESTIONS

1. What drugs are we looking at in this order?
2. What class(es) of drugs do these drugs fall into?
3. What are the trade names for the drugs listed in the order?
4. How long will 50 cc of the amphotericin B mixture last if it is running at 0.9 cc/hr?
5. How much does the patient weigh in kilograms?
6. How much does the patient weigh in pounds?
7. Was the total dose calculated correctly for amphotericin B?
8. What are the directions for using each drug?

PATIENT:
AGE:
SEX:
RACE:
CHART NO.

MEMORIAL HOSPITAL
BALTIMORE, MARYLAND
PHYSICIAN'S ORDER RECORD

BEAR DOWN ON HARD SURFACE WITH BALL POINT PEN

GENERIC EQUIVALENT IS AUTHORIZED UNLESS CHECKED IN THIS COLUMN

ALLERGY OR SENSITIVITY
TO
NONE KNOWN ☐ SIGNED:

DIAGNOSIS

COMPLETED OR DISCONTINUED

DATE	TIME	ORDERS	PHYSICIAN'S SIG.		NAME	DATE	TIME
		(1) D/C metronidazole					
		(2) Gentamycin 140mg IV loading dose					
		Gentamycin 70mg IV Q8°					
		√ Peak and trough with third dose.					

PHARMACY COPY

Exhibit 7

EXHIBIT 7 QUESTIONS

1. What drug is being discontinued?
2. What is the primary indication for the drug that is being discontinued?
3. What drug is replacing the drug that is being discontinued?
4. What is the primary indication for the drug replacing the discontinued drug?
5. How will the new drug be dosed?
6. What is a loading dose?
7. What is the brand name for the drug being discontinued?
8. What is a peak and trough?

PATIENT:
AGE:
SEX:
RACE:
CHART NO.

MEMORIAL HOSPITAL
BALTIMORE, MARYLAND
PHYSICIAN'S ORDER RECORD

BEAR DOWN ON HARD SURFACE WITH BALL POINT PEN

GENERIC EQUIVALENT IS AUTHORIZED UNLESS CHECKED IN THIS COLUMN

ALLERGY OR SENSITIVITY
TO ____
NONE KNOWN ☐ SIGNED: ____

DIAGNOSIS

COMPLETED OR DISCONTINUED

DATE	TIME	ORDERS	PHYSICIAN'S SIG.		NAME	DATE	TIME
		Meds: Verapamil 240mg PO QD					
		Rantac 50mg IV q8°					
		Ativan 1mg PO q8°					
		Demerol 25mg IM q6° prn					
		Compazine 10mg IV q8° prn nausea					
		Labs: EKG on arrival to floor ✓					
		IBC q6° x 24° ✓					
		AM L 8/3/97 CBC, Chem7, Ca, Mg ✓					

PHARMACY COPY

Exhibit 8

EXHIBIT 8 QUESTIONS

1. List all the medications on the order by:
   brand name
   generic name
   therapeutic action
2. What are the directions for use for each drug?
3. Which of the drugs are ordered to be given parenterally and which ones enterally?
4. What type of length of action formulations are available for verapamil?

PATIENT:
AGE:
SEX:
RACE:
CHART NO.

MEMORIAL HOSPITAL
BALTIMORE, MARYLAND
PHYSICIAN'S ORDER RECORD

BEAR DOWN ON HARD SURFACE WITH BALL POINT PEN

GENERIC EQUIVALENT IS AUTHORIZED UNLESS CHECKED IN THIS COLUMN

ALLERGY OR SENSITIVITY TO___ NONE KNOWN ☐ SIGNED:___	DIAGNOSIS		COMPLETED OR DISCONTINUED

DATE	TIME	ORDERS	PHYSICIAN'S SIG.	NAME	DATE	TIME
		Admit to ICU				
		Dx: AIDS				
		ΔMS				
		Cond: grave				
		Vitals: routine				
		Allergies: sulfa – hives				
		Diet: soft mechanical				
		Act: bedrest ē BR privileges				
		Meds. Zantac 50 mg IV q 8°				
		IVF D5 ½ NS @ 150 cc/hr x 2L				
		pyrimethamine 200 mg per NGT x 1				
		then 75 mg per NGT q d				
		~~clindamycin 600 mg IV q 6°~~ error				
		folinic acid 10 mg per NGT q d				
		azithromycin 1 gm per NGT x 1 then				
		500 mg per NGT q d				
		cefotaxime 1.0 gm IV q 8°				
		heparin 5000 u SQ bid				
		Call HO T > 101.5				
		SBP < 90 > 160				
		P < 60 > 120				
		AM labs 10/27: CBC, Chem-20, PT/PTT				
		O2 4L NC				

PHARMACY COPY

Exhibit 9

EXHIBIT 9 QUESTIONS

1. What type of health-care unit is the patient being admitted to?
2. Does this patient have any allergies or sensitivities? If so, list them.
3. What designation or acronym represents the *diagnosis?*
4. List all the medications being prescribed for this patient.
5. List each medication and its use.
6. Identify the brand name and generic name for each medication.
7. What is the route of administration for pyrimethamine?
8. How do folic acid and folinic acid differ?
9. How would you determine if the physician meant folic acid or folinic acid?
10. Which are the anti-infective drugs?
11. How is heparin written in this order to be given?
12. Write out the "Sig" for each medication in this order.
13. What large volume intravenous fluids are being ordered?

PATIENT:
AGE:
SEX:
RACE:
CHART NO.

MEMORIAL HOSPITAL
BALTIMORE, MARYLAND
PHYSICIAN'S ORDER RECORD

BEAR DOWN ON HARD SURFACE WITH BALL POINT PEN

GENERIC EQUIVALENT IS AUTHORIZED UNLESS CHECKED IN THIS COLUMN

ALLERGY OR SENSITIVITY
TO________
NONE KNOWN ☐ SIGNED:________

DIAGNOSIS

COMPLETED OR DISCONTINUED

DATE	TIME	ORDERS	PHYSICIAN'S SIG.	NAME	DATE	TIME
		Pen G 5 mu ~~then~~ IV now then 2.4 mu IV q4°				

PHARMACY COPY

Exhibit 10

EXHIBIT 10 QUESTIONS

1. Write this order so that it is fully understandable.
2. Is this a drug? If so, what is it used for?
3. If this is a drug, what allergy would preclude its use?

PATIENT:
AGE:
SEX:
RACE:
CHART NO.

MEMORIAL HOSPITAL
BALTIMORE, MARYLAND
PHYSICIAN'S ORDER RECORD

BEAR DOWN ON HARD SURFACE WITH BALL POINT PEN

GENERIC EQUIVALENT IS AUTHORIZED UNLESS CHECKED IN THIS COLUMN

ALLERGY OR SENSITIVITY

TO

NONE KNOWN ☐ SIGNED:

DIAGNOSIS

COMPLETED OR DISCONTINUED

DATE	TIME	ORDERS	PHYSICIAN'S SIG.	NAME	DATE	TIME
		① ↑ HEPARIN TO 1300 u/hr, ✓PTT p̄ 6°				
		② ~~[illegible]~~ ACETAMINOPHEN TO TYLENOL ES				
		650mg q4° PRN PAIN				
		③ AM CHEM 7 Ca/Mg ↑ß,				
		SERUM OSM, CBC, PT/PTT				
		④ D5NS @ 100 cc/hr × TL				

PHARMACY COPY

Exhibit 11

EXHIBIT 11 QUESTIONS

1. What drugs are being ordered?
2. What drug is being discontinued?
3. What drug is replacing the discontinued drug?
4. Write out the directions for item numbers one and two on the order.
5. What does item number four on the order say?
6. List the use for each drug ordered and the drug being replaced.

PATIENT:
AGE:
SEX:
RACE:
CHART NO.

MEMORIAL HOSPITAL
BALTIMORE, MARYLAND
PHYSICIAN'S ORDER RECORD

BEAR DOWN ON HARD SURFACE WITH BALL POINT PEN

GENERIC EQUIVALENT IS AUTHORIZED UNLESS CHECKED IN THIS COLUMN

ALLERGY OR SENSITIVITY	DIAGNOSIS	COMPLETED OR DISCONTINUED
TO. ___ NONE KNOWN ☐ SIGNED: ___		

DATE	TIME	ORDERS	PHYSICIAN'S SIG.	NAME	DATE	TIME

(3) Cond: Stable
(4) Vitals: routine
(5) ACT: Bed rest c̄ bedside commode
(6) ALL: NKDA
(7) Diet: Cardiac
(8) IVF: IV to heplock – saline flush Q shift
(9) O_2 2L NC
(10) Dig 0.25 mg po QD
(11) Captopril 25 mg po Q8
(12) Lasix 40 mg IVP QD (today's dose given in ICU)
(13) Nitropaste 1" Q6 (hold 12 MN dose)
(14) Zantac 150 mg po BID
(15) Maalox 30 cc between meals & h/s
(16) Colace 100 mg po QD
(17) EKG in AM
(18) I's & O's please (Foley in place)
(19) guiac stools & record in nurse's notes
(20) warm compresses to lower legs prn cramps
(21) ECHO c̄ color doppler → ordered by ICU staff
(22) AM labs: CBC, SMA-7, Ca, Mg, Phos, Dig level
(23) pulse ox QAM
(24) Call HO: (BP) >150/100, <80/60 (HR) >120, <50
(RR) >25, <10 (T) >101
(U.O) <30 cc/hr
(25) tylenol ii tabs po PRN pain

[signature]

Exhibit 12

EXHIBIT 12 QUESTIONS

1. What is meant by ALL:NKDA?
2. Is Dig a drug? If so, which one?
3. Is captopril a generic or brand name?
4. What is Nitropaste?
5. What is Zantac used for?
6. Is Maalox a prescription (i.e., legend) drug?
7. What is the generic name for Colace?
8. By looking at this selection of drugs, what can we surmise about the ailment of the patient?
9. What drug is listed, but not included with all the drugs listed?
10. For each drug listed give the:
    trade name
    generic name
    directions

PATIENT:
AGE:
SEX:
RACE:
CHART NO.

MEMORIAL HOSPITAL
BALTIMORE, MARYLAND
PHYSICIAN'S ORDER RECORD

BEAR DOWN ON HARD SURFACE WITH BALL POINT PEN

GENERIC EQUIVALENT IS AUTHORIZED UNLESS CHECKED IN THIS COLUMN

ALLERGY OR SENSITIVITY TO Morphine (hives)
NONE KNOWN ☐ SIGNED:

DIAGNOSIS

COMPLETED OR DISCONTINUED

DATE	TIME	ORDERS	PHYSICIAN'S SIG.	NAME	DATE	TIME
		- FULL LIQUID DIET. ADVANCE TO REGULAR AS TOLERATED ✓				
		- ✓ LOWER EXTREMITY STRENGTH + SENSATION ✓				
		q½° x 4. q1° x 4. THEN q4° ✓				
		- IVF: RL @ 100cc/hr. ✓				
		D/C IV WHEN TOLERATING PO WELL ✓				
		- INCENTIVE SPIROMETRY q2° WHILE AWAKE ✓				
		- MEDS MSO4 8-10mg. s.q. q3° PRN PAIN ✓				
		OR				
		PERCOCET TAB i - ii PO q3° PRN PAIN				
		MOM 30cc p.o hs PRN ✓				
		DALMANE 15mg. p.o. hs PRN SLEEP ✓				
		PERICOLACE TAB i ~~po~~ BID ✓				
		[signature]				
		D/C MSO4				
		DEMEROL 100mg } IM q3° PRN PAIN				
		VISTARIL 25mg }				

PHARMACY COPY

Exhibit 13

EXHIBIT 13 QUESTIONS

1. What is the patient's allergy?
2. What class of drugs does the drug to which the patient shows an allergic response belong to?
3. Do you see a problem with the allergy and any of the drugs ordered? If yes, what is the problem?
4. Why would MOM and Peri-Colace seem to be a good idea to use with this patient?
5. Is there more than one strength of Dalmane? If so, what are they?
6. What drug was discontinued? Why do you think it was discontinued?
7. What drug(s) is replacing the discontinued drug?
8. What is the rationale for the Demerol/Vistaril combination?
9. List each drug by trade name (if available), generic name, and the directions for use.

PATIENT:
AGE:
SEX:
RACE:
CHART NO.

MEMORIAL HOSPITAL
BALTIMORE, MARYLAND
PHYSICIAN'S ORDER RECORD

BEAR DOWN ON HARD SURFACE WITH BALL POINT PEN

GENERIC EQUIVALENT IS AUTHORIZED UNLESS CHECKED IN THIS COLUMN

ALLERGY OR SENSITIVITY TO ____ | DIAGNOSIS | COMPLETED OR DISCONTINUED

NONE KNOWN ☐ SIGNED: ____

DATE	TIME	ORDERS	PHYSICIAN'S SIG.	NAME	DATE	TIME

Dx: Fever, AMS, CML
Cond: Stable
Vitals: q 6° c̄ neurocheck
Allergy: NKDA
Activity: Bedrest
Nursing: NHO T > 100.4, P > 105 < 55 SBP > 160 < 100 DBP > 105
RR > 25 < 10
Diet: Cardiac, ~~soft mech~~
Meds: Titrate O₂ to keep sats > 94%
Amiodarone 200 mg PO QD Cefepime 2 gm IV q 12°
Digoxin 0.125 mg PO QD
Allopurinol 300 mg PO qAM
Hydroxyurea 3000 mg PO QD
Megace 40mg/ml 20cc PO QD
Oxycontin i PO q 12°
Roxicet i - ii PO q4-6° PRN
AML: CBC, Chem 7, Ca, Mg, Ph
for 8/31: Chest CT, Abd CT c̄ oral + IV contrast
Give pt oral contrast prior to CT study

PHARMACY COPY

Exhibit 14

EXHIBIT 14 QUESTIONS

1. What is NHO?
2. What is ">" and "<" in the order?
3. List all the drugs ordered by the doctor.
4. What is the difference between Oxycontin and Roxicet?
5. Do you see any reason to call the doctor about Oxycontin and/or Roxicet?
6. How many grams of Hydroxyurea are in 3,000 mg?
7. How many milligrams of Megace will the patient get with each daily dose?
8. List the routes of administration for each drug ordered.
9. List each drug by:
   trade name
   generic name
   directions
10. What is the most likely use for Hydroxyurea and Megace?

PATIENT:
AGE:
SEX:
RACE:
CHART NO.

MEMORIAL HOSPITAL
BALTIMORE, MARYLAND
PHYSICIAN'S ORDER RECORD

BEAR DOWN ON HARD SURFACE WITH BALL POINT PEN

GENERIC EQUIVALENT IS AUTHORIZED UNLESS CHECKED IN THIS COLUMN

ALLERGY OR SENSITIVITY TO	DIAGNOSIS		COMPLETED OR DISCONTINUED
NONE KNOWN ☐ SIGNED:			

DATE	TIME	ORDERS	PHYSICIAN'S SIG.		NAME	DATE	TIME

Meds. Glucotrol XL 5mg PO qd
Zantac 150mg PO bid
Zestril 10mg PO qd
Premarin 0.625mg PO qd
Dilaudid 1-2mg IV q4-6 prn pain
Compazine 5mg IV q4-6 prn nausea/vomiting
Tylenol 650mg PO q4-6 prn pain/fever >1..
Labs: CBC c diff, Chem 7, Mg, Ca, amylase, lipase
RUQ ultrasound in AM: R/O cholelithiasis, biliary duct obstruction
MOM 30cc PO qhs

PHARMACY COPY

Exhibit 15

EXHIBIT 15 QUESTIONS

1. List the drugs ordered by the physician.
2. Which of the drugs ordered is the pain medication?
3. What is the difference between Zantac and Zestril?
4. Which drug is most likely being used for nausea?
5. What are the directions for each drug ordered?
6. What is the brand name, generic name, and use for each drug ordered?

PATIENT:
AGE:
SEX:
RACE:
CHART NO.

MEMORIAL HOSPITAL
BALTIMORE, MARYLAND
PHYSICIAN'S ORDER RECORD

BEAR DOWN ON HARD SURFACE WITH BALL POINT PEN

GENERIC EQUIVALENT IS AUTHORIZED UNLESS CHECKED IN THIS COLUMN

ALLERGY OR SENSITIVITY
TO
NONE KNOWN ☐ SIGNED:

DIAGNOSIS

COMPLETED OR DISCONTINUED

DATE	TIME	ORDERS	PHYSICIAN'S SIG.	NAME	DATE	TIME
		FS AC + HS				
		SSI 200 – 250 → 2 units				
		251 – 300 → 4 units				
		301 – 350 → 6 units				
		351 – 400 → 8 units				
		>400 → 10 units				
		1800 diabetic ADA diet				
		Timentin 3.1 gm IV q6°				
		CBC & Chem-7 in AM				
		NS + 20 KCl @ 80 cc/h				
		NPH 37 units in AM				
		17 units in pm				
		Demerol 50 mg IV q3-4° prn				
		Vistaril 50 mg IV q3-4° prn				

PHARMACY COPY

Exhibit 16

EXHIBIT 16 QUESTIONS

1. What is FS AC & HS in the order?
2. What, if any, drug(s) is associated with FS AC & HS in the order?
3. What is SSI in the order?
4. What do the numbers in SSI represent? (e.g., 200–250 → 2 units)
5. What drugs are being ordered?
6. What is the use for each drug?
7. Do you see the need to call the doctor for any reason? If so, why?
8. Can you spot any liter size volumes that are ordered? If so, what are they?
9. How many different kinds of insulin will be needed to fill the order? What are they?

PATIENT:
AGE:
SEX:
RACE:
CHART NO.

MEMORIAL HOSPITAL
BALTIMORE, MARYLAND
PHYSICIAN'S ORDER RECORD

BEAR DOWN ON HARD SURFACE WITH BALL POINT PEN

GENERIC EQUIVALENT IS AUTHORIZED UNLESS CHECKED IN THIS COLUMN

ALLERGY OR SENSITIVITY
TO________
NONE KNOWN ☐ SIGNED:________

DIAGNOSIS

COMPLETED OR DISCONTINUED

DATE	TIME	ORDERS	PHYSICIAN'S SIG.		NAME	DATE	TIME
		Cefotaxime 1g IV q8°					
		↓ FiO_2 50%. Δ IMV 8					
		Lasix 100mg IV x T					
		Zaroxolyn 10mg N x T					
		✓ABGs 1 hr.					

PHARMACY COPY

Exhibit 17

EXHIBIT 17 QUESTIONS

1. What drugs are being ordered?
2. List the drugs by brand name, generic name, and directions.
3. Which of the medications warrants a call to the practitioner and why?

PATIENT:
AGE:
SEX:
RACE:
CHART NO.

MEMORIAL HOSPITAL
BALTIMORE, MARYLAND
PHYSICIAN'S ORDER RECORD

BEAR DOWN ON HARD SURFACE WITH BALL POINT PEN

GENERIC EQUIVALENT IS AUTHORIZED UNLESS CHECKED IN THIS COLUMN

ALLERGY OR SENSITIVITY	DIAGNOSIS	COMPLETED OR DISCONTINUED
TO		
NONE KNOWN ☐ SIGNED:		

DATE	TIME	ORDERS	PHYSICIAN'S SIG.		NAME	DATE	TIME
		Meds:					
		IVF NS @ 100 cc/hr x 2 Liters					
		Insulin Sliding Scale					
		FS <200 Give 0 units Insulin (Regular)					
		201-250 " 2 "					
		251-300 " 4 "					
		301-350 " 6 "					
		351-400 " 8 "					
		>400 " 10 "					
		Clonidine 0.2 mg PO QD BID					
		Prinivil 20 mg PO QD					
		ECASA 325 mg PO QD					
		Metoprolol 50 mg PO BID					

PHARMACY COPY

Exhibit 18

EXHIBIT 18 QUESTIONS

1. What kind and how much intravenous fluid is being ordered?
2. List the drugs by:
   brand name
   generic name
3. Write out the directions for each drug.

PATIENT:
AGE:
SEX:
RACE:
CHART NO.

MEMORIAL HOSPITAL
BALTIMORE, MARYLAND
PHYSICIAN'S ORDER RECORD

BEAR DOWN ON HARD SURFACE WITH BALL POINT PEN

GENERIC EQUIVALENT IS AUTHORIZED UNLESS CHECKED IN THIS COLUMN

ALLERGY OR SENSITIVITY
TO
NONE KNOWN ☐ SIGNED:

DIAGNOSIS

COMPLETED OR DISCONTINUED

DATE	TIME	ORDERS	PHYSICIAN'S SIG.	NAME	DATE	TIME
		Solucortef 100mg IV q8°				
		Flagyl 500mg IV q8°				
		Demerol 50/Vistaril 50mg IM q3-4° prn pain				
		AM labs: CBC/diff, BMP				
		IVFs: D5RL at 100cc/hr				
		Diet: NPO				
		ZANTAC 50mg q12°				

PHARMACY COPY

Exhibit 19

EXHIBIT 19 QUESTIONS

1. What is NPO on the order?
2. Which drugs are written in their generic form?
3. Which drugs are written in their brand name form?
4. Write out the directions for each drug.
5. List each drug with its use.

PATIENT:
AGE:
SEX:
RACE:
CHART NO.

MEMORIAL HOSPITAL
BALTIMORE, MARYLAND
PHYSICIAN'S ORDER RECORD

BEAR DOWN ON HARD SURFACE WITH BALL POINT PEN

GENERIC EQUIVALENT IS AUTHORIZED UNLESS CHECKED IN THIS COLUMN

ALLERGY OR SENSITIVITY TO ______ NONE KNOWN ☐ SIGNED: ______	DIAGNOSIS		COMPLETED OR DISCONTINUED

DATE	TIME	ORDERS	PHYSICIAN'S SIG.		NAME	DATE	TIME
		Graposon 50mg BD					
		Oprilosc 20mg BD					

PHARMACY COPY

Exhibit 20

EXHIBIT 20 QUESTIONS

1. What does this combination of drugs suggest?
2. What class of drugs does each drug belong to?
3. Does drug item number two require any special handling?
4. Are there any special instructions for the patient when taking drug item number one?
5. What strength of each drug is being ordered?
6. What is BD in the order? Is this the same as QD or BID?

PATIENT: AGE: SEX: RACE: CHART NO.	MEMORIAL HOSPITAL BALTIMORE, MARYLAND PHYSICIAN'S ORDER RECORD BEAR DOWN ON HARD SURFACE WITH BALL POINT PEN

GENERIC EQUIVALENT IS AUTHORIZED UNLESS CHECKED IN THIS COLUMN

ALLERGY OR SENSITIVITY TO NONE KNOWN ☐ SIGNED:	DIAGNOSIS	COMPLETED OR DISCONTINUED

DATE	TIME	ORDERS	PHYSICIAN'S SIG.	NAME	DATE	TIME
		Meds: TORADOL 30mg IV q6°				
		PHENOBARBITONE 30mg PO BID				
		DILANTIN 100mg PO TID				
		DILANTIN 300mg PO stat				
		DILANTIN 300mg PO qHS				
		GENTAMICIN 550mg IV qD.				
		UNASYN 1.5gm IV q6°				
		LABS: AM CBC + diff } both 4/14				
		Chem 20 + Mg } , 4/15.				
		IV Fluids - NS + 20mEq KCl at 100cc/hr x 4 liters -				

PHARMACY COPY

Exhibit 21

Exhibit 21 Questions

1. List each drug by trade name, generic name, and directions.
2. What is the use for each drug?
3. What class of drugs does each drug belong to?
4. How many total milliliters will satisfy the order for large volume IV fluids?
5. Why would the doctor order a large stat dose of Dilantin and then have the patient take a smaller dose more often?

PATIENT:
AGE:
SEX:
RACE:
CHART NO.

MEMORIAL HOSPITAL
BALTIMORE, MARYLAND
PHYSICIAN'S ORDER RECORD

BEAR DOWN ON HARD SURFACE WITH BALL POINT PEN

GENERIC EQUIVALENT IS AUTHORIZED UNLESS CHECKED IN THIS COLUMN

ALLERGY OR SENSITIVITY
TO
NONE KNOWN ☐ SIGNED:

DIAGNOSIS

COMPLETED OR DISCONTINUED

DATE	TIME	ORDERS	PHYSICIAN'S SIG.		NAME	DATE	TIME
		(1) 30cc mom + 15cc cascara today					

PHARMACY COPY

Exhibit 22

EXHIBIT 22 QUESTIONS

1. What drugs are being ordered?
2. How much of each drug is ordered?
3. How often is each drug being given?

PATIENT:
AGE:
SEX:
RACE:
CHART NO.

MEMORIAL HOSPITAL
BALTIMORE, MARYLAND
PHYSICIAN'S ORDER RECORD

BEAR DOWN ON HARD SURFACE WITH BALL POINT PEN

GENERIC EQUIVALENT IS AUTHORIZED UNLESS CHECKED IN THIS COLUMN

ALLERGY OR SENSITIVITY
TO________
NONE KNOWN ☐ SIGNED:________

DIAGNOSIS

COMPLETED OR DISCONTINUED

	DATE	TIME	ORDERS	PHYSICIAN'S SIG.		NAME	DATE	TIME

① Cardizem CD 180 mg po q d or equivalent
② Norvasc 5 mg po q d
③ Atrovent 6 puffs q 6°
③ Azmt – CBG chem 7, Mg
④ Prilosec 20 mg po q d

PHARMACY COPY

Exhibit 23

EXHIBIT 23 QUESTIONS

1. What drug(s) would be classified as cardiovascular agents?
2. What is the term "equivalent" referring to in item number one?
3. What do you think is the route of administration for the drug in item number three?
4. Do you think the directions for drug in item number three are excessive?
5. Is Prilosec a brand or generic name?
6. Is Atrovent a brand or generic name?
7. What is Prilosec used for?
8. What other forms are available for Atrovent?

PATIENT: AGE: SEX: RACE: CHART NO.	**MEMORIAL HOSPITAL** BALTIMORE, MARYLAND **PHYSICIAN'S ORDER RECORD** BEAR DOWN ON HARD SURFACE WITH BALL POINT PEN

GENERIC EQUIVALENT IS AUTHORIZED UNLESS CHECKED IN THIS COLUMN

ALLERGY OR SENSITIVITY TO____ NONE KNOWN ☐ SIGNED:____	DIAGNOSIS		COMPLETED OR DISCONTINUED

DATE	TIME	ORDERS	PHYSICIAN'S SIG.		NAME	DATE	TIME

Medn :-

① Minoxidil 7.5 mg 1 tb by mouth qd

② . Hold Coumadin 5 mg 1 tb .

③ . Tenormin 50 mg 1 tb ~~bid~~ qd

④ . Lanoxin Tab 0.125 mg 1 tb daily

⑤ Nirozal 2% oint (ringworm area)

⑥ Propine 0.1% eyedrop → bid

Timoptic 0.5% " → bid

Pilocar 4% → qid .

⑦ Procardia XL 60mg 1 tb bid .

Lab :- ① CBC c̄ diff , CHEM 20 in AM

PHARMACY COPY

Exhibit 24

EXHIBIT 24 QUESTIONS

1. What strength of Minoxidil is being ordered?
2. Which drugs listed have routes of administration other than oral?
3. List the brand name, generic name, and directions for each drug being ordered.

PATIENT:
AGE:
SEX:
RACE:
CHART NO.

MEMORIAL HOSPITAL
BALTIMORE, MARYLAND
PHYSICIAN'S ORDER RECORD

BEAR DOWN ON HARD SURFACE WITH BALL POINT PEN

GENERIC EQUIVALENT IS AUTHORIZED UNLESS CHECKED IN THIS COLUMN

ALLERGY OR SENSITIVITY
TO
NONE KNOWN ☐ SIGNED:

DIAGNOSIS

COMPLETED OR DISCONTINUED

	DATE	TIME	ORDERS	PHYSICIAN'S SIG.		NAME	DATE	TIME
			① COLACE 100mg 2 tabs PO BID. X 1 DAY.					
			② SENOKOTT I-II tabs PO BID x 1 DAY.					

PHARMACY COPY

Exhibit 25

EXHIBIT 25 QUESTIONS

1. What are the names of the drugs being ordered?
2. Does anything seem strange about this combination of drugs?
3. What is the generic name for each drug?
4. What is the Sig for each drug?

PATIENT:
AGE:
SEX:
RACE:
CHART NO.

MEMORIAL HOSPITAL
BALTIMORE, MARYLAND
PHYSICIAN'S ORDER RECORD

BEAR DOWN ON HARD SURFACE WITH BALL POINT PEN

GENERIC EQUIVALENT IS AUTHORIZED UNLESS CHECKED IN THIS COLUMN

ALLERGY OR SENSITIVITY TO ____ DIAGNOSIS

NONE KNOWN ☐ SIGNED: ____

COMPLETED OR DISCONTINUED

DATE	TIME	ORDERS	PHYSICIAN'S SIG.		NAME	DATE	TIME
		Please send Cruel Lotion one tube					

PHARMACY COPY

Exhibit 26

EXHIBIT 26 QUESTIONS

1. Do you think the physician really wants the pharmacy to fill an order for a "Cruel Lotion?"
2. What do you think the doctor wants?
3. How many will you dispense?
4. What ancillary label would be proper for this medication?
5. What is the use for this lotion?

PATIENT: AGE: SEX: RACE: CHART NO.	**MEMORIAL HOSPITAL** BALTIMORE, MARYLAND **PHYSICIAN'S ORDER RECORD** BEAR DOWN ON HARD SURFACE WITH BALL POINT PEN

GENERIC EQUIVALENT IS AUTHORIZED UNLESS CHECKED IN THIS COLUMN

ALLERGY OR SENSITIVITY TO NONE KNOWN ☐ SIGNED:	DIAGNOSIS	COMPLETED OR DISCONTINUED

DATE	TIME	ORDERS	PHYSICIAN'S SIG.	NAME	DATE	TIME
		(1) Paxil 20mg po Qd				
		(2) Rhthmol 150mg po TID				
		(3) NitroBid 2.5mg po Q12°.				

PHARMACY COPY

Exhibit 27

EXHIBIT 27 QUESTIONS

1. Are all the drugs spelled correctly? If not, which one(s) is incorrect and what is the correct spelling?
2. Which drug(s) is cardiovascular?
3. What is the difference between Paxil and Taxol?

PATIENT:
AGE:
SEX:
RACE:
CHART NO.

MEMORIAL HOSPITAL
BALTIMORE, MARYLAND
PHYSICIAN'S ORDER RECORD

BEAR DOWN ON HARD SURFACE WITH BALL POINT PEN

GENERIC EQUIVALENT IS AUTHORIZED UNLESS CHECKED IN THIS COLUMN

ALLERGY OR SENSITIVITY TO ___ NONE KNOWN ☐ SIGNED: ___ | DIAGNOSIS | COMPLETED OR DISCONTINUED

DATE	TIME	ORDERS	PHYSICIAN'S SIG.	NAME	DATE	TIME
		I's ē O's				
		NKDA				
		Bedrest, can get OOB → chair				
		if tol ambulate this pm				
		ē assistance				
		Diet . Reg – low residue				
		HL IV				
		Provachol 40 mg po q HS				
		Zestril 40 mg po q D				
		Norvasc 10 mg po BID				
		Lasix 40 mg po q D				
		Nitrodur 0.6 mg q po q D				
		Clonidine 0.3 mg po q D				
		Lescol 40 mg po q D				
		Terental 400 mg po q AC				
		Beclovent 2 puffs q 6°				
		Albuterol 2 puffs q 6° prn				
		Percocet i-ii po q 4° prn pain				
		IS @ bedside; 10×/° while awake				
		(B) Venodynes				

PHARMACY COPY

Exhibit 28

EXHIBIT 28 QUESTIONS

1. What is NKDA on this order?
2. What are I's & O's in the order?
3. What is HL in the order?
4. Is Provachol a drug?
5. Would you have questions to ask the doctor about this order? If so, what would they be?
6. What are strengths that are available for clonidine? How would you fill the doctor's request for clonidine 0.3 mg in this order?
7. What drug do you think the doctor is looking for by ordering Terental?
8. List the drugs on the basis of brand name, generic name, directions, and drug class.

PATIENT: AGE: SEX: RACE: CHART NO.	**MEMORIAL HOSPITAL** BALTIMORE, MARYLAND **PHYSICIAN'S ORDER RECORD** BEAR DOWN ON HARD SURFACE WITH BALL POINT PEN

GENERIC EQUIVALENT IS AUTHORIZED UNLESS CHECKED IN THIS COLUMN

ALLERGY OR SENSITIVITY TO NONE KNOWN ☐ SIGNED:	DIAGNOSIS		COMPLETED OR DISCONTINUED		

	DATE	TIME	ORDERS	PHYSICIAN'S SIG.		NAME	DATE	TIME
			D/C Regranex cream					
			use santy cream BID x 3 days					
			Continue whirlpool BID					

PHARMACY COPY

Exhibit 29

EXHIBIT 29 QUESTIONS

1. What drug is being discontinued?
2. Is the name of the discontinued drug a brand or generic name?
3. What drug is replacing the discontinued drug?
4. How long does the doctor want to use the replacement drug?
5. What are the directions for use for the replacement drug?

PATIENT: AGE: SEX: RACE: CHART NO.	**MEMORIAL HOSPITAL** BALTIMORE, MARYLAND **PHYSICIAN'S ORDER RECORD** BEAR DOWN ON HARD SURFACE WITH BALL POINT PEN

GENERIC EQUIVALENT IS AUTHORIZED UNLESS CHECKED IN THIS COLUMN

ALLERGY OR SENSITIVITY TO. NONE KNOWN ☐ SIGNED:	DIAGNOSIS		COMPLETED OR DISCONTINUED

DATE	TIME	ORDERS	PHYSICIAN'S SIG.		NAME	DATE	TIME
		KDUR 30 mEq po BID today					
		MgOxide 40 mg po x i today ←					
		d/c PCA					
		percocet i-ii po q 4-6 hrs prn pain					
		decrease IVF to 42cc/hr					

PHARMACY COPY

Exhibit 30

EXHIBIT 30 QUESTIONS

1. How many drugs are mentioned in the order?
2. How many drugs are being ordered? What are they?
3. How many drugs are being discontinued? Which ones?
4. What is PCA in the order?
5. Do PCA and percocet have the same therapeutic use? If so, what is it?
6. What is the K in KDUR in the order?
7. What is the Mg in MgOxide in the order?
8. What are the directions for use for the KDUR?
9. Do any strengths need questioning? If so, which one(s)?
10. What are the directions for the percocet?

PATIENT:
AGE:
SEX:
RACE:
CHART NO.

MEMORIAL HOSPITAL
BALTIMORE, MARYLAND
PHYSICIAN'S ORDER RECORD

BEAR DOWN ON HARD SURFACE WITH BALL POINT PEN

GENERIC EQUIVALENT IS AUTHORIZED UNLESS CHECKED IN THIS COLUMN

ALLERGY OR SENSITIVITY
TO
NONE KNOWN ☐ SIGNED:

DIAGNOSIS

COMPLETED OR DISCONTINUED

	DATE	TIME	ORDERS	PHYSICIAN'S SIG.		NAME	DATE	TIME
			ECASA i tab PO qd					
			Motrin 650mg q6° prn PO					

PHARMACY COPY

Exhibit 31

EXHIBIT 31 QUESTIONS

1. What are the names of the drugs listed?
2. What are the strengths for each drug?
3. Does anything written in the order warrant a call for clarification?
4. What is ECASA in this order?
5. Would there be a reason for ordering these drugs together? If so, why?
6. What class of drugs does Motrin belong to?
7. Is there any auxillary label that would be important for Motrin?

PATIENT:
AGE:
SEX:
RACE:
CHART NO.

MEMORIAL HOSPITAL
BALTIMORE, MARYLAND
PHYSICIAN'S ORDER RECORD

BEAR DOWN ON HARD SURFACE WITH BALL POINT PEN

GENERIC EQUIVALENT IS AUTHORIZED UNLESS CHECKED IN THIS COLUMN

ALLERGY OR SENSITIVITY

TO________

NONE KNOWN ☐ SIGNED:________

DIAGNOSIS

COMPLETED OR DISCONTINUED

DATE	TIME	ORDERS	PHYSICIAN'S SIG.		NAME	DATE	TIME
		Naproxen 200mg po BID prn for HA					

PHARMACY COPY

Exhibit 32

EXHIBIT 32 QUESTIONS

1. Is naproxen a brand or generic name of a drug?
2. What class of drugs does this drug belong to?
3. What is the usual indication for this drug?
4. What are the directions as stated in the order?
5. How should this drug be taken?

PATIENT:
AGE:
SEX:
RACE:
CHART NO.

MEMORIAL HOSPITAL
BALTIMORE, MARYLAND
PHYSICIAN'S ORDER RECORD

BEAR DOWN ON HARD SURFACE WITH BALL POINT PEN

GENERIC EQUIVALENT IS AUTHORIZED UNLESS CHECKED IN THIS COLUMN

ALLERGY OR SENSITIVITY | DIAGNOSIS | COMPLETED OR DISCONTINUED

TO

NONE KNOWN ☐ SIGNED:

DATE	TIME	ORDERS	PHYSICIAN'S SIG.	NAME	DATE	TIME
		Allergy - PCN.				
		I.V Hep lock c̄ Flush.				
		Labs.				
		CBC, chem 7, cal, mg, Phosp in am.				
		- Chest xray in am F/u infiltrate.				
		- EKG in am.				
		- Urine Analysis.				
		- CPK c̄ mb q 8hrs x 3				
		Lopressor 175mg Po qd. Tylenol 650mg				
		Zocar 40 mg Po qd.				
		Premarin 0.625 mg Po qd.				
		Provera 5mg Po qd.				
		Albuterol nebs q4hrs.				
		Atrovent MDI 2puff q6hrs.				
		Solumedrol 40 mg IVPB q6hrs.				
		Cefuroxime 750mg IVPB q8hrs.				
		ASA 325mg Po qd.				

PHARMACY COPY

Exhibit 33

EXHIBIT 33 QUESTIONS

1. Are any cephalosporins ordered among the drugs? If so, what?
2. What should the prescriber be made aware of?
3. List the analgesics being ordered.
4. Are there any allergies that we should be concerned with?
5. Do the dosages of any drugs appear strange? If so, which ones?
6. List the drugs used to control hypercholesteremia.
7. List the drugs used to control hypertension.
8. What is the difference between Albuterol in the neb form and the Atrovent in the MDI form?

PATIENT:
AGE:
SEX:
RACE:
CHART NO.

MEMORIAL HOSPITAL
BALTIMORE, MARYLAND
PHYSICIAN'S ORDER RECORD

BEAR DOWN ON HARD SURFACE WITH BALL POINT PEN

GENERIC EQUIVALENT IS AUTHORIZED UNLESS CHECKED IN THIS COLUMN

ALLERGY OR SENSITIVITY
TO
NONE KNOWN ☐ SIGNED:

DIAGNOSIS

COMPLETED OR DISCONTINUED

DATE	TIME	ORDERS	PHYSICIAN'S SIG.		NAME	DATE	TIME
		DIAGNOSIS RLL PNEUMONIA					
		LUNG CA					
		CONDITION: Stable					
		NKDA					
		Regular diet					
		Room Air (Confirm Sats ≥ 90% q4H)					
		IV KVO.					
		TIMENTIN 3.1 G IV q6H					
		GENTAMICIN 70 mg IV q8H					
		(PEAK & TROUGH c̄ am)					
		ALBUTEROL NEBS UNIT DOSE q6H					

PHARMACY COPY

Exhibit 34

EXHIBIT 34 QUESTIONS

1. What antibiotics are listed?
2. What strength for each antibiotic is listed?
3. How often is each antibiotic to be given?
4. What other drug(s) is listed?
5. What are the directions for those drugs other than the antibiotics?

PATIENT:
AGE:
SEX:
RACE:
CHART NO.

MEMORIAL HOSPITAL
BALTIMORE, MARYLAND
PHYSICIAN'S ORDER RECORD

BEAR DOWN ON HARD SURFACE WITH BALL POINT PEN

GENERIC EQUIVALENT IS AUTHORIZED UNLESS CHECKED IN THIS COLUMN

ALLERGY OR SENSITIVITY
TO
NONE KNOWN ☐ SIGNED:

DIAGNOSIS

COMPLETED OR DISCONTINUED

DATE	TIME	ORDERS	PHYSICIAN'S SIG.		NAME	DATE	TIME
		MAAlux 60 mg P.O x ī now					
		Carafate ī gm p.o. x ī now					
		EKG now [illegible]					

PHARMACY COPY

Exhibit 35

EXHIBIT 35 QUESTIONS

1. For the drugs ordered, list the trade name, generic name, and strengths for each.
2. Do you have any questions that need clarification? If so, what?

PATIENT: AGE: SEX: RACE: CHART NO.	MEMORIAL HOSPITAL BALTIMORE, MARYLAND PHYSICIAN'S ORDER RECORD BEAR DOWN ON HARD SURFACE WITH BALL POINT PEN

GENERIC EQUIVALENT IS AUTHORIZED UNLESS CHECKED IN THIS COLUMN

ALLERGY OR SENSITIVITY TO NONE KNOWN ☐ SIGNED:	DIAGNOSIS		COMPLETED OR DISCONTINUED		
DATE	TIME	ORDERS	PHYSICIAN'S SIG.	NAME	DATE	TIME

DATE	TIME	ORDERS	PHYSICIAN'S SIG.		NAME	DATE	TIME
		② Vit B12 1000 u now IM					
		+ repeat in am					

PHARMACY COPY

Exhibit 36

EXHIBIT 36 QUESTIONS

1. What is another name for Vit B_{12} as written in the order?
2. What strength is ordered?
3. What is wrong with the strength ordered?
4. What strengths are available for this drug?
5. What is this drug used for?
6. What is the route of administration ordered?
7. Are there other routes of administration for this drug? If yes, what are they?

PATIENT:
AGE:
SEX:
RACE:
CHART NO.

MEMORIAL HOSPITAL
BALTIMORE, MARYLAND
PHYSICIAN'S ORDER RECORD

BEAR DOWN ON HARD SURFACE WITH BALL POINT PEN

GENERIC EQUIVALENT IS AUTHORIZED UNLESS CHECKED IN THIS COLUMN

ALLERGY OR SENSITIVITY TO	DIAGNOSIS	COMPLETED OR DISCONTINUED
NONE KNOWN ☐ SIGNED:		

DATE	TIME	ORDERS	PHYSICIAN'S SIG.	NAME	DATE	TIME
		① MILK OF MAGNESIUM 30cc x1 PO				
		② CASCARA 30cc x1 PO				
		③ STAT CT ABDOMEN				
		④ STAT CT PELVIS				
		⑤ CBC STAT AT 6:00 AM				
		⑥ TYPE & CROSS 2 U BLOOD				

PHARMACY COPY

Exhibit 37

EXHIBIT 37 QUESTIONS

1. What drugs are being ordered?
2. What dosages are being ordered?
3. Are the dosages acceptable? If not, what is wrong?
4. What is PO on the order?
5. How often does the physician want the drugs to be given?

PATIENT:
AGE:
SEX:
RACE:
CHART NO.

MEMORIAL HOSPITAL
BALTIMORE, MARYLAND
PHYSICIAN'S ORDER RECORD

BEAR DOWN ON HARD SURFACE WITH BALL POINT PEN

GENERIC EQUIVALENT IS AUTHORIZED UNLESS CHECKED IN THIS COLUMN

ALLERGY OR SENSITIVITY TO ___
NONE KNOWN ☐ SIGNED: ___

DIAGNOSIS

COMPLETED OR DISCONTINUED

DATE	TIME	ORDERS	PHYSICIAN'S SIG.		NAME	DATE	TIME
	11[36] am	Telephone order to give Sudafed 60mg q4-6° PRN & Robitussin q4-6° PRN for cold symptoms					

PHARMACY COPY

Exhibit 38

EXHIBIT 38 QUESTIONS

1. What is Sudafed used for?
2. What is Robitussin used for?
3. What are the generic names for the drugs listed in the order?
4. What are the directions for each drug?

PATIENT:
AGE:
SEX:
RACE:
CHART NO.

MEMORIAL HOSPITAL
BALTIMORE, MARYLAND
PHYSICIAN'S ORDER RECORD

BEAR DOWN ON HARD SURFACE WITH BALL POINT PEN

GENERIC EQUIVALENT IS AUTHORIZED UNLESS CHECKED IN THIS COLUMN

ALLERGY OR SENSITIVITY TO
NONE KNOWN ☐ SIGNED:

DIAGNOSIS

COMPLETED OR DISCONTINUED

DATE	TIME	ORDERS	PHYSICIAN'S SIG.	NAME	DATE	TIME
		Give i colace BID today				
		Start psyllium on 11/22				
		i teaspoon Tid c meals				

PHARMACY COPY

Exhibit 39

EXHIBIT 39 QUESTIONS

1. What is the purpose for using the drugs listed in the order?
2. Are you able to dispense the drugs as written? If not, why not?
3. What class of drugs do the drugs listed in the order belong to?
4. How are these drugs different?
5. Write out the directions for each drug.

PATIENT:
AGE:
SEX:
RACE:
CHART NO.

MEMORIAL HOSPITAL
BALTIMORE, MARYLAND
PHYSICIAN'S ORDER RECORD

BEAR DOWN ON HARD SURFACE WITH BALL POINT PEN

GENERIC EQUIVALENT IS AUTHORIZED UNLESS CHECKED IN THIS COLUMN

ALLERGY OR SENSITIVITY
TO
NONE KNOWN ☐ SIGNED:

DIAGNOSIS

COMPLETED OR DISCONTINUED

DATE	TIME	ORDERS	PHYSICIAN'S SIG.		NAME	DATE	TIME
		① Keflex ṫ PO QID x 14 da.					
		② Soak both ft. 1T Epsom salt or Domboro soltn. per quart warm H_2O x 15 min. QD x 14 da.					
		Thouroughly dry b/w toes c̄ re-apply a small amount of abx ointment to 1 Bil, 2,3,5 Ⓡ, 5 Ⓛ. c̄ DSD.					

PHARMACY COPY

Exhibit 40

EXHIBIT 40 QUESTIONS

1. What is wrong with the Keflex order?
2. What is Epsom salt and Domboro solt'n listed in the order?
3. What is abx ointment?
4. What is the generic name for Keflex?
5. What generation cephalosporin is Keflex?
6. What is the designation 1T in the order?
7. What is H_2O a symbol for in the order?

PATIENT:
AGE:
SEX:
RACE:
CHART NO.

MEMORIAL HOSPITAL
BALTIMORE, MARYLAND
PHYSICIAN'S ORDER RECORD

BEAR DOWN ON HARD SURFACE WITH BALL POINT PEN

GENERIC EQUIVALENT IS AUTHORIZED UNLESS CHECKED IN THIS COLUMN

ALLERGY OR SENSITIVITY
TO
NONE KNOWN ☐ SIGNED:

DIAGNOSIS

COMPLETED OR DISCONTINUED

DATE	TIME	ORDERS	PHYSICIAN'S SIG.	NAME	DATE	TIME
		MOM 30ml +				
		Cascara 5mg P.O. now				
		+ then MOM 30ml P.O. qhs				
		prn for constipation				

PHARMACY COPY

Exhibit 41

EXHIBIT 41 QUESTIONS

1. Write out the order for the medications.

2. Is there a problem with the cascara dose? If so, what?

PATIENT:
AGE:
SEX:
RACE:
CHART NO.

MEMORIAL HOSPITAL
BALTIMORE, MARYLAND
PHYSICIAN'S ORDER RECORD

BEAR DOWN ON HARD SURFACE WITH BALL POINT PEN

GENERIC EQUIVALENT IS AUTHORIZED UNLESS CHECKED IN THIS COLUMN

ALLERGY OR SENSITIVITY
TO: Sulfa, Demerol, Seconal, Tegretol, Procardia, Talwin,
NONE KNOWN ☐ SIGNED:

DIAGNOSIS

COMPLETED OR DISCONTINUED

DATE	TIME	ORDERS	PHYSICIAN'S SIG.	NAME	DATE	TIME

Admit
Stable.
Vitals per routine
All as above
Act. as tol.
Strict I/O's.
Daily wts.
call HO if UOP < 60cc/°.
T&C x 4 units. CBC, chem 20, Mg, Φ,
PT, PTT, EKG, CXR now please.
Clear liquid diet
NPO p midnight. x meds.
Golytely 2L (12oz q15min).
Erythromycin 500mg po @ 11, 1, 5PM.
Neomycin 500mg po @ 11, 1, 5PM.
Fleets enema x 3
then tap water enemas x 3 until stool ru
D5 1/2NS @ 125cc/° after midnight.
Start on heparin 1000U I.V. q h° (no bolus).
Please obtain PT/PTT in 6hrs.
Meds: Synthroid 0.25mg po QD.
✓ Normodyne 200mg ii q AM, i q PM.
✓ Xanax 0.25mg i po TID
Tiazac 360mg i po QD
✓ Vasotec 5mg i po BID.
✓ Colace 100mg i po BID.
✓ Catapres TTS 2 patch i q wk.

Exhibit 42

EXHIBIT 42 QUESTIONS

1. What is the patient allergic to?
2. List all the drugs as written in the order.
3. Which of the drugs acts as a gastrointestinal cleansing agent?
4. Which of the drugs are antibiotics? Are any of them sulfa drugs?
5. What types of Fleets enemas are available?
6. List each drug by its trade name, generic name, use, dosage, and the directions listed.

PATIENT: AGE: SEX: RACE: CHART NO.	MEMORIAL HOSPITAL BALTIMORE, MARYLAND PHYSICIAN'S ORDER RECORD BEAR DOWN ON HARD SURFACE WITH BALL POINT PEN

GENERIC EQUIVALENT IS AUTHORIZED UNLESS CHECKED IN THIS COLUMN

ALLERGY OR SENSITIVITY TO ___ NONE KNOWN ☐ SIGNED: ___	DIAGNOSIS		COMPLETED OR DISCONTINUED

DATE	TIME	ORDERS	PHYSICIAN'S SIG.		NAME	DATE	TIME
		(1) Coumadin 5mg Po tonight					
		(2) Am Lab · CBC, PT/PTT/INR					
		(3) Albuterol nebs q4°					
		(4) Δ BP meds to Am	[signature], MD				
		(5) Triamcinolone Cream					
		to areas BID	/ Strain				

PHARMACY COPY

Exhibit 43

EXHIBIT 43 QUESTIONS

1. What is Coumadin used for?
2. What cream is the doctor prescribing?
3. What are the directions for the use of the cream?
4. What drug is used for respiratory purposes?

PATIENT: AGE: SEX: RACE: CHART NO.	**MEMORIAL HOSPITAL** BALTIMORE, MARYLAND **PHYSICIAN'S ORDER RECORD** BEAR DOWN ON HARD SURFACE WITH BALL POINT PEN

GENERIC EQUIVALENT IS AUTHORIZED UNLESS CHECKED IN THIS COLUMN

ALLERGY OR SENSITIVITY TO NONE KNOWN ☐ SIGNED:	DIAGNOSIS		COMPLETED OR DISCONTINUED

DATE	TIME	ORDERS	PHYSICIAN'S SIG.		NAME	DATE	TIME

DIAGNOSIS: COPD/CHF - TELEMETRY BED
vitals routine + FS bid + Pulsox q 6°
Activity bedrest / Fall risk c̄ bedside commode
Nursing: Strict I's + O's, NHO T>101, SBP >170 or P>130 or <60
Daily wts - 1st one upon Arrival, Bipap 10/5 mmHg @ night only
Diet 2gm Na/day
IV: Heplock
meds. • Lasix 40mg IV upon arrival to floor
• ASA 325mg po qd
• Zocor 10mg po qd
• Albuterol/Atrovent nebs q 4° } 1st one upon arrival to floor!
• Albuterol MDI to bedside
• Prednisone ~~40mg~~ 20mg po qd
• ~~Levo flo Bactrim DS~~ Levofloxacin 500mg po qd
• Humibid 1200mg po bid
• Depakote 500mg po tid • Haldol 2mg IM/IV q4° prn agitation
• Buspar 40mg po tid
• Pepcid 20mg po qday
• Loxapine 25mg po tid
• Maalox 30cc po q6° prn indigestion
• O2 NC 2Liters/hr - Do NOT increase s̄ NHO
• Thiamine 100mg IV qday
labs • CPK c̄ MB q8° x3 • RPR
• valproate serum level • ~~[illegible]~~ NA
• Troponin I + Troponin T level
• 12 lead EKG
• urinalysis
• urine Tox screen

PHARMACY COPY

Exhibit 44

EXHIBIT 44 QUESTIONS

1. What is the patient's diagnosis?
2. Which of the drugs listed have respiratory indications?
3. What is ASA?
4. Why is Albuterol listed twice?
5. What drug is used for hypercholesteremia?
6. Is prednisone ordered for the COPD or CHF?
7. Which drug is indicated for loosening respiratory congestion?
8. Which of the drugs ordered work on the central nervous system?
9. What class of drugs does Levofloxacin belong to?
10. Which of the medications are available as over-the-counter drugs?
11. Which drug is indicated primarily for seizures?
12. Which drug(s) is used for anxiety?
13. Is there a potential problem using Loxapine and the central nervous system drugs together?
14. Which of the drugs may help in managing gastric irritation?

PATIENT:
AGE:
SEX:
RACE:
CHART NO.

MEMORIAL HOSPITAL
BALTIMORE, MARYLAND
PHYSICIAN'S ORDER RECORD

BEAR DOWN ON HARD SURFACE WITH BALL POINT PEN

GENERIC EQUIVALENT IS AUTHORIZED UNLESS CHECKED IN THIS COLUMN

ALLERGY OR SENSITIVITY

TO__________

NONE KNOWN ☐ SIGNED:__________

DIAGNOSIS

DATE	TIME	ORDERS	PHYSICIAN'S SIG.		NAME	DATE	TIME
		8Ø cc po Q6° Simethicone PRN gas pain repeated & verified -					

COMPLETED OR DISCONTINUED

PHARMACY COPY

Exhibit 45

EXHIBIT 45 QUESTIONS

1. What is the drug being ordered by the doctor?
2. In what form is the drug being ordered?
3. What are the directions for its use?
4. What is the dose and how often?
5. How many teaspoonsful makes up each dose?

PATIENT:
AGE:
SEX:
RACE:
CHART NO.

MEMORIAL HOSPITAL
BALTIMORE, MARYLAND
PHYSICIAN'S ORDER RECORD

BEAR DOWN ON HARD SURFACE WITH BALL POINT PEN

GENERIC EQUIVALENT IS AUTHORIZED UNLESS CHECKED IN THIS COLUMN

ALLERGY OR SENSITIVITY
TO
NONE KNOWN ☐ SIGNED:

DIAGNOSIS

COMPLETED OR DISCONTINUED

DATE	TIME	ORDERS	PHYSICIAN'S SIG.		NAME	DATE	TIME
		D/c home 12/6/98 if stable					
		Lansinoh cream to bedside					
		Pt is a thosan candidate					

PHARMACY COPY

Exhibit 46

EXHIBIT 46 QUESTIONS

1. Do you feel clarification is needed for this order?
2. When asked to clarify the order, what do you think the doctor prescribed?

PATIENT:
AGE:
SEX:
RACE:
CHART NO.

MEMORIAL HOSPITAL
BALTIMORE, MARYLAND
PHYSICIAN'S ORDER RECORD

BEAR DOWN ON HARD SURFACE WITH BALL POINT PEN

GENERIC EQUIVALENT IS AUTHORIZED UNLESS CHECKED IN THIS COLUMN

ALLERGY OR SENSITIVITY
TO
NONE KNOWN ☐ SIGNED:

DIAGNOSIS

COMPLETED OR DISCONTINUED

DATE	TIME	ORDERS	PHYSICIAN'S SIG.	NAME	DATE	TIME
		10) Medication: ECASA 325 mg PO qD				
		HCTZ 25 mg PO qD				
		Univasc 7.5 mg BID				
		Claforan 1 gram IV q6°				
		Entex LA PO BID				
		11) CXR PA + LAT please / EKG 12 lead				
		12) LABS CBC w/ man diff, Chem 20, Mg, coags				
		UA, Ctx sputum & Gram stain				
		& Blood Ctx × 2				
		AML (2/15) CBC, Chem 7, Ca, Mg, Ø				
		13) NHO. if SBP>180<90 DBP>110<40				
		P>110<40 R>30<8				
		Temp>101.5°F UO<30 cc/hr × 2 hrs.				
		14) Benadryl 25 mg IV q8° PRN Insomnia				
		15) Tylenol 625 mg PO q4-6° PRN pain				

PHARMACY COPY

Exhibit 47

EXHIBIT 47 QUESTIONS

1. Of the drugs listed in the order, which are antibiotics?
2. Which drug is used primarily to relieve edema?
3. Why is Benadryl, an antihistamine drug, used for insomnia?
4. What is ECASA on the order?
5. What is HCTZ on the order?
6. What is the primary indication for Univasc?
7. Which of the drugs is a combination of two drugs?
8. Which drug is an antibiotic? What class antibiotic is the drug? What class generation is this antibiotic?
9. What is wrong with the Tylenol strength?
10. Write out the directions for each drug.

PATIENT:
AGE:
SEX:
RACE:
CHART NO.

MEMORIAL HOSPITAL
BALTIMORE, MARYLAND
PHYSICIAN'S ORDER RECORD

BEAR DOWN ON HARD SURFACE WITH BALL POINT PEN

GENERIC EQUIVALENT IS AUTHORIZED UNLESS CHECKED IN THIS COLUMN

ALLERGY OR SENSITIVITY
TO
NONE KNOWN ☐ SIGNED:

DIAGNOSIS

COMPLETED OR DISCONTINUED

DATE	TIME	ORDERS	PHYSICIAN'S SIG.		NAME	DATE	TIME
		Prednisone 40mg P.O on 10/26					
		30mg P.o on 10/27					
		20 mg Po on 10/28					
		15mg P.o on 10/29					
		10mg P.o on 10/30					
		5mg Po on 10/31, then D/C					
		Give with food					
		Dietary Consult					
		d/c HIV Viral Load - not in lab, please					
		in process please redraw					
		PPD					

PHARMACY COPY

Exhibit 48

Exhibit 48 Questions

1. What is the drug prescribed by the physician?
2. Why is the dosing written like this?
3. How should this medication be given?
4. What is PPD?

PATIENT: AGE: SEX: RACE: CHART NO.	**MEMORIAL HOSPITAL** BALTIMORE, MARYLAND **PHYSICIAN'S ORDER RECORD** BEAR DOWN ON HARD SURFACE WITH BALL POINT PEN

GENERIC EQUIVALENT IS AUTHORIZED UNLESS CHECKED IN THIS COLUMN

ALLERGY OR SENSITIVITY TO ___ NONE KNOWN ☐ SIGNED: ___	DIAGNOSIS	COMPLETED OR DISCONTINUED

DATE	TIME	ORDERS	PHYSICIAN'S SIG.	NAME	DATE	TIME
		① Multivitamin tablet i tab po qd.				
		② Pentoxifylline 400 mg PO tid				
		③ Zincsulfate 220 mg Po qd.				
		④ Becaplermin 0.01% gel apply sparingly once a day Keep refrigerate				

PHARMACY COPY

Exhibit 49

EXHIBIT 49 QUESTIONS

1. List each drug, its use, and the directions.
2. How should drug item number four be stored?

PATIENT:
AGE:
SEX:
RACE:
CHART NO.

MEMORIAL HOSPITAL
BALTIMORE, MARYLAND
PHYSICIAN'S ORDER RECORD

BEAR DOWN ON HARD SURFACE WITH BALL POINT PEN

GENERIC EQUIVALENT IS AUTHORIZED UNLESS CHECKED IN THIS COLUMN

ALLERGY OR SENSITIVITY	DIAGNOSIS		COMPLETED OR DISCONTINUED
TO			
NONE KNOWN ☐ SIGNED:			

DATE	TIME	ORDERS	PHYSICIAN'S SIG.		NAME	DATE	TIME
① Prilosec 20 mg per KEO ~~po~~ QD - please slurry tablet in orange juice							

PHARMACY COPY

Exhibit 50

Exhibit 50 Questions

1. What is the drug name listed? What is the generic name for this drug?
2. What is the route of administration?
3. What is wrong with the way the drug is to be given?

PATIENT:
AGE:
SEX:
RACE:
CHART NO.

MEMORIAL HOSPITAL
BALTIMORE, MARYLAND
PHYSICIAN'S ORDER RECORD

BEAR DOWN ON HARD SURFACE WITH BALL POINT PEN

GENERIC EQUIVALENT IS AUTHORIZED UNLESS CHECKED IN THIS COLUMN

ALLERGY OR SENSITIVITY	DIAGNOSIS	COMPLETED OR DISCONTINUED
TO____		
NONE KNOWN ☐ SIGNED:____		

DATE	TIME	ORDERS	PHYSICIAN'S SIG.	NAME	DATE	TIME
		Meds: Heparin 5000 U Bolus				
		Heparin Drip @ 1000 U/hr.				
		Tylenol 650 mg po q6° PRN T>101				
		Nifedepine 10 mg SL q6° PRN SBP>180 DBP>100				
		Zantac 50 mg po BID				
		Benadryl 25 mg po q6° + qHS prn insomnia & itching				
		NHO T>101, SBP>180/DBP>100, UO<30cc/hr x4°				

PHARMACY COPY

Exhibit 51

EXHIBIT 51 QUESTIONS

1. What is a bolus of heparin?
2. Why is a bolus of heparin ordered?
3. What other drugs are listed?
4. What is SL?
5. What is the problem with the Zantac order?
6. Write out the directions for each drug.

EXHIBIT 1 ANSWERS

1. ethyl alcohol
2. no known drug allergies
3. notify house officer
   systolic blood pressure
   diastolic blood pressure
   nothing by mouth
   intravenous fluids

EXHIBIT 2 ANSWERS

1. discontinue Unasyn
   increase dopamine to 3 micrograms per drop
   Zofran 8 milligrams intravenous every 8 hours as needed for nausea and vomiting
   Senokot one orally twice a day
2. unasyn—anti-infective to treat susceptible pathogenic organisms
   dopamine—cardiovascular agent used to stimulate receptors of the sypathomimetic nervous system. Indicated for shock caused by hypotensive condition. The drug improves blood flow to vital organs and increases cardiac output.
   Zofran—an antiemetic drug used to prevent nausea and vomiting associated with chemotherapy treatments.
   Senokot—laxative used to stimulate peristalsis in the intestines, thereby resulting in fecal evacuation.
3. Trade names begin in capital letters and generic names in lowercase letters
   Unasyn—ampicillin and sulbactam
   Intropin—dopamine
   Zofran—ondansetron
   Senokot—senna concentrate

EXHIBIT 3 ANSWERS

1. **& 2.** (Brand name drugs listed, followed by their primary indication)
   Toprol XL—hypertension
   Premarin—hormone replacement
   Coumadin—blood thinning agent used in conjunction with deep vein thrombosis (DVT) and cardiovascular conditions such as myocardial infarction (MI)
   Neupogen—stimulates proliferation of neutrophils (a type of white blood cell)
   Procrit—stimulates the production of red blood cells (RBCs)
   Oscal—a calcium supplement
   Compazine—an antiemetic, antinauseant
   Ativan—sedative agent
3. Toprol XL—metoprolol succinate (long acting)
   Premarin—conjugated estrogens
   Coumadin—warfarin
   Neupogen—filgrastim
   Procrit—epoetin alpha, erythropoietin (*Note:* another brand name is Epogen)
   Oscal—calcium carbonate
   Compazine—prochlorperazine
   Ativan—lorazepam
4. sulfa and codeine
5. IV—intravenous
   po—oral
   SQ—subcutaneous
   PR—rectal
6. Vit B_6—pyridoxine
7. MVI is a **M**ultiple **V**itamin **I**nfusion. MVI is often written to represent a multiple vitamin. The route of administration is usually listed such as the oral form (po) in this instance.
8. Procrit is to be given as 10,000 units subcutaneously every Monday, Wednesday, and Friday.
9. The dosage for Neupogen is 480 micrograms (subcutaneously every day).

EXHIBIT 4 ANSWERS

1. Pamelor
   KCl (potassium chloride)
   Tums
2. Pamelor
3. Central nervous system (CNS) drugs, antidepressant agent
4. Tums—Take 500 mg (or one tablet) by mouth (or orally) one time.
5. nortriptyline
6. calcium carbonate
7. Tablets, capsules, and as an oral solution
8. Pamelor—Take one capsule (or tablet) orally 1 hour before sleep.
9. 40 milliequivalents (mEq) (*Note:* This order was verified with the doctor before dispensing the KCl.)
10. KCl—Take 40 milliequivalents by mouth one time.
11. Antacid and calcium supplement

EXHIBIT 5 ANSWERS

1. Complete Blood Count
2. Viscous lidocaine
   Maalox
3. Yes. The order is requesting 5 cc of Viscous lidocaine in 15 cc of Maalox. Each dose will result in a volume of 20 cc.
4. Each 20 cc dose is given four times a day (i.e., every 6 hours) for a total of 80 cc per day. Three days dosing will require 240 cc (80 cc per day times 3 days).
5. The order will require 60 cc of Viscous lidocaine (5 cc every 4 hours for 3 days) and 180 cc of Maalox (15 cc every 4 hours for 3 days).
6. Viscous lidocaine is a topical anesthetic for irritated and inflammed mucosa (mouth and pharynx).
7. Use 20 cc (of the prepared mixture) orally every 6 hours as needed for sore throat.
8. Xylocaine

EXHIBIT 6 ANSWERS

1. Vancomycin
   Cefotaxime
   Amphotericin B
2. Anti-infective agents
3. vancomycin—Vancocin
   cefotaxime—Claforan
   amphotericin B—Fungizone
4. 55.5 hours
5. The patient weighs .940 Kg. The weight should be written as 0.940 Kg to preclude a potential error. We know by our conversion to pounds that the patient does not weigh 940 Kg. Further examination of the original order identified the patient as a premature birth.
6. The patient weighs 2.07 pounds. As noted in question 5, the patient is a premature birth. We could surmise that the doctor did not intend the weight to be 940 Kg because this would make the patient over 2,000 pounds which is extremely unlikely.
7. According to the order, the patient is to receive 0.5 cc per kilogram weight per day (0.5 times 0.940) which equals 0.47 cc per day. Running at 0.9 cc per hour, the total time to run 0.47 cc should be one-half hour. The confusion in the writing of this order prompted a call to the practitioner who subsequently discontinued the order.
8. Vancomycin—Give 14.1 mg intravenously every 18 hours.

   Cefotaxime—Give 47 mg intravenously every 12 hours.

   Amphotericin B—run 0.9 cc per hour for 5 hours.

EXHIBIT 7 ANSWERS

1. metronidazole
2. This anti-infective agent has properties against amoebic organisms, trichomona organisms, and bacterial organisms that cause bacterial vaginosis. This drug also has properties against bacterial anaerobic organisms.
3. Gentamycin (*Note:* Correct spelling is gentamicin.)
4. Serious infections caused by susceptible strains of Pseudomonas aeruginosa, Escherichia coli, Proteus, Klebsiella, Enterobacter, and Staphylococcus.
5. There will be an initial intravenous loading dose of 140 mg, followed by 70 mg intravenously every 8 hours.
6. A loading dose is a priming or first dose given to reduce the time it takes to reach the minimum effective dose for the particular drug. The loading dose is normally a larger amount than the maintenance doses.
7. metronidazole—Flagyl
8. Peak is the maximum drug concentration in the plasma and trough is the low drug concentration in the plasma.

EXHIBIT 8 ANSWERS

(Drug trade names start with capital letters.)

1. verapamil—Calan, Isoptin—antianginal, antiarrhythmic, antihypertensive
   Zantac—ranitidine—histamine H_2-blocker, anti-ulcer agent
   Ativan—lorazepam—antianxiety agent
   Demerol—meperidine—opiate analgesic
   Compazine—prochlorperazine—antinauseant, antiemetic
2. Verapamil—Take 240 mg orally every day. (*Note:* The dosage warranted a call to the practitioner to determine if he or she wanted two tablets of 120 mg each, or a single 240 mg extended release formulation. The result was the single 240 mg extended release capsule every day.)
   Zantac—Give 50 mg intravenously every 8 hours.
   Ativan—Take 1 mg (one tablet) orally every 8 hours.
   Demerol—Give 25 mg intramuscularly every 6 hours as needed.
   Compazine—Give 10 mg intravenously every 8 hours as needed for nausea.
3. Parenterally: Zantac, Demerol, Compazine
   Enterally: verapamil, Ativan
4. short-acting and long-acting (also referred to as sustained release)

EXHIBIT 9 ANSWERS

1. ICU is the Intensive Care Unit
2. Yes. The patient has an allergy to sulfa.
3. "Dx" is a designation for diagnosis.
4. Zantac, pyrimethamine, folinic acid, azithromycin, cefotaxime, heparin
5. Zantac—histamine H_2-blocker indicated for heartburn and ulcers (duodenal and gastric)
   pyrimethamine—antimalarial
   folinic acid—a folic acid derivative that is used, in this case, to prevent hematologic toxicity caused by pyrimethamine. The drug is indicated for any overdose of a folic acid antagonist such as methotrexate or trimethoprim.
   azithromycin—bacterial anti-infective agent of the macrolide variety.
   cefotaxime—bacterial anti-infective agent of the cephalosporin variety (third generation).
   heparin—anticoagulant
6. Zantac—ranitidine
   pyrimethamine—Daraprim
   folinic acid—Leucovorin

azithromycin—Zithromax
cefotaxime—Claforan
heparin—no branded products

7. In this order pyrimethamine is ordered to be given via **N**aso**G**astric **T**ube (NGT).
8. Folinic acid is a form of folic acid that is easily converted in the body to other folic acid compounds. Folic acid (Folvite) is vitamin B_9.
9. Look at the dose. Folic acid is available in doses up to 1 mg. Folinic acid is available in oral form in preparations up to 25 mg and parenteral forms up to 350 mg. Also, the use of pyrimethamine is an indication that there may be a need for folinic acid.
10. The anti-infective drugs are pyrimethamine (malaria), azithromycin (bacteria), and cefotaxime (bacteria).
11. Heparin, in this order, is written to be given subcutaneously (SQ for sub Q). You may also see it written as SC (SubCutaneously).
12. Zantac—Give 50 mg intravenously every 8 hours.
    pyrimethamine—Give 200 mg per nasogastric tube one time, then give 75 mg per nasogastric tube every day.
    folinic acid—Give 10 mg per nasogastric tube every day.
    azithromycin—Give 1 Gm per nasogastric tube for one dose, then give 500 mg per nasogastric tube every day.
    cefotaxime—Give 1 Gm intravenously every 8 hours.
    heparin—Give 5,000 units subcutaneously twice a day.
13. Two liters of 5 percent dextrose in one-half normal saline. *Note:* normal saline is 0.9% saline. Therefore, one-half normal (also called "half" normal saline) is 0.45 percent saline.

EXHIBIT 10 ANSWERS

1. Penicillin 5 million units intravenously now, then 2.4 million units intravenously every 4 hours.
2. Yes, penicillin is a drug that is a bacterial anti-infective. Penicillin belongs to the beta-lactam variety.
3. Penicillin allergy along with a potential for cephalosporin cross-allergenicity.

EXHIBIT 11 ANSWERS

1. Heparin, Tylenol
2. Motrin
3. Tylenol ES (*Note:* ES = extra strength. However, ES is 500 mg, *not* the 650 mg that is being ordered.)
4. (1) Increase heparin to 1,300 units per hour.
   (2) Change Motrin to Tylenol ES 650 mg every 4 hours as needed for pain.
5. Dextrose 5% in normal saline [to run] at 100 cc per hour for 1 liter. (*Note:* At 100 cc per hour, 1 liter should last for 10 hours.)
6. Heparin—anticoagulant drug
   Motrin—analgesic and anti-inflammatory (*Note:* This drug belongs to a class of drugs called nonsteroidal anti-inflammatory drugs or NSAIDs. This class of drugs is very irritating to the stomach lining and may cause ulceration.)
   Tylenol ES—analgesic drug used for pain and an antipyretic used to lower body temperature. (*Note:* As noted, the ES is 500 mg.)

EXHIBIT 12 ANSWERS

1. Allergy: **N**o **K**nown **D**rug **A**llergies
2. Yes. Dig (pronounced "dij") is the shortened version of digoxin.
3. Generic name
4. Nitropaste is nitroglycerin in an ointment formulation.

5. Zantac is a histamine H_2-blocking agent used to suppress gastric acids and thereby prevent heartburn and to prevent duodenal or gastric ulcers.
6. Maalox is an **o**ver-**t**he-**c**ounter (OTC) drug obtainable without a prescription.
7. Colace—docusate sodium
8. The patient appears to have a cardiovascular ailment. The bulk of drugs ordered (dig, captopril, Lasix, and nitropaste) support this conclusion.
9. Tylenol is a drug that is listed, but not included with all the other drugs on the order.
10. dig (or digoxin)—Lanoxin—Take 0.25 mg (one tablet) every day.
    captopril—Capoten—Take 25 mg (one tablet) every 8 [*hours* is understood]
    Lasix—furosemide—Give 40 mg intravenously every day. (Today's dose given in the intensive care unit)
    nitropaste—NITROL—Apply 1 inch [of ointment] every 6 [*hours* is understood]. (Hold 12 midnight dose)
    Zantac—ranitidine—Take 150 mg (one capsule) orally twice a day.
    Maalox—aluminum hydroxide, magnesium hydroxide—Take 30 cc (2 tablespoonsful) between meals and at bedtime.
    Colace—docusate—Take 100 mg (one capsule) orally every day.
    Tylenol—acetaminophen—Take two tablets orally as needed for pain. (*Note:* No strength is listed.)

EXHIBIT 13 ANSWERS

1. The patient is allergic to morphine.
2. Morphine is an opiate analgesic. It is a narcotic.
3. Yes. Morphine was ordered for the patient although the patient has an allergy to morphine.
4. Milk of magnesia and Peri-Colace will prevent the constipating effects associated with narcotics.
5. Yes. Dalmane is available in 15 mg and 30 mg strengths.
6. Morphine sulfate was discontinued because the patient is allergic to the drug.
7. Morphine is being replaced with Demerol and Vistaril.
8. This combination is common because Vistaril enhances the analgesic effects of Demerol.
9. morphine sulfate—multiple trade names—Give 8 to 10 mg subcutaneously every 3 hours as needed for pain.
   Percocet—oxycodone + acetaminophen—Take one or two tablets orally every 3 hours as needed for pain.
   Milk of magnesia (MOM)—milk of magnesia—Take 30 cc (2 tablespoonsful) orally at bedtime as needed.
   Dalmane—flurazepam—Take 15 mg (one capsule) by mouth at bedtime as needed for sleep.
   Peri-Colace—docusate sodium + casanthranol—Take one tablet (actually in capsule form) orally twice a day.
   Demerol—meperidine—Give 100 mg intramuscularly every 3 hours as needed for pain.
   Vistaril—hydroxyzine—Give 25 mg intramuscularly every 3 hours as needed for pain.

EXHIBIT 14 ANSWERS

1. NHO is an acronym to **N**otify **H**ouse **O**fficer.
2. The symbol ">" means "greater than" and "<" means "less than."
3. Amiodarone, cefepime, Digoxin, Allopurinol, Hydroxyurea, Megace, Oxycontin, and Roxicet
4. Oxycontin is a brand name version for oxycodone, an opiate analgesic.
   Roxicet is a brand name version for a combination drug comprised of **oxy**codone + **acet**aminophen.
5. The doctor has ordered Oxycontin with directions for every 12 hours. The usual dose for short acting Oxycontin is every 6 hours. The short acting form of the drug is available in only one strength while the long acting (i.e., controlled-release) form is available in a variety of strengths ranging from 10 mg to 80 mg. Clarify the doctor's intent by calling to determine what form (short acting or controlled-release), the strength, and verification of the directions. Also, since

both drugs contain oxycodone, does the doctor want both drugs? The answer is probably yes because Roxicet is on an "as needed" regime to supplement the Oxycontin if it falls short of its analgesic effect.

6. There are 3 grams in 3,000 mg.
7. The drug is written on the order as 40 mg per milliliter. Therefore, each 20 cc will contain 800 mg of Megace. The daily dose is 20 cc orally every day. Therefore, the daily dose will be 800 mg.
8. amiodarone—oral
cefepime—intravenous
digoxin—oral
allopurinol—oral
hydroxyurea—oral
Megace—oral
Oxycontin—oral
Roxicet—oral
9. amiodarone—Cordarone—Take 200 mg (one tablet) orally every day.
cefepime—Maxipime—Give 2 grams intravenously every 12 hours.
digoxin—Lanoxin—Take 0.125 mg (one tablet) orally every day.
allopurinol—Zyloprim—Take 300 mg (one tablet) orally every morning.
hydroxyurea—Hydrea—Take 3,000 mg (six capsules at 500 mg per capsule) orally every day.
Megace—megestrol acetate (*Note:* **Meg**estrol + **ace**tate)—Take 20 cc (4 teaspoonsful) orally every day.
Oxycontin—oxycodone—Take one tablet orally every 12 hours.
Roxicet—oxycodone + acetaminophen—Take one or two tablets orally every 4 to 6 hours as needed.
10. At the dose ordered for Megace, the use may be as an appetite stimulant in AIDS patients. Megace is also an antineoplastic drug which may be the more likely use in this case because the drug is being used in conjunction with hydroxyurea which is another antineoplastic drug.

EXHIBIT 15 ANSWERS

1. Glucotrol XL, Zantac, Zestril, Premarin, Dilaudid, Compazine, Tylenol, MOM
2. Dilaudid and Tylenol
3. Zantac is a histamine H_2-blocking agent used to suppress gastric acidity. Zestril is a cardiovascular drug of the ACE-inhibitor variety used for hypertension and as adjunctive treatment in heart failure.
4. Compazine is indicated for nausea.
5. Glucotrol—Take 5 mg (one tablet) orally every day.
Zantac—Take 150 mg (one tablet) orally twice a day.
Zestril—Take 10 mg (one tablet) orally every day. (*Note:* Prinivil is another brand name product for lisinopril.)
Premarin—Take 0.625 mg (one tablet) orally every day.
Dilaudid—Give 1 mg intravenously every 4 to 6 hours as needed for pain.
Compazine—Give 5 mg intravenously every 4 to 6 hours as needed for nausea and vomiting.
Tylenol—Take 650 mg (two tablets) orally every 4 to 6 hours as needed for pain and fever greater than 101 degrees.
MOM—Take 30 cc (2 tablespoonsful) orally every day.
6. Glucotrol XL—glipizide extended release—hypoglycemic agent used for diabetes. (*Note:* Do not confuse drug with another hypoglycemic agent named glyburide [Diabeta, Micronase, Glynase Prestab])
Zantac—ranitidine—used to suppress gastric acid production
Zestril—lisinopril—used primarily to control hypertension
Premarin—conjugated estrogens—hormone supplementation
Dilaudid—hydromorphone—used to suppress pain (*Note:* hydromorphone is a controlled drug, C-II)
Compazine—prochlorperazine—used to control nausea and vomiting
Tylenol—acetaminophen—used to eleviate pain (analgesic) and to reduce fever (antipyretic)
MOM—milk of magnesia or magnesium hydroxide—used as a laxative

EXHIBIT 16 ANSWERS

1. FS AC & HS is a series of acronyms for **F**asting **S**ugar before meals and at bedtime.
2. NPH represents a long-acting type of insulin.
3. SSI stands for Sliding Scale Insulin.
4. The first numbers such as 200–250 and 251–300 indicate blood glucose readings. The units numbers (e.g., 2 units, 4 units) represent the amount of insulin needed to be administered for the associated blood glucose level.
5. The order is written for Timentin, insulin (NPH type), Demerol, and Vistaril.
6. Timentin—bacterial anti-infective (beta-lactam type) used to treat infection caused by susceptible bacterial organisms.
   NPH (insulin)—used to treat high blood sugar (glucose) levels.
   Demerol—an opiate analgesic used to eleviate pain.
   Vistaril—a sedative and anti-anxiety agent used in conjunction with Demerol to achieve a better response to relieving pain.
7. Yes, because Vistaril is written to be given intravenously. Vistaril should be administered only by the intramuscular route.
8. Yes. Normal saline with 20 milliequivalents of potassium chloride added is a liter (also referred to as large volume) bottle.
9. Two. Regular insulin will be needed for the sliding scale insulin treatments (if needed) and the long-acting NPH insulin has a regular schedule of 37 units in the morning and 17 units in the evening. (*Note:* insulin measurement is in units and the drug is administered through an insulin syringe specifically designed to accommodate the unit measurement.)

EXHIBIT 17 ANSWERS

1. cefotaxime, Lasix, Zaroxolyn
2. cefotaxime—Claforan—Give 1 gram intravenously every 8 hours.
   Lasix—furosemide—Give 100 milligrams intravenously one time.
   Zaroxolyn—metolazone—Give 10 mg intravenously one time.
3. Call the practitioner to clarify the route of administration for Zaroxolyn which is available only by mouth.

EXHIBIT 18 ANSWERS

1. Two liters (also, 2,000 milliliters or cc's) of normal saline (also known as physiologic saline and 0.9 percent saline) are being ordered.
2. insulin (regular)—Regular Iletin II, Humulin R, Novolin R
   clonidine—Catapres (oral route of administration) (*Note:* There is a Catapres-TTS which is a transdermal route of administration)
   Prinivil—lisinopril
   ECASA (This is an acronym for **e**nteric **c**oated **a**cetyl**s**alicylic **a**cid or enteric coated aspirin)—Ecotrin
   metoprolol—Lopressor
3. insulin (regular)—Insulin Sliding Scale
   clonidine—Take 0.2 mg (one tablet) orally every day twice a day. (*Note:* After clarification of the confusing directions with the physician, it was understood that the physician meant the patient to take the medication twice a day, every day, and not to miss any days.)
   Prinivil—Take 20 mg (one tablet) orally every day.
   ECASA—Take 325 mg (one tablet) orally every day.
   metoprolol—Take 50 mg (one tablet) orally twice a day.

EXHIBIT 19 ANSWERS

1. NPO is nothing by mouth.
2. None. All the drugs are brand or trade names for generics.
3. All the drugs are a brand name for the generic: Solu-Cortef, Flagyl, Demerol, Vistaril, Zantac
4. Solu-Cortef—Give 100 milligrams intravenously every 8 hours.
   Flagyl—Give 500 milligrams intravenously every 8 hours.
   Demerol—Give 50 [milligrams] intramuscularly every 3 to 4 hours as needed for pain.
   Vistaril—Give 50 milligrams intramuscularly every 3 to 4 hours as needed for pain.
   Zantac—Give 50 milligrams every 12 hours. (*Note:* We can be assured that the practitioner wants the parenteral route of administration because the parenteral form is available as 50 mg, the prescription oral form is available as 150 mg, all the other medications are in the parenteral form, and finally, the order explicitly notes "NPO."
5. Solu-Cortef—a corticosteroid has properties to reduce inflammation. Other uses include treatment for shock and adrenal insufficiency.
   Flagyl—an amoebic and protozoal anti-infective agent used to treat infections caused by susceptible organisms.
   Demerol—an opiate narcotic analgesic used to eleviate pain
   Vistaril—a sedative and antianxiety agent often used as an adjunct to Demerol in order to achieve a better response to pain treatment.
   Zantac—a histamine H_2-blocker used to suppressive the production of gastric acid, thereby used to treat or prevent duodenal or gastric ulcers

EXHIBIT 20 ANSWERS

1. This combination suggests that one drug potentially causes gastric ulceration and the other drug has the role to prevent the unwanted side effect of the first drug.
2. Naprosyn (correct spelling)—**N**on-**S**teroidal **A**nti-**I**nflammatory **D**rug (NSAID)
   Prilosec (correct spelling)—gastric acid (proton) pump inhibitor
3. Prilosec must be swallowed whole. The capsules should not be opened, crushed, or chewed.
4. Patients should take NSAIDs, such as Prilosec, with food or milk to prevent gastric upset. Each dose should be taken with a full glass of water.
5. Naprosyn 500 mg
   Prilosec 20 mg
6. BD is the designation for twice a day. BD is the same as BID.

EXHIBIT 21 ANSWERS

1. Toradol—ketorolac—Give 30 mg intravenously every 6 hours.
   phenobarbitone (*Note:* same as phenobarbital)—Luminal—Take 30 mg (one tablet) orally twice a day.
   Dilantin—phenytoin—Take 100 mg (one capsule) orally 3 times a day.
   Dilantin—phenytoin—Take 300 mg (three capsules) orally immediately.
   Dilantin—phenytoin—Take 300 mg (three capsules) orally every bedtime.
   gentamicin—Garamycin—Give 550 mg intravenously every day.
   Unasyn—ampicillin + sulbactam—Give 1.5 grams intravenously every 6 hours.
2. Toradol—relieve pain and reduce inflammation
   phenobarbitone—sedation
   Dilantin—seizures
   gentamicin—bacterial anti-infective (aminoglycoside variety) used to treat infecitons by susceptible organisms
   Unasyn—bacterial anti-infective (beta lactam variety) used to treat infections by susceptible organisms

3. Toradol—nonsteroidal anti-inflammatory drugs (NSAIDs)
   phenobarbitone—sedative/hypnotics
   Dilantin—antiseizures, antiepileptic
   gentamicin—anti-infective
   Unasyn—anti-infective
4. Four liters of the large volume intravenous fluids will provide 4,000 milliliters.
5. The large stat dose is a loading dose prescribed to reduce the onset time to achieve the minimum effective dose of the drug. The smaller dose is the usual maintenance dose for the drug.

EXHIBIT 22 ANSWERS

1. Milk of magnesia ("MOM") and cascara (also written as cascara sagrada)
2. MOM—30 cc (2 tablespoonsful)
   cascara—15 cc (1 tablespoonful)
3. Each drug will be given only once.

EXHIBIT 23 ANSWERS

1. Cardizem CD and Norvasc belong to the cardiovascular group of drugs.
2. Equivalent refers to any drug that will provide the same therapeutic outcome. For example, Cardizem CD is a calcium channel blocker. Norvasc (amlodipine) is also a calcium channel blocker. The order is confusing since two therapeutically equivalent drugs have been ordered. The prescriber should be contacted for clarification.
3. Atrovent puffs refer to inhalation orally.
4. Yes. Six puffs every 6 hours provides 24 puffs in a 24-hour peroid. The total number of inhalations for Atrovent should not exceed 12 inhalations during a 24-hour peroid. The prescriber should be called to clarify the directions.
5. Prilosec is the brand name for omeprazole.
6. Atrovent is the brand name for ipratropium
7. Prilosec is a gastric acid (proton) pump inhibitor used as an antiulcer agent.
8. Atrovent is available as an aerosol, solution (for nebulizers), and nasal spray.

EXHIBIT 24 ANSWERS

1. minoxidil 7.5 mg (3 × 2.5 mg tablets)
2. Tenormin (intravenous)
   Lanoxin (intravenous)
3. minoxidil—Loniten—Take 7.5 mg (3 × 2.5 mg tablets) by mouth every day.
   Coumadin—warfarin—Hold Coumadin 5 mg one tablet.
   Tenormin—atenolol—Take 50 mg (one tablet) every day. (*Note:* bid was crossed out.)
   Lanoxin—digoxin—Take 0.125 mg (one tablet) daily.
   Nizoral—ketoconazole—no directions other than "ringworm area." Usual directions would be "Apply to ringworm area XX times a day." An "External Use Only" auxiliary label should be placed on the dispensed prescription. Contact the prescriber to clarify the directions.
   Propine—dipivefrin—Instill eyedrop twice a day. (*Note:* How many drops and to which eye or eyes? Contact the prescriber for clarification.)
   Timoptic—timolol—Instill eyedrop twice a day. See note under Propine.
   Pilocar—pilocarpine—Instill four times a day. See note under Propine.
   Procardia XL—nifedipine extended release—Take 60 mg (one tablet) twice a day.

EXHIBIT 25 ANSWERS

1. Colace and Senokot (correct spelling for Sinokott)
2. Both drugs are laxatives. Why are two laxatives being ordered before seeing if either one will work?
3. Colace—docusate (sodium)
   Senokot—senna concentrate
4. Colace—Take two tablets of 100 mg each orally twice a day for 1 day. More appropriately written as: Take two capsules orally twice a day for 1 day.
   Senokot—Take one or two tablets orally twice a day for 1 day.

EXHIBIT 26 ANSWERS

1. No.
2. The physician really meant Curel therapeutic moisturizing lotion.
3. Dispense one tube.
4. The preparation should have a "For External Use Only" auxiliary label attached to the product.
5. Curel is an emollient/moisturizing preparation which helps to rehydrate and soften dry skin. The product is over-the-counter (OTC) and does not require a prescription.

EXHIBIT 27 ANSWERS

1. No. Rythmol (propafenone) is the correct spelling for Rhthmol.
2. Rythmol (antiarrhythmic agent) and Nitro-bid (anti-anginal) are cardiovascular drugs.
3. Paxil (paroxetine) is an antidepressant drug and includes uses for **O**bsessive-**C**ompulsive **D**isorders (OCD), panic disorder, and social anxiety disorder.
   Taxol (paclitaxel) is an antineoplastic drug indicated for ovarian cancer and breast cancer. (*Note:* Poor legibility of the drugs may cause confusion. Be careful.)

EXHIBIT 28 ANSWERS

1. NKDA is the acronym for **N**o **K**nown **D**rug **A**llergies.
2. I's is the intake. This refers to the amount of fluid intake measured for a patient. O's refer to the output or the measurement of fluid (urine) eliminated by the patient.
3. HL is the acronym for **H**eparin **L**ock. Heparin locks are heparin flushes (blood anticoagulating agents) to clean blood from intravenous tubes hooked to patients.
4. Yes. The correct spelling for the drug is Pravachol.
5. Yes. I would be curious to know why both Pravachol and Lescol were ordered for the same patient. Both drugs are hypolipidemic agents.
6. Clonidine is available in 0.1 mg, 0.2 mg, and 0.3 mg tablets. Clonidine is also available as transdermal patches that provide 0.1 mg/24 hours, 0.2 mg/24 hours, and 0.3 mg/24 hours. The order calls for a clonidine 0.3 mg tablet.
7. Trental is the correct spelling for Terental.
8. Pravachol—pravastatin—Take 40 mg (one tablet) orally every bedtime. (hypolipidemic agent)
   Zestril—lisinopril—Take 40 mg (one tablet) orally every day. (antihypertensive agent)
   Norvasc—amlodipine—Take 10 mg (one tablet) orally twice a day. (antihypertensive, anti-anginal agent)
   Lasix—furosemide—Take 40 mg (one tablet) orally every day. (diuretic)
   Nitro-dur—nitroglycerin—0.6 mg orally every day. (anti-anginal agent) (*Note:* This order was written incorrectly. Nitroglycerin is

available as 0.6 mg patch in strength for daily use. The 0.6 mg transdermal patch provides a release rate for nitroglycerin of 0.6 mg per hour. Nitroglycerin sublingual tablets are scheduled very differently and not used in a maintenance manner. Oral nitroglycerin is available as tablets and capsules in doses ranging from 2.5 mg to 13 mg. The prescriber surely meant to write for the nitroglycerin 0.6 mg patch.)
clonidine—Catapres—Take 0.3 mg (one tablet) orally every day. (antihypertensive agent)
Lescol—fluvastatin—Take 40 mg (one capsule) orally every day. (hyplipidemic agent)
Trental—pentoxifylline—Take 400 mg (one tablet) orally before each meal. (hemorrheologic agent—improves capillary blood flow)
Beclovent—beclomethasone—Take two puffs every 6 hours. (respiratory corticosteroid agent)
albuterol—Proventil, Ventolin—Take two puffs every 6 hours as needed. (bronchodilator)
Percocet—oxycodone + acetaminophen—Take one or two tablets orally every 4 hours as needed for pain. (analgesic)

EXHIBIT 29 ANSWERS

1. Regranex cream is discontinued. (*Note:* Regranex is actually a gel.)
2. Regranex is a brand name for the generic drug becaplermin.
3. Santy cream is replacing the Regranex. (*Note:* The correct spelling is Santyl and the product is an ointment.)
4. Santyl ointment (collangenase) is ordered for 3 days.
5. Santyl ointment—Apply twice a day for 3 days.

EXHIBIT 30 ANSWERS

1. Three.
2. Three. K-Dur, Mg Oxide, and Percocet
3. Only the PCA (**p**atient **c**ontrolled **a**nalgesia) is being discontinued. PCA is a pump containing an analgesic such as morphine or meperidine. However, we do not know what analgesic is being used for the pump.
4. PCA is **p**atient-**c**ontrolled **a**nalgesia, which is administered through a pump.
5. Yes. The PCA and Percocet are used therapeutically to relieve pain.
6. The K in KDUR represents potassium.
7. The Mg in MgOxide represents magnesium.
8. K-DUR—Take 30 milliequivalents (3 × 10 mEq tablets) orally twice a day today.
9. Yes. The MgOxide requires clarification because the dosages available are 140 mg capsules, 400 mg tablets, 420 tablets, and 500 mg tablets.
10. Percocet—Take one or two tablets orally every 4 to 6 hours as needed for pain.

EXHIBIT 31 ANSWERS

1. ECASA and Motrin
2. The strength has been omitted for ECASA. Motrin 650 mg.
3. Yes. We need to know the strength the prescriber for ECASA. We must also clarify the strength for Motrin because there is no 650 mg dose available.
4. ECASA is the acronym for **E**nteric **C**oated **A**cetyl**S**alicylic **A**cid.
5. Both drugs are anti-inflammatory analgesics. However, ECASA in low doses seems to prevent the aggregation of blood platelets. ECASA also has an antipyretic action (lowering of body temperature).

6. Motrin is a **n**on-**s**teroidal **a**nti-**i**nflammatory **d**rug (NSAID).
7. Yes. Motrin should be taken with food or milk. An auxiliary label to this effect should be attached to the dispensed product.

EXHIBIT 32 ANSWERS

1. Naproxen is the generic name for the trade product, Naprosyn.
   Naproxen sodium can be found under the trade names of Aleve and Anaprox.
2. Naproxen belongs to the class of **n**on-**s**teroidal **a**nti-**i**nflammatory **d**rugs (NSAIDs).
3. The drug is used for inflammatory conditions (e.g., arthritis, bursitis, tendinitis) and pain.
4. Naproxen—Take 200 mg orally twice a day as needed for headache. (*Note:* Naproxen is a prescription drug available in strengths of 250 mg, 375 mg, and 500 mg. However, naproxen "sodium," under the brand name Aleve, is an over-the-counter (OTC) product containing 220 mg of naproxen sodium of which there is 200 mg of naproxen. Clarify what the prescriber intended.
5. This drug should be taken after meals or with milk to prevent gastric irritation and potential ulceration.

EXHIBIT 33 ANSWERS

1. Yes. Cefuroxime (Zinacef, Kefurox) is a second generation cephalosporin.
2. The patient has a penicillin (PCN, acronym for penicillin) allergy. Cephalosporins should be used cautiously in patients with penicillin sensitivity or allergy because of a potential for cross-allergenicity between penicillin and cephalosporins.
3. Tylenol (acetaminophen) and ASA (**a**cetyl**s**alicylic **a**cid or aspirin) are the only listed medications with analgesic properties.
4. The patient has a penicillin (PCN) allergy.
5. At first glance, Lopressor seems to have a strange dose at 175 mg. However, the effective dose range is between 100 mg and 400 mg daily.
6. Zocor (simvastatin) is a hypolipidemic agent.
7. Lopressor (metoprolol) is an antihypertensive agent.
8. Albuterol (Proventil, Ventolin) in neb (abbreviated for nebule) form must be mixed in a vehicle such as saline and administered through an inhalation machine called a nebulizer. Atrovent (ipratropium) in an MDI (**m**etered **d**ose **i**nhaler) form requires no mixing of the drug in any vehicle. The drug is self-contained in an aerosolized container that emits a premeasured amount of drug with each spray or puff.

EXHIBIT 34 ANSWERS

1. Timentin (ticarcillin/clavulanate) (beta-lactam variety), gentamicin (Garamycin) (aminoglycoside variety)
2. Timentin 0.15 (*Note:* Order requires clarification. Timentin is available as a 3.1 gram product. The 0.15 has no meaning in this order without clarification. A follow-up was done with the practitioner verifying the 0.15 actually being poor legibility for 3.1G which is the traditional dose for the drug.)
   gentamicin—70 mg
3. Timentin—Give intravenously every 6 hours.
   gentamicin—Give 70 mg intravenously every 8 hours.
4. The practitioner has also ordered albuterol nebs.
5. Albuterol nebs—Use one unit dose every 6 hours.

EXHIBIT 35 ANSWERS

1. Maalox—magnesium hydroxide/aluminum hydroxide—60 mg (*Note:* Maalox suspension is measured by volume such as 15 cc or ml, 30 cc or ml. In each teaspoonful or 5 cc, there is 200 mg of magnesium hydroxide and 225 mg of aluminum hydroxide.)
   Carafate—sucralfate—1 gram
2. Yes. A call to the prescriber is needed to clarify the dose for Maalox.

EXHIBIT 36 ANSWERS

1. Vit B_{12} is also known as cyanocobalamine (Rubramin PC).
2. The doctor ordered 1,000 units.
3. Cyanocobalamine is measured in micrograms (mcg).
4. Cyanocobalamine is available in a variety of doses for the tablet form from 25 mcg to 1,000 mcg and in injection form as 1,000 mcg.
5. The primary indications for Vit B_{12} are deficiency of the vitamin, malabsorption of the vitamin, and pernicious anemia.
6. The route of administration is intramuscularly.
7. The drug may also be administered subcutaneously. Tablets indicate that the drug may also be taken orally.

EXHIBIT 37 ANSWERS

1. Milk of magnesia (MOM) and cascara are being ordered.
2. The practitioner is requesting 30 cc (2 tablespoonsful) of milk of magnesia and 50 cc of cascara.
3. No. The milk of magnesia is an appropriate dose. However, 50 cc of cascara is 10 times the usual dose. (*Note:* A follow-up clarification call revealed that the order which was faxed to the pharmacy did not pick up the decimal point after the number 5. The prescriber in fact did order 5.0 cc.)
4. The PO is the acronym for the Latin phrase meaning "by mouth."
5. The physician wants only a one-time dose for each drug.

EXHIBIT 38 ANSWERS

1. Sudafed is used as a nasal decongestant.
2. Robitussin is used as an expectorant.
3. Sudafed—pseudoephedrine
   Robitussin—guaifenesin, glyceryl guaiacolate (sometimes referred to as GG.)
4. Sudafed—Take 60 mg (one tablet) every 4 to 6 hours as needed.
   Robitussin—Take ?? every 4 to 6 hours as needed for cold symptoms. (*Note:* No dose was provided. Therefore, a clarification call is required. The usual dose for Robitussin is 100 mg to 400 mg orally every 4 hours. The syrup contains 100 mg per 5 ml (5 ml or 5 cc = 1 teaspoonful). There is also a solid long-acting capsule form known by the brand name Humibid. Humibid is available in 300 mg and 600 mg capsules. The usual schedule is 600 mg to 1,200 mg every 12 hours by mouth.

EXHIBIT 39 ANSWERS

1. Both Colace and psyllium are used to relieve constipation.
2. No. Colace does not have a dose listed. The drug is available as a 50 mg and 100 mg strength capsule. Also, the instructions do not make clear if a capsule or liquid form is wanted.
3. Both drugs are laxativs. Colace is a stool softener. Psyllium is a bulk laxative.
4. Colace acts to soften stools by reducing surface tension of the liquid contents of the bowel. Psyllium works by absorbing water, thereby expanding the bulk content which stimulates peristalsis (bowel movement).
5. Colace—Give one Colace twice a day today. psyllium—Take 1 teaspoonful three times a day with meals. (*Note:* Each teaspoonful should be added to a full glass of water before ingestion. Also, follow with a full glass of water.)

EXHIBIT 40 ANSWERS

1. Keflex has no dose associated with it.
2. Epsom salts is magnesium sulfate. Epsom salts has multiple uses such as a saline laxative and a soak. As a soak, the magnesium sulfate provides a soothing feeling for relief of minor irritations of the skin. Epsom salts can be purchased without a prescription.
   Domeboro solution contains the active ingredient aluminum acetate. The solution is an astringent. The solution is used for temporary relief of minor skin irritations. The product is sold over-the-counter (OTC).
3. The abx ointment refers to antibiotic ointment.
4. Keflex—cephalexin
5. Keflex is a first generation cephalosporin.
6. The practitioner is requesting *one tablespoonful* (1 T).
7. The H_2O is the symbol for water.

EXHIBIT 41 ANSWERS

1. Milk of magnesia 30 ml and cascara 5 mg orally now. And then milk of magnesia 30 ml orally every bedtime as needed for constipation. The appropriate version for the patient states:

   Take 2 tablespoonsful of milk of magnesia and 1 teaspoonful of cascara orally now. Then, take 2 tablespoonsful of milk of magnesia by mouth before every bedtime when needed for constipation.
2. Yes. The order has the dose in mg when cascara is measured by volume such as cc or ml.

EXHIBIT 42 ANSWERS

1. The patient is allergic to sulfa, Demerol, Seconal, Tegretol, Procardia, and Talwin.
2. Golytely, erythromycin, neomycin, heparin, Synthroid, Normodyne, Xanax, Tiazac, Vasotec, Colace, Catapres
3. Golytely (polyethylene glycol and electrolyte solution) (*Note:* erythromycin and neomycin scheduled in this manner will provide a gut sterilization prior to an intestinal surgery. The Fleets enema and tap water enema will also assist in cleaning out the bowel.)
4. erythromycin (*Note:* There is a variety of brand name drugs depending on the erythromycin salt.) and neomycin
5. Fleet enemas are available without a prescription as disposable enemas containing monobasic

sodium phosphate and dibasic sodium biphosphate, and as a mineral oil-containing enema. The former ready-to-use enema functions as a laxative and bowel cleanser. The latter ready-to-use enema is used to soften and lubricate the bowel content. Other enemas are available that contain stool softeners such as docusate sodium or bisacodyl.

6. Golytely—polyethylene glycol + electrolyte solution—osmotic laxative agent used to prepare a bowel before a gastrointestinal examination—2 liters, Drink 12 ounces every 15 minutes.
   erythromycin—multiple brand names—bacterial anti-infective agent (macrolide variety)—bactericidal to susceptible organisms—500 mg—Take 500 mg (one tablet) orally at 11 A.M., 1 P.M., and 5 P.M. (*Note:* The erythromycin base is the form of choice for gut sterilization.)
   neomycin—primarily generic versions—bacterial anti-infective agent (aminoglycoside variety)—bactericidal to susceptible organisms—500 mg—Take 500 mg (one tablet) orally at 11 A.M., 1 P.M., and 5 P.M. (*Note:* Neomycin is used in conjunction with erythromycin for gut sterilization.)
   heparin—only generic versions—anticoagulation therapy—dosage depends on the results of prothrombin time lab results (measure of clotting time)—Run 1,000 units intravenously every hour (no bolus). (*Note:* No bolus is required because the physician determined that there is no need to achieve a minimum effective dose as soon as possible.)
   Synthroid—levothyroxine—thyroid hormone replacement therapy—doses are available ranging from 25 mcg (micrograms) to 300 mcg. (*Note:* A parenteral form is also available.)—Take 0.25 mg (2 × 125 mcg tablets) orally every day. (*Note:* The dose should be clarified to be assured that the prescriber intends the patient to take 250 mcg which is equivalent to 0.25 mg.)
   Normodyne (also Trandate)—labetalol—antihypertensive agent—tablets are available in 100 mg, 200 mg, and 300 mg. Parenteral form is available as 5 milligrams per 1 milliliter (5 mg/ml)—Take 400 mg (2 × 200 mg tablets) every morning and 200 mg (1 × 200 mg tablet) every evening.
   Xanax—alprazolam—antianxiety agent—tablets are available as 0.25 mg, 0.5 mg, 1 mg, and 2 mg—Take 0.25 mg (one tablet) orally three times a day.
   Tiazac (various other brand names)—diltiazem—antihypertensive agent—available as extended release capsules in doses of 120 mg, 180 mg, 240 mg, 300 mg, 360 mg, and 420 mg—Take 360 mg (one capsule) orally every day.
   Vasotec—enalapril—antihypertensive agent—Tablets are available in 2.5 mg, 5 mg, 10 mg, and 20 mg doses—Take 5 mg (one tablet) orally every day.
   Colace—docusate—stool softening agent—Capsules in 50 mg and 100 mg doses are available—Take 100 mg (one capsule) orally twice a day.
   Catapres (tablet), Catapres-TTS (transdermal patches)—clonidine—antihypertensive agent—Tablets are available in 0.1 mg, 0.2 mg, and 0.3 mg strengths. Transdermal patches are available as 0.1, 0.2, and 0.3 mg release rates per 24 hours—Apply 0.2 patch (1 × 0.2 mg patch) every night.

EXHIBIT 43 ANSWERS

1. Coumadin (warfarin) is an anticoagulation agent used to thin blood.
2. The doctor is writing for triamcinolone cream. (*Note:* The strength of the cream has been omitted. The cream is available in strengths of 0.025%, 0.1%, and 0.5%. Call the doctor for a strength.)
   Triamcinolone is also available in other forms. You can find triamcinolone as an inhalation aerosol (Azmacort), 1 mg, 2 mg, 4 mg, and 8 mg tablets (variety of brand names including Aristocort and Kenacort), injectable suspension (variety of brand names including Kenalog-10 and Kenalog-40), and as a nasal aerosol (Nasacort and Nasacort AQ).
3. Apply triamcinolone cream to areas twice a day.
4. Albuterol nebs. (every 4 hours)

EXHIBIT 44 ANSWERS

1. COPD is **c**hronic **o**bstructive **p**ulmonary **d**isease.
   CHF is **c**ongestive **h**eart **f**ailure.
2. albuterol (Proventil, Ventolin)/Atrovent (ipratropium) nebs albuterol MDI
   Humibid (guaifenesin) (*Note:* respiratory indications as an expectorant)
3. ASA is the acronym for **a**cetyl**s**alicylic **a**cid or aspirin.
4. Albuterol is written twice to accommodate the nebs (nebules) that are required every 4 hours and the MDI (**m**etered **d**ose **i**nhaler) form that is available for the patient as needed (but not to exceed the manufacturer's dosing requirements).
5. Zocor (simvastatin) is a hypolipidemic agent used for hypercholesteremia.
6. The prednisone (Deltasone) is most likely prescribed for the COPD.
7. Humibid (guaifenesin), an expectorant, is indicated for loosening respiratory congestion.
8. Depakote (divalproex) as an antiepileptic agent, antimigraine, and antimania agent
   Haldol (haloperidol) as an antipsychotic agent.
   Buspar (buspirone) as an antianxiety agent.
   loxapine (Loxitane) as an antipsychotic agent.
9. Levofloxacin (Levaquin) is a bacterial anti-infective agent that belongs to the fluoroquinolone class of drugs.
10. ASA (aspirin), Pepcid (famotidine) Pepcid AC 10 mg strength, Maalox (magnesium hydroxide + aluminum hydroxide), and thiamine (vitamin B_1) oral form are available as over-the-counter (OTC) drugs.
11. Depakote (divalproex) is indicated primarily for seizures.
12. Buspar (buspirone) is indicated primarily for anxiety whereas a number of the other CNS (central nervous system) drugs are used primarily as antipsychotic agents. The dose requested by the doctor requires clarification because the maximum recommended dose per day is 60 mg. Written as 40 mg orally three times a day will provide 120 mg or twice the recommended daily dose.
13. Loxapine has the potential to interact with other CNS depressants resulting in an increased CNS depression. Concomitant use should be avoided, but ultimately the situation is determined by the state and condition of the patient.
14. Maalox and Pepcid will help to manage gastric irritation especially because the patient is taking gastric irritating drugs such as the prednisone and ASA (aspirin).

EXHIBIT 45 ANSWERS

1. The doctor ordered simethicone (Mylicon, Phazyme) an antiflatulant.
2. The liquid form of simethicone was ordered.
3. The drug is to be used for gas pain.
4. Take 80 cc orally every 6 hours as needed (for gas pain).
5. The 80 cc dose is made up of 16 teaspoonsful. (*Note:* A clarification call to the doctor revealed that the prescriber wanted 80 mg of simethicone which was subsequently dispensed in tablet form. The order was rewritten for Simethicone 80 mg (one tablet) every 6 hours.

EXHIBIT 46 ANSWERS

1. Yes. Never dispense guesswork.
2. The order was clarified with a call to the prescriber. The prescriber wanted the patient to have lanolin ointment.

EXHIBIT 47 ANSWERS

1. Claforan (cefotaxime) is an antibiotic.
2. "HCTZ" (an acronym) (Hydrodiuril, Esidrix (hydrochlorothiazide)—diuretic (thiazide variety)
3. One of the side effects for Benadryl (diphenhydramine) is drowsiness, which is very useful for treating insomnia.
4. "ECASA" is the acronym for enteric-coated aspirin (Ecotrin). The acronym is derived from **e**nteric **c**oated **a**cetyl**s**alicylic **a**cid. Acetylsalicylic acid is the chemical name for aspirin.
5. "HCTZ" on the order is the acronym for **h**ydro**c**hloro**t**hia**z**ide, a thiazide diuretic.
6. Univasc (moexipril) is an antihypertensive agent (ACE inhibitor variety) indicated for hypertension.
7. Entex LA is a combination of phenylpropanolamine (nasal decongestant) and guaifenesin (expectorant).
8. Claforan (cefotaxime) is an antibiotic. Claforan is a bacterial anti-infective. Claforan is a representative of the third generation cephalosporins.
9. Tylenol (acetaminophen) is available as a 325 mg tablet as one of its strengths. There is no way to make 625 mg from 325 mg tablets. A clarification call is needed to determine if the prescriber wanted one tablet of 325 mg or two tablets of 325 mg each to equal a 650 mg dose.
10. ECASA—Take 325 mg (one tablet) orally every day.

    HCTZ—Take 25 mg (one tablet) orally every day.

    Univasc—Take 7.5 mg (one tablet) twice a day.

    Claforan—Give 1 gram intravenously every 6 hours.

    Entex LA—Take one tablet orally twice a day. (*Note:* The prescriber neglected to indicate how many tablets the patient should take. However, in this case we could comfortably assume that the prescriber wanted one tablet.)

    Benadryl—Give 25 mg intravenously every 8 hours as needed for insomnia.

    Tylenol—Take 650 mg [subsequent to a clarification call to doctor] (two tablets) orally every 4 to 6 hours as needed for pain.

EXHIBIT 48 ANSWERS

1. The physician prescribed prednisone (Deltasone), a corticosteroid drug.
2. The prescriber has written the directions in a declining dosing pattern to avoid a sudden withdrawal from prednisone which could have negative effects and even be fatal.
3. As indicated on the order, the medication should be given with food that will reduce the potential for gastric irritation associated with prednisone.
4. PPD is **p**urified **p**rotein **d**erivative. This is a tuberculin diagnostic test to determine an individual's exposure to tuberculosis and his or her sensitivity to the organism.

EXHIBIT 49 ANSWERS

1. multiple vitamin (many varieties)—supplementation—Take one tablet every day.

   pentoxifylline (Trental)—hemorrheologic agent used to improve capillary blood flow in chronic occlusive vascular conditions—Take 400 mg (1 tablet) orally three times a day.

   zinc sulfate—zinc (trace element) supplementation—Take 220 mg (one capsule) orally every day.

   becaplermin 0.01% (100 micrograms [mcg] per gram) gel (Regranex gel)—promotes wound repair and formation of new tissue—Apply sparingly once a day. *Keep Refrigerated.*
2. Becaplermin should be stored in the regrigerator.

EXHIBIT 50 ANSWERS

1. The drug listed is the brand name Prilosec. The generic name is omeprazole.
2. The route of administration is oral. However, oral administration is through a feeding tube.
3. Prilosec capsules should not be chewed, opened, or crushed. The instructions are to make a slurry in orange juice which is contradictory to the manufacturer's information.

EXHIBIT 51 ANSWERS

1. A bolus of heparin is a single, one-time, large amount of drug given as an initial dose.
2. The bolus of heparin is administered to achieve a minimum effective dose as quickly as possible.
3. Tylenol (acetaminophen), nifedipine (Procardia, Adalat), Zantac (ranitidine), and Benadryl (diphenhydramine).
4. SL is an acronym for **s**ub**l**ingual.
5. The oral form of Zantac is available as a 150 mg dose.
6. Heparin—Give a 5,000 units bolus.
   Heparin drip—Run at 1,000 units per hour.
   Tylenol—Take 650 mg (2 × 325 mg tablets) orally every 6 hours as needed for temperature greater than 101 degrees.
   Nifedipine—Take 10 mg (one capsule) sublingually every 6 hours as needed for a systolic blood pressure greater than 180, diastolic blood pressure greater than 100.
   Zantac—Take 50 mg orally twice a day. (*Note:* A clarification call to the physician is needed to change the order to the usual oral tablet dose of 150 mg.)

Glossary

Admixture preparation of an intravenous fluid containing a drug or electrolyte that has been added to a larger volume solution

Anatomy refers to the body's parts, structure, and systems

Antibiotic drug used to treat infection caused by bacteria, virus, fungus, and other living microscopic organisms

ANS acronym for autonomic nervous system

Antilipemics cholesterol-reducing agents

Aseptic pertaining to the methods used to minimize infiltration of pyrogenic and pathogenic contamination

Automatic stop order (ASO) refers to a time limit for the use of specific drugs in the hospital setting

Bolus one mass injection as opposed to a continuous administration over a period of time

Bradycardia abnormally slow heart rate

Catecholamines body biochemicals; serotonin, dopamine, norepinephrine, and epinephrine

Catheter a hollow tube

Cell membrane covering that surrounds each cell; permits only selected substances to pass through

Central venous system vascular system directly entering and leaving the heart

Cerumen ear wax

Chronotropic referring to the effect on heart rate

CNS acronym for central nervous system

Collagen diseases a collective term that refers to disorders affecting the body's connective tissue; includes arthritis, rheumatism, scleroderma, and systemic lupus erythematosus (SLE)

Compromised term used to indicate a patient with a dysfunction

Coombs test a laboratory test used to determine hemolytic anemia

Cytology study of cell structure and function

Cytoplasm living substance in a cell which surrounds the nucleus

DEA acronym for the Drug Enforcement Agency

Dehydration a condition characterized by excessive water loss

Diffusion process by which molecules disperse themselves equally throughout an available space

Digitalization individual adjustment of digoxin to achieve an effective dosage

Diluent fluid used to dissolve drugs in solid form

Diuresis urination

DNA acronym for desoxyribonucleic acid; an essential part of the gene makeup

Drip slow administration of an intravenous fluid dropwise

Endocrine glands organs that pass their secretions directly into the blood system

Epilepsy a disorder characterized by seizures

Equilibrium a state of equality

Exacerbate a worsening condition

Exocrine glands organs that secrete substances via ducts

Filtration process by which larger-sized substances are strained out of liquids

Formulary a list of drugs acceptable for dispensing; usually found in the hospital

Glossitis inflammation of the tongue

Half-life the time it takes for one half of the drug to be metabolized

Homeostasis a state of physiologic equilibrium

Hormones chemical substances produced by the body that elicit responses with only minute amounts

Hypercalcemia state in which the body's calcium level is abnormally high

Hyperkalemia state in which the body's potassium level is abnormally high

Hypermagnesemia state in which the body's magnesium level is abnormally high

Hypernatremia an above-normal level of serum sodium

Hypertension high blood pressure

Hypertonic a salt solution with a concentration greater than 0.5%

Hypocalcemia state in which the body's calcium level is very low

Hypokalemia state in which the body's potassium level is very low

Hypomagnesemia state in which the body's magnesium level is very low

Hyponatremia a below-normal level of serum sodium

Hypotonic a salt solution with a concentration less than 0.9%

Icterus jaundice; yellow complexion

Inflammation a condition characterized by redness, heat, and swelling

Infusion a drug administered into the body by way of a vein for therapeutic purposes

Inotropic pertains to the effect on muscular contractility especially referring to the heart muscle

Integumentary pertains to skin, hair, and nails

Laminar flow hood a specialized workspace designed to prepare intravenous fluids in a pyrogen-free and pathogen-free environment

Loading dose an initial amount of drug used in a procedure to determine an effective dosage

Maintenance dose a drug dosage that provides therapeutic effect with minimal risk of toxicity

Miosis constriction of the eye's pupil

Morphogenetic pertaining to structural development

Mydriasis dilation of the eye's pupil

Nosocomial pertaining to the hospital setting as in nosocomial infections

NSAIA acronym for nonsteroidal anti-inflammatory agents

Nucleus the component of the cell responsible for all activities' coordination

Osmosis a special type of diffusion that relies on a semipermeable membrane separating two solutions of unequal concentrations

Palpitations pulsations or throbbing, usually referring to the beat of the heart

Paradoxical responses drug effects completely opposite to the expected effect

Parenteral pertaining to the injectable route directly or indirectly into blood vessels, outside the gastrointestinal tract

Particulate matter undissolved substances present in parenteral products

Pathogens disease-producing organisms

Peripheral pertaining to areas on the body surface

Peristalsis progressive wave motion as in the intestines

Permeability selective passage through a membrane

Photosensitivity sensitivity to sunlight

Physiology refers to the functions of the body's systems, responsibilities, and how it works

Piggyback term used to define the delivery of a secondary IV medication from an outside source into an existing large-volume IV solution

PNS acronym for peripheral nervous system

Posology study of drug dosages

Presents term used to indicate that a patient has a problem, found in journal case entries

PRN acronym for *pro re nata,* meaning "when needed"

Protocol a set of steps that are to be followed

Pruritus itching

Pyrogens fever-producing organisms

Rebound a paradoxical phenomenon in which a drug causes the effect opposite to the one intended

RNA acronym for ribonucleic acid; an essential part of the gene makeup

Salt sodium chloride

Script prescription

Sepsis a condition characterized by fever and caused by pyrogenic or pathogenic microorganisms or their toxins

Spasms painful muscle contractions

Sterile free of all living organisms

Steroids a group of compounds that include D vitamins, certain hormones, and some human-made products

System groups of organs joined to perform a specialized function

Tachycardia abnormally fast heart rate

Titration process used to slowly build up a drug dosage to an effective or maintenance level

Tolerance a time-related reduction in drug effectiveness

Toxins poison

USP acronym for *United States Pharmacopeia*

Vasodilation a response representing an increasing diameter of the blood vessels

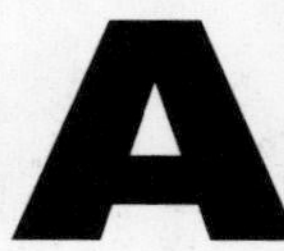

The National Pharmacy Technician Certification Examination

As the role of the pharmacy technician becomes increasingly important, the need for standardized training is essential. A national certification was initiated as a step to ensure the consistency and uniformity of pharmacy technician knowledge and abilities. The certification acknowledges that the individual who has successfully completed the examination has met predetermined qualifications in performing pharmacy activities.

The Pharmacy Technician Certification Board (PTCB) certification program is a voluntary program designed to establish the pharmacy technician as a well-defined position in pharmacy. The PTCB administers the National Pharmacy Technician Certification Examination.

The examination covers three broad functional areas. They are:

I. Assisting the pharmacist in serving patients (50% of the examination)

II. Medication distribution and inventory control systems (35% of the examination)

III. Operations (15% of the examination)

The first functional area includes the activities related to traditional distributive pharmacy dispensing functions. The second functional area focuses on purchasing, inventory control, and policy and procedures to control the preparation and distribution of drugs. The final functional area deals with activities related to administrative processes, which include procedures for operations, the facilities and equipment, and information systems.

The PTCB is located at the following address:
Pharmacy Technician Certification Board
2215 Constitution Avenue, NW
Washington, DC 20037-2985
Telephone: 202/429-7578

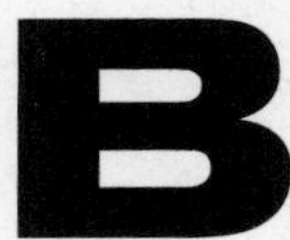

The Professional Pharmacy Technician

A professional is an individual qualified to perform the activities of a specific occupation. Professionalism exceeds the knowledge, skills, and abilities required to perform those activities.

Professionalism encompasses character, professional standards, and ethical standards. The pharmacy technician, as a professional, represents the profession of pharmacy. Your presentation is essential to establish a foundation for credibility. This will be evident in your mannerisms, your dress, your hygiene, and your presentation.

Establish a dress code that represents both your profession and your organization. Regardless of the attire, personal clothing or uniform, be sure it is conservative, is clean, fits appropriately, and is not in need of alteration or fixing. Be sure your shoes are clean, polished, and quiet.

A professional is always courteous and listens with focus. As a health-care professional, you must respect the privacy of patients and keep all information confidential. Confidentiality is a prime responsibility of each health-care professional. Respond to questions with answers that are clear and concise. Never be hesitant to say you do not know. Your image is enhanced with honesty.

Finally, one of the most important facets of being a professional is being current with knowledge. Keep up-to-date by reading journals, taking continuing education classes, and talking with other professionals. Pharmacy is a dynamic field. New drugs enter the market often, established drugs get new indications, new research provides new approaches to treating illnesses, and new laws change the way health care is practiced. You are a resource to the patient, you assist the pharmacist, and you interact with other health-care providers. Constantly think of yourself as a professional. Remember, *you are a professional.*

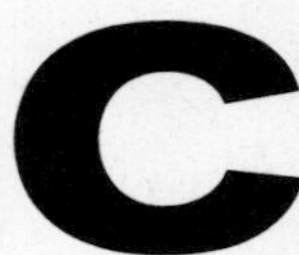

Practice Prescriptions

Review each of the following practice prescriptions (Figures C.1 to C.26). For each drug, give the *generic name,* the *trade name, strength, dosage form,* the *amount* to be *dispensed,* and the *directions to the patient.* Answers may be found following the prescriptions.

PAT SMITH, M.D.
27 Oak Leaf Lane
Baltimore, MD 12121
Phone: 322 -7890

Name________________________

Address______________________

Age______

Rx Lotrimin 1% Cream
15 Gm
Sig. apply to affected area BID in AM & PM

[ ] Contents are labeled unless checked

May be refilled 1 2 3 4

Signed____________________ M.D.

Date__________ 20___ DEA No.__________

FIGURE C.1

PAT SMITH, M.D.
27 Oak Leaf Lane
Baltimore, MD 12121
Phone: 322 -7890

Name__________
Address__________
Age__________

Rx Transderm - Nitro Patch
5 cm² (2.5 mg/24 H)
#30
Sig. i q 24°

[ ] Contents are labeled unless checked

May be refilled 0 1 2 3 4

Signed__________ M.D.

Date__________ 20___ DEA No.__________

FIGURE C.2

PAT SMITH, M.D.
27 Oak Leaf Lane
Baltimore, MD 12121
Phone: 322 -7890

Name__________
Address__________
Age__________

Rx Timoptic 0.25%
Ophthalmic drops
#1
S. gtts i o.u. BID

[ ] Contents are labeled unless checked

May be refilled 0 1 2 3 4

Signed__________ M.D.

Date__________ 20___ DEA No.__________

FIGURE C.3

PAT SMITH, M.D.
27 Oak Leaf Lane
Baltimore, MD 12121
Phone: 322 –7890

Name ______________________

Address ______________________

Age __________

Rx alupent metered Dose (225mg)
#1

Inhale ii puffs q 3-4°
No more than 12 per day

[ ] Contents are labeled unless checked

May be refilled 0 1 2 3 4

Signed ______________________ M.D.

Date __________ 20___ DEA No. __________

FIGURE C.4

PAT SMITH, M.D.
27 Oak Leaf Lane
Baltimore, MD 12121
Phone: 322 –7890

Name ______________________

Address ______________________

Age __________

Rx Caps Lopid 300mg
#C

ii ½h ā breakfast, ii ½h ā dinner

[ ] Contents are labeled unless checked

May be refilled 0 1 2 3 4

Signed ______________________ M.D.

Date __________ 20___ DEA No. __________

FIGURE C.5

PAT SMITH, M.D.
27 Oak Leaf Lane
Baltimore, MD 12121
Phone: 322 -7890

Name____________________
Address____________________
Age________

Rx Premarin Tabs 1.25mg
#40
i AM & PM for 20 d, rest 10 d,
resume schedule. Dispense
PPI

[ ] Contents are labeled unless checked

May be refilled 0 1 2 3 4

Signed____________________ M.D.

Date__________ 20__ DEA No.__________

FIGURE C.6

PAT SMITH, M.D.
27 Oak Leaf Lane
Baltimore, MD 12121
Phone: 322 -7890

Name____________________
Address____________________
Age________

Rx Inderal 40mg
#50
S. 80 mg daily (i AM and i PM)

[ ] Contents are labeled unless checked

May be refilled 0 1 2 3 4

Signed____________________ M.D.

Date__________ 20__ DEA No.__________

FIGURE C.7

PAT SMITH, M.D.
27 Oak Leaf Lane
Baltimore, MD 12121
Phone: 322 -7890

Name ______________________

Address ______________________

Age __________

Rx Synthroid 100 mcg tablets
#C
Take 1 tablet d

[ ] Contents are labeled unless checked

May be refilled 0 1 2 3 4

Signed ______________________ M.D.

Date __________ 20___ DEA No. __________

FIGURE C.8

PAT SMITH, M.D.
27 Oak Leaf Lane
Baltimore, MD 12121
Phone: 322 -7890

Name ______________________

Address ______________________

Age __________

Rx Zantac 150 mg Tablets
#100
i BID

[ ] Contents are labeled unless checked

May be refilled 0 1 2 3 4

Signed ______________________ M.D.

Date __________ 20___ DEA No. __________

FIGURE C.9

PAT SMITH, M.D.
27 Oak Leaf Lane
Baltimore, MD 12121
Phone: 322 -7890

Name______________________________

Address____________________________

Age________

Rx Tagamet 300 mg/5ml
Disp 480 ml
Sig. 800 mg hs

[ ] Contents are labeled unless checked

May be refilled 0 1 2 3 4

Signed__________________________ M.D.

Date__________ 20___ DEA No.__________

FIGURE C.10

PAT SMITH, M.D.
27 Oak Leaf Lane
Baltimore, MD 12121
Phone: 322 -7890

Name______________________________

Address____________________________

Age________

Rx Xanax 0.5 mg Tabs.
#30
S. 0.5mg TID - no more than 4 mg per day. No ETOH

[ ] Contents are labeled unless checked

May be refilled 0 1 2 3 4

Signed__________________________ M.D.

Date__________ 20___ DEA No.__________

FIGURE C.11

PAT SMITH, M.D.
27 Oak Leaf Lane
Baltimore, MD 12121
Phone: 322 -7890

Name____________________
Address____________________
Age________

Rx Tabs. Coumadin 5mg
d.t.d. 30
S. 5mg daily – DO NOT TAKE ASA

[ ] Contents are labeled unless checked

May be refilled 0 1 2 3 4

Signed____________________ M.D.

Date__________ 20___ DEA No.__________

FIGURE C.12

PAT SMITH, M.D.
27 Oak Leaf Lane
Baltimore, MD 12121
Phone: 322 -7890

Name____________________
Address____________________
Age________

Rx Cardizem 30mg tablets
120
$\dot{T}$ QID ac and hs

[ ] Contents are labeled unless checked

May be refilled 0 1 2 3 4

Signed____________________ M.D.

Date__________ 20___ DEA No.__________

FIGURE C.13

PAT SMITH, M.D.
27 Oak Leaf Lane
Baltimore, MD 12121
Phone: 322 -7890

Name __________
Address __________
Age __________

Rx Darvocet-N 50 Tabs
#XXX
S: i q 4° prn pain

[ ] Contents are labeled unless checked

May be refilled 0 1 2 3 4

Signed __________ M.D.

Date __________ 20___ DEA No. __________

FIGURE C.14

PAT SMITH, M.D.
27 Oak Leaf Lane
Baltimore, MD 12121
Phone: 322 -7890

Name __________
Address __________
Age __________

Rx Valium 5mg
Tabs # XX
S: ss tab 3-4 x d. May have 1 tab
hs prn muscle spasms.
NO ETOH

[ ] Contents are labeled unless checked

May be refilled 0 1 2 3 4

Signed __________ M.D.

Date __________ 20___ DEA No. __________

FIGURE C.15

PAT SMITH, M.D.
27 Oak Leaf Lane
Baltimore, MD 12121
Phone: 322 -7890

Name__________
Address__________
Age__________

Rx Motrin 400 mg Tabs
#40
Sig: 400 mg to 800 mg TID
w/food prn pain

[ ] Contents are labeled unless checked

May be refilled 0 1 2 3 4

Signed __________ M.D.

Date__________ 20___ DEA No.__________

FIGURE C.16

PAT SMITH, M.D.
27 Oak Leaf Lane
Baltimore, MD 12121
Phone: 322 -7890

Name__________
Address__________
Age__________

Rx Sumycin Caps 0.250 Gm
#40
Sig: Open 1 cap in 1 oz. H_2O and
rinse mouth QID

[ ] Contents are labeled unless checked

May be refilled 0 1 2 3 4

Signed __________ M.D.

Date__________ 20___ DEA No.__________

FIGURE C.17

PAT SMITH, M.D.
27 Oak Leaf Lane
Baltimore, MD 12121
Phone: 322 -7890

Name____________________
Address____________________
Age________

Rx Theo-Dur tablets
#100 X 300mg
S: 450mg Q12H for wheezing

[ ] Contents are labeled unless checked

May be refilled 0 1 2 3 4

Signed____________________ M.D.

Date__________ 20__ DEA No.__________

FIGURE C.18

PAT SMITH, M.D.
27 Oak Leaf Lane
Baltimore, MD 12121
Phone: 322 -7890

Name____________________
Address____________________
Age________

Rx Tabs Halcion 0.25mg
XXX
Sig: Take i hs prn sleep

[ ] Contents are labeled unless checked

May be refilled 0 1 2 3 4

Signed____________________ M.D.

Date__________ 20__ DEA No.__________

FIGURE C.19

PAT SMITH, M.D.
27 Oak Leaf Lane
Baltimore, MD 12121
Phone: 322 -7890

Name____________________
Address____________________
Age________

Rx Dilantin 100mg Caps.
dtd #100
Sig: 400mg stat, 100 mg BD 1st day,
then 100mg TID thereafter.

[ ] Contents are labeled unless checked

May be refilled 0 1 2 3 4

Signed____________________ M.D.
Date__________ 20___ DEA No.__________

FIGURE C.20

PAT SMITH, M.D.
27 Oak Leaf Lane
Baltimore, MD 12121
Phone: 322 -7890

Name____________________
Address____________________
Age________

Rx Monistat Vaginal Cr. 2%
45 Gm.
Sig: i applicatorful vaginally
daily hs X 7d

[ ] Contents are labeled unless checked

May be refilled 0 1 2 3 4

Signed____________________ M.D.
Date__________ 20___ DEA No.__________

FIGURE C.21

PAT SMITH, M.D.
27 Oak Leaf Lane
Baltimore, MD 12121
Phone: 322 -7890

Name ____________________
Address ____________________
Age ________

Rx Slow-K (8 mEq)
\# sixty
Sig: ii d. Swallow whole.

[ ] Contents are labeled unless checked

May be refilled 0 1 2 3 4

Signed ____________________ M.D.
Date __________ 20___ DEA No. __________

FIGURE C.22

PAT SMITH, M.D.
27 Oak Leaf Lane
Baltimore, MD 12121
Phone: 322 -7890

Name ____________________
Address ____________________
Age ________

Rx Caps. Feldene 20 mg
\#30
Sig. i q d w/food or milk.

[ ] Contents are labeled unless checked

May be refilled 0 1 2 3 4

Signed ____________________ M.D.
Date __________ 20___ DEA No. __________

FIGURE C.23

PAT SMITH, M.D.
27 Oak Leaf Lane
Baltimore, MD 12121
Phone: 322 -7890

Name________________
Address________________
Age________

Rx Ortho-Novum 2mg
d. i pack
i tab daily days 5-25 of
menstrual cycle.

[ ] Contents are labeled unless checked

May be refilled 0 1 2 3 4

Signed ________________ M.D.

Date__________20___ DEA No.__________

FIGURE C.24

PAT SMITH, M.D.
27 Oak Leaf Lane
Baltimore, MD 12121
Phone: 322 -7890

Name________________
Address________________
Age________

Rx Nicorette 2mg gum
Disp. i box of 96
Sig: ut dict per instructions. No
more than 30 pieces per day.

[ ] Contents are labeled unless checked

May be refilled 0 1 2 3 4

Signed ________________ M.D.

Date__________20___ DEA No.__________

FIGURE C.25

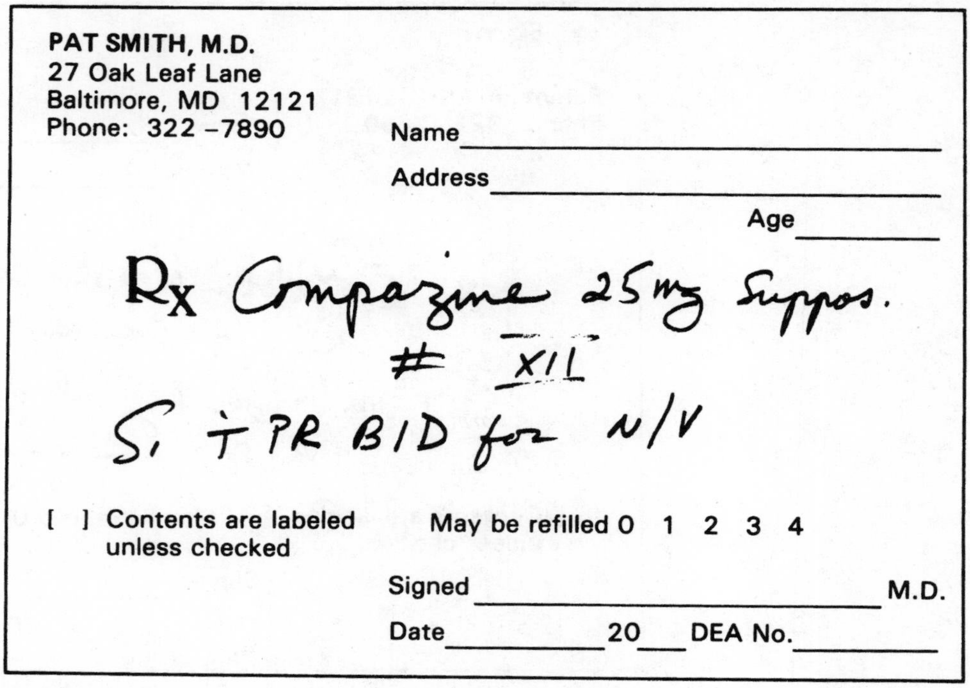

PAT SMITH, M.D.
27 Oak Leaf Lane
Baltimore, MD 12121
Phone: 322 -7890

Name ____________________

Address ____________________

Age ________

Rx Compazine 25mg Suppos.
XII
S. i PR BID for N/V

[ ] Contents are labeled unless checked

May be refilled 0 1 2 3 4

Signed ____________________ M.D.

Date __________ 20___ DEA No. __________

FIGURE C.26

FIGURE C.1

Generic name: clotrimazole

Trade name: Lotrimin

Strength: 1%

Dosage form: cream

Amount dispensed: 15 grams

Directions to the patient: Apply to affected area twice a day, morning and evening.

FIGURE C.2

Generic name: nitroglycerin

Trade name: Transderm-Nitro

Strength: 2.5 mg.

Dosage form: patch

Amount dispensed: 30

Directions to the patient: Apply one patch every 24 hours.

FIGURE C.3

Generic name: timolol

Trade name: Timoptic

Strength: 0.25 %

Dosage form: ophthalmic drops

Amount dispensed: one bottle

Directions to the patient: Instill one drop to both eyes twice a day.

FIGURE C.4

Generic name: metaproterenol

Trade name: Alupent

Strength: 225 mg per inhaler

Dosage form: inhalant

Amount dispensed: one inhaler unit

Directions to the patient: Inhale two puffs every 3 to 4 hours. Use no more than 12 puffs per day.

FIGURE C.5

Generic name: gemfibrozil

Trade name: Lopid

Strength: 300 mg

Dosage form: capsule (oral)

Amount dispensed: 100

Directions to the patient: Take two capsules one-half hour before breakfast and two capsules one-half hour before dinner.

FIGURE C.6

Generic name: conjugated estrogens

Trade name: Premarin

Strength: 1.25 mg

Dosage form: tablet (oral)

Amount dispensed: 40

Directions to the patient: Take one tablet in the morning and evening for 20 days, rest 10 days, and resume schedule.

(*Note:* This drug is to be dispensed with a patient package insert—PPI.)

FIGURE C.7

Generic name: propranolol

Trade name: Inderal

Strength: 40 mg

Dosage form: tablet (oral)

Amount dispensed: 50

Directions to the patient: Take two tablets daily (one tablet in the morning and one tablet in the evening).

FIGURE C.8

Generic name: levothyroxine

Trade name: Synthroid

Strength: 100 micrograms (or 0.1 mg)

Dosage form: tablet (oral)

Amount dispensed: 100

Directions to the patient: Take one tablet daily.

FIGURE C.9

Generic name: ranitidine

Trade name: Zantac

Strength: 150 mg

Dosage form: tablet (oral)

Amount dispensed: 100

Directions to the patient: Take one tablet twice a day.

FIGURE C.10

Generic name: cimetidine

Trade name: Tagamet

Strength: 300 mg per teaspoonful

Dosage form: liquid (oral)

Amount dispensed: 480 ml or 1 pint

Directions to the patient: Take $2\frac{1}{2}$ teaspoonsful at bedtime.

(*Note:* Actual calculations indicate 2.6 teaspoonsful at bedtime. However, patients understand $2\frac{1}{2}$ teaspoonsful, which measure within an accurate dosage.)

FIGURE C.11

Generic name: alprazolam

Trade name: Xanax

Strength: 0.5 mg

Dosage form: tablet (oral)

Amount dispensed: 30

Directions to the patient: Take one tablet three times a day. Do *not* take more than 8 tablets per day. *No alcohol.*

FIGURE C.12

Generic name: warfarin

Trade name: Coumadin

Strength: 5 mg

Dosage form: tablet (oral)

Amount dispensed: 30

Directions to the patient: Take one tablet daily. *Do not take aspirin.*

FIGURE C.13

Generic name: diltiazem

Trade name: Cardizem

Strength: 30 mg

Dosage form: tablet (oral)

Amount dispensed: 120

Directions to the patient: Take one tablet four times a day before meals and at bedtime.

FIGURE C.14

Generic name: propoxyphene/acetaminophen

Trade name: Darvocet-N

Strength: propoxyphene 50 mg/acetaminophen 325 mg

Dosage form: tablet (oral)

Amount dispensed: 30

Directions to the patient: Take one tablet every 4 hours as needed for pain.

FIGURE C.15

Generic name: diazepam

Trade name: Valium

Strength: 5 mg

Dosage form: tablet (oral)

Amount dispensed: 20

Directions to the patient: Take one-half tablet three or four times a day. May have one tablet at bedtime as needed for muscle spasms. *No alcohol.*

FIGURE C.16

Generic name: ibuprofen

Trade name: Motrin (or Rufen)

Strength: 400 mg

Dosage form: tablet (oral)

Amount dispensed: 40

Directions to the patient: Take one or two tablets three times a day with food as needed for pain.

FIGURE C.17

Generic name: tetracycline

Trade name: Sumycin (or Achromycin V)

Strength: 250 mg

Dosage form: capsule (oral)

Amount dispensed: 40

Directions to the patient: Open one capsule in 1 ounce of water and rinse mouth four times a day.

FIGURE C.18

Generic name: theophylline

Trade name: Theo-Dur (or Slo-Bid, Slo-Phyllin)

Strength: 300 mg

Dosage form: tablet (oral)

Amount dispensed: 100

Directions to the patient: Take $1\frac{1}{2}$ tablets every 12 hours for wheezing.

FIGURE C.19

Generic name: triazolam

Trade name: Halcion

Strength: 0.25 mg

Dosage form: tablet (oral)

Amount dispensed: 30

Directions to the patient: Take one tablet at bedtime as needed for sleep.

FIGURE C.20

Generic name: phenytoin

Trade name: Dilantin

Strength: 100 mg

Dosage form: capsule (oral)

Amount dispensed: 100

Directions to the patient: Take four capsules at once, one capsule twice a day for the first day, then one capsule three times a day thereafter.

FIGURE C.21

Generic name: miconazole

Trade name: Monistat

Strength: 2%

Dosage form: vaginal cream

Amount dispensed: 45 grams

Directions to the patient: Insert one applicatorful vaginally daily at bedtime for 7 days.

FIGURE C.22

Generic name: potassium

Trade name: Slow-K (or Micro-K, K-Tab, Klotrix, K-Lyte, Kaon)

(*Note:* Strengths vary for each product.)

Strength: 8 milliequivalents

Dosage form: tablet (oral)

Amount dispensed: 60

Directions to the patient: Take two tablets daily. *Swallow whole.*

FIGURE C.23

Generic name: piroxicam

Trade name: Feldene

Strength: 20 mg

Dosage form: capsule (oral)

Amount dispensed: 30

Directions to the patient: Take one capsule every day with food or milk.

FIGURE C.24

Generic name: norethindrone/mestranol

Trade name: Ortho-Novum

Strength: norethindrone 2 mg/mestranol 0.10 mg

Dosage form: tablet (oral)

Amount dispensed: one pack (contains 21 tablets)

Directions to the patient: Take one tablet daily, days 5-25 of the menstrual cycle.

FIGURE C.25

Generic name: nicotine

Trade name: Nicorette

Strength: 2 mg

Dosage form: gum (oral)

Amount dispensed: 96

Directions to the patient: Chew as directed per instructions. Chew no more than 30 pieces per day.

FIGURE C.26

Generic name: prochlorperazine

Trade name: Compazine

Strength: 25 mg

Dosage form: suppository (rectal)

Amount dispensed: 12

Directions to the patient: Insert one suppository rectally twice a day for nausea and vomiting.

APPENDIX D

Practice Hospital Orders

The Physician's Order Record is the primary method used to communicate a hospitalized patient's medication needs to the pharmacy. Therefore, you must be able to review the order and highlight the information needed by pharmacy staff to complete the physician's request for drugs. This appendix contains actual hospital orders that have been rewritten with special highlights (lettered arrows) added to emphasize practice with phrases, abbreviations, and special terminology.

Read each practice hospital order (Physician's Order Record) entirely (Figures D.1 to D.10). Note the items highlighted by lettered arrows. Interpret each of these highlighted items. Answers follow the practice orders.

PATIENT:
AGE:
SEX:
RACE:
CHART NO.

MEMORIAL HOSPITAL
BALTIMORE, MARYLAND
PHYSICIAN'S ORDER RECORD

BEAR DOWN ON HARD SURFACE WITH BALL POINT PEN

GENERIC EQUIVALENT IS AUTHORIZED UNLESS CHECKED IN THIS COLUMN

ALLERGY OR SENSITIVITY TO none
NONE KNOWN ☐ SIGNED:

DIAGNOSIS S/P (R) wrist FX ← A

COMPLETED OR DISCONTINUED

DATE	TIME	ORDERS	PHYSICIAN'S SIG.		NAME	DATE	TIME
6/22	6:15 P	Admit to Med C					
		condition: stable					
		diet 4Gm Na+					
		activity - bedrest					
		vitals Q4°					
		Med:					
		Capoten 12.5mg P.O. BID ← B					
		C → Colace 100mg P.O. QD					
		D → HCTZ 50mg PO QD					
		E → clonidine - 1 patch i a week					
		F → Tylenol with codeine (#3) PO Q4-6° prn					
		G → heparin SQ 5000u q 12°					
		IVF D5½NS KVO ← H					
		schedule for AM { (1) holter (2) cat scan (3) EEG (4) Echo					
		[illegible] MD					
6/23	9A	Prepare for OR					
		NPO					
		I → Scrub wrist c̄ povidone-iodine scrub					
		Diazepam 10mg IV ← J					
		[illegible] MD					

PHARMACY COPY

FIGURE D.1

PATIENT:
AGE:
SEX:
RACE:
CHART NO.

MEMORIAL HOSPITAL
BALTIMORE, MARYLAND
PHYSICIAN'S ORDER RECORD

BEAR DOWN ON HARD SURFACE WITH BALL POINT PEN

GENERIC EQUIVALENT IS AUTHORIZED UNLESS CHECKED IN THIS COLUMN

ALLERGY OR SENSITIVITY TO NKA
NONE KNOWN ☐ SIGNED:

DIAGNOSIS ASHD

DATE	TIME	ORDERS	PHYSICIAN'S SIG.		COMPLETED OR DISCONTINUED NAME	DATE	TIME
2/7	4p	TNG s.l. 1/150 gr. i̇ NOW ← A					
		May repeat Q5' X 3 doses					
		B → Maalox 30cc alternate c̄ AMPHOGEL 30cc					
		Q2° w.a.					
		Isosorbide L.A. 40 MG. P.O. Q8° ← C					
		D → Verapamil s.r. 240 mg. ½ tab QD (P.O.)					
		Zantac 150 MG P.O. Q12 H ← E					
		F → Lubriderm at bedside PRN USE					
		APAP ii tabs. P.O. Q4° PRN HA					
		(or i̇ SUPPOS (650 MG)) ← G					
		H → Halcion 0.25 MG PO QHS PRN					
		Baby ASA i̇ P.O. QD ← I					
		lactulose 15 cc PO QD ← J					
		Dietary Consult in AM.					
		MD					

PHARMACY COPY

FIGURE D.2

PATIENT:
AGE:
SEX:
RACE:
CHART NO.

MEMORIAL HOSPITAL
BALTIMORE, MARYLAND
PHYSICIAN'S ORDER RECORD

BEAR DOWN ON HARD SURFACE WITH BALL POINT PEN

GENERIC EQUIVALENT IS AUTHORIZED UNLESS CHECKED IN THIS COLUMN

ALLERGY OR SENSITIVITY TO: ibuprofen, diflunisal, PCN
NONE KNOWN ☐ SIGNED:

DIAGNOSIS: UGI bleeding (A)

COMPLETED OR DISCONTINUED

DATE	TIME	ORDERS	PHYSICIAN'S SIG.	NAME	DATE	TIME
7/2	1645	Admit to MED A DRS P/C/N				
		Condition: fair				
		Vitals: Q4° X3, then Q shift.				
		Act: Bedrest tonight, then ad lib				
		I and O please				
		Diet: CLD tonite (C)				
		NPO p̄ MN				
		Schedule upper endoscopy in AM.				
		Meds –				
		Maalox 30 cc PO q 4° (D)				
		(E) Zantac 50 mg IV q 8°				
		Folic acid i mg PO QD (F)				
		(G) KCl 20 mEq in O.J. QD X 2 days				
		Labs: Stat CBC tonite p̄ i unit PRBCs				
		AM Labs: CBC, SMA 7, PT, PTT				
		Call H.O. systolic BP < 100, > 180				
		(H) HR < 60, > 100				
		IVF ½ NS @ 100 cc / hr x 3 l				
		(I) O₂ NC 2 l				
		Vit K 10 mg IM QD X 3 d				
		(J)	MD			

PHARMACY COPY

FIGURE D.3

PATIENT:
AGE:
SEX:
RACE:
CHART NO.

MEMORIAL HOSPITAL
BALTIMORE, MARYLAND
PHYSICIAN'S ORDER RECORD

BEAR DOWN ON HARD SURFACE WITH BALL POINT PEN

GENERIC EQUIVALENT IS AUTHORIZED UNLESS CHECKED IN THIS COLUMN

ALLERGY OR SENSITIVITY TO: Φ
NONE KNOWN ☐ SIGNED: [signature]

DIAGNOSIS: UTI

COMPLETED OR DISCONTINUED

DATE	TIME	ORDERS	PHYSICIAN'S SIG.	NAME	DATE	TIME
7/15	8A	Admit to Dr. [signature] /urology				
		S/P Ⓡ ureteral stone extraction				
		Cond: stable				
		Vitals: Per routine				
		Act: Bedrest				
		Diet: CLD				
		A → IVF: D5 ½ NS c̄ 20 mEq KCl @ 100 ml/H				
		Meds:				
		AMPICILLIN 500MG IV Q6° ← B				
		C → GENT 80 MG IV Q8°				
		Percocet ı̄-ı̄ı̄ PO Q4° PRN ← D				
		E → (-OR- DEMEROL 50MG & VISTARIL 50MG IM Q4° PRN)				
		Lasix 20mg IV now ← F				
		Labs: CBC c̄ diff				
			[signature] MD			
		CAPTOPRIL 25MG PO BID ← G				
		H → HCTZ 25MG PO QAM				
		Trental 400 MG PO BID ← I				
		J → Halcion 0.25 MG PO Q HS PRN				
			[signature] MD			

PHARMACY COPY

FIGURE D.4

PATIENT:
AGE:
SEX:
RACE:
CHART NO.

MEMORIAL HOSPITAL
BALTIMORE, MARYLAND
PHYSICIAN'S ORDER RECORD

BEAR DOWN ON HARD SURFACE WITH BALL POINT PEN

GENERIC EQUIVALENT IS AUTHORIZED UNLESS CHECKED IN THIS COLUMN

ALLERGY OR SENSITIVITY TO Ragweed, fish
NONE KNOWN ☐ SIGNED:

DIAGNOSIS Pneumonia

COMPLETED OR DISCONTINUED

DATE	TIME	ORDERS	PHYSICIAN'S SIG.		NAME	DATE	TIME
6/14	10:30 P	Admit to Med A					
		Cond. Fair					
		Vitals. Q shift					
		Act: UP AD LIB ← A					
		DIET: REGular					
		B → IVF: D5 ½ NS c̄ 10 mEq/L. @ 50 cc/h. x3L.					
		Meds:					
		C → Cefuroxime 0.75 gm. IV Q 8° – 1st dose STAT					
		Alupent inhaler ii puffs Q 6° ← D					
		Tonite: ABG ← E					
6/15	8:15 A	40 mEq KCl RTS ← F					
		G → 10 mEq KCl in 100 cc NS X 4 runs over 1° ea.					
		portable CXR in AM					
		H → Temp PR. APAP ii (650 mg) T > 101.5					
6/16	1 AM	Halcion 0.125 mg. PO now ← I					
		V.O.					
6/17	7 A	Start gent. 55 mg Q 8 H ← J					

PHARMACY COPY

FIGURE D.5

PATIENT:
AGE:
SEX:
RACE:
CHART NO.

MEMORIAL HOSPITAL
BALTIMORE, MARYLAND
PHYSICIAN'S ORDER RECORD

BEAR DOWN ON HARD SURFACE WITH BALL POINT PEN

GENERIC EQUIVALENT IS AUTHORIZED UNLESS CHECKED IN THIS COLUMN

ALLERGY OR SENSITIVITY TO: NKDA ← A

NONE KNOWN ☐ SIGNED: [illegible signature]

DIAGNOSIS: ASCVD ← B

COMPLETED OR DISCONTINUED

DATE	TIME	ORDERS	PHYSICIAN'S SIG.		NAME	DATE	TIME
7/5		Admit to 10th Floor					
		Cond. Fair					
		VS: Q4H x 24H Then Q SHIFT					
		Act: OOB c̄ ASSISTANCE ← C					
		DIET: 4 Gm Na^+ diet					
		EKG QAM x 3 D					
		O_2 2L/min. via NC ← D					
		Meds:					
		Digox 0.25 mg. po. qam ← E					
		F → Kondremul 15cc po q hs on M.W.F					
		Tylenol ii Q4H PRN ← G P.O. ← I					
		Xanax 0.25 mg q hs prn					
		H → Dig. level in am					
			Dr [illegible] MD.				
		J → D/c Xanax. give flurazepam 15mg					
		q hs prn. V.O. Dr [illegible]					

PHARMACY COPY

FIGURE D.6

PATIENT:
AGE:
SEX:
RACE:
CHART NO.

MEMORIAL HOSPITAL
BALTIMORE, MARYLAND
PHYSICIAN'S ORDER RECORD

BEAR DOWN ON HARD SURFACE WITH BALL POINT PEN

GENERIC EQUIVALENT IS AUTHORIZED UNLESS CHECKED IN THIS COLUMN

ALLERGY OR SENSITIVITY TO ASA ← A
NONE KNOWN ☐ SIGNED: [signature]

DIAGNOSIS: chest pain
CHF ← B

COMPLETED OR DISCONTINUED

DATE	TIME	ORDERS	PHYSICIAN'S SIG.	NAME	DATE	TIME
1/14	715	Admit to Telemetry				
		Cond: Fair				
		Activity: Bedrest				
		Diet: NPO except Meds				
		VS q 4 h				
		Meds:				
		① Dig. 0.25 mg IV q 6° x 2 doses ← C				
		then Dig. 0.25 mg PO QAM				
		D → ② Demerol 25 mg IM c̄ Hydroxyzine 25 mg IM				
		q 6 H prn				
		E → ③ Heparin SQ 5000 u Q 12 H				
		F → ④ Thiamine 100 mg IM Tonite and QD x 3D				
		G → ⑤ mgSO4 1 gm IM to each buttocks				
		H → IVF: D5NS c̄ 30 MEq KCl at 250 cc/hr. x 2 L.				
		then ↓ rate to 125 cc per h				
		add i amp MVI } to bottle #2 ← I				
		add i mg folate }				
		Labs: SMA-7, amylase in AM				
		Dig. Level in AM				
		Echocardiogram				
		EKG QAM x 3d ← J				
		[signature], MD				

PHARMACY COPY

FIGURE D.7

PATIENT:
AGE:
SEX:
RACE:
CHART NO.

MEMORIAL HOSPITAL
BALTIMORE, MARYLAND
PHYSICIAN'S ORDER RECORD

BEAR DOWN ON HARD SURFACE WITH BALL POINT PEN

GENERIC EQUIVALENT IS AUTHORIZED UNLESS CHECKED IN THIS COLUMN

ALLERGY OR SENSITIVITY TO PCN ← A
NONE KNOWN ☐ SIGNED: [signature]

DIAGNOSIS Acute exacerbation of COPD, Bronchitis

COMPLETED OR DISCONTINUED

DATE	TIME	ORDERS	PHYSICIAN'S SIG.	NAME	DATE	TIME
7/9	8AM	Admit to Med C				
		Cond - guarded				
		VS per floor routine				
		Activities as tolerated				
		Diet: 1800 Kcal ADA, 4 g Na				
		Meds:				
		Aminophylline 500 mg. in 500cc NS at 40 cc/hr. ← C				
		B → Lasix 40 mg po BID				
		D → nitroglycerin patch 10 cm² QD				
		E → tolazamide 250 mg po QD				
		F → Slow-K ╫ 9 AM				
		G → alupent nebulizers 0.3cc/3cc NS q4°				
		H → ampicillin 250 mg po TID				
		Labs:				
		Aminophylline level tonight and in AM ← I				
		J → Call H.O. for T > 100.5				
		Systolic BP > 200				
		Diastolic BP < 60				
		[signature] MD				

PHARMACY COPY

FIGURE D.8

PATIENT:
AGE:
SEX:
RACE:
CHART NO.

MEMORIAL HOSPITAL
BALTIMORE, MARYLAND
PHYSICIAN'S ORDER RECORD

BEAR DOWN ON HARD SURFACE WITH BALL POINT PEN

GENERIC EQUIVALENT IS AUTHORIZED UNLESS CHECKED IN THIS COLUMN

ALLERGY OR SENSITIVITY TO Codeine, Darvocet-N
NONE KNOWN ☐ SIGNED:

DIAGNOSIS Syncope

COMPLETED OR DISCONTINUED

DATE	TIME	ORDERS	PHYSICIAN'S SIG.	NAME	DATE	TIME
12/3	1p	① Admit to Med A				
		② Cond. – stable				
		③ Diet – CL diet × 2d				
		④ ACT – OOB ad lib				
		⑤ Vitals – q 4° × 24°, then per routine				
		⑥ MEDS:				
		phenytoin 100mg q8° ← A				
		B → KCl 25 mEq po now, then qd.				
		Thiamine 100mg po qd ← C				
		D → folic acid i mg q A.M.				
		MVI i po qd ← E				
		F → ⑦ IVF – D5·NS @ 75cc/hr × 2L				
		⑧ G → V.O. MD –				
		H → 1g mg SO4 each buttock × 1				
		I → triazolam 0.125mg q hs prn sleep				
		⑨ AM Labs. CBC, SMA, phenytoin level				
		⑩ EKG, EEG in AM				
		⑪ J → Call H/O if SOB or seizing				
		[signature], MD				

PHARMACY COPY

FIGURE D.9

PATIENT:
AGE:
SEX:
RACE:
CHART NO.

MEMORIAL HOSPITAL
BALTIMORE, MARYLAND
PHYSICIAN'S ORDER RECORD

BEAR DOWN ON HARD SURFACE WITH BALL POINT PEN

GENERIC EQUIVALENT IS AUTHORIZED UNLESS CHECKED IN THIS COLUMN

ALLERGY OR SENSITIVITY TO: Ø ← A
NONE KNOWN ☐ SIGNED:

DIAGNOSIS: S/P hernia repair

COMPLETED OR DISCONTINUED

DATE	TIME	ORDERS	PHYSICIAN'S SIG.	NAME	DATE	TIME
11/8	pm	Post Op Orders				
		Admit to RR				
		Condition - stable				
		VS: q 4° x 2, then q shift ← B				
		Diet: Regular				
		D5 1/2 NS w/20 mEq KCl/L ← C				
		run @ 100 cc/hr.				
		D/C when taking PO well ← D				
		Meds:				
		E → Meperidine 50 mg IM q 3° h prn pain				
		F → Vistaril 25 mg IM q3H prn pain				
		G → Halcion 0.25 mg PO q hs prn				
		H → LOC prn				
		Lancefoot sore in AM				
		I → cefazolin 1 Gm IV in RR				
		J → Call H.O. T > 101.5				
		BP > 180/100 or				
		< 80/60				
		, MD				

PHARMACY COPY

FIGURE D.10

FIGURE D.1

A. Diagnosis-condition: fracture of the right wrist.

B. Capoten, 12.5 mg orally twice a day.

C. Colace, 100 mg. orally every day.

D. Hydrochlorothiazide, 50 mg orally every day.

E. Clonidine-1 patch, one patch per week.

F. Tylenol with codeine (number 3 refers to 30 mg of codeine in this product), one tablet orally every 4 to 6 hours as needed.

G. Heparin, 5,000 units every 12 hours subcutaneously.

H. Intravenous fluids, dextrose 5% in $\frac{1}{2}$ normal saline, keep vein open.

I. Scrub wrist with povidone-iodine scrub.

J. Diazepam, 10 mg intravenously.

FIGURE D.2

A. Nitroglycerin sublingual $\frac{1}{150}$ grain, one now and may repeat every 5 minutes for three doses.

B. Maalox 30 cc., alternate with Amphogel 30 cc. every 2 hours while awake.

C. Isosorbide long acting 40 mg, one orally every 8 hours.

D. Verapamil sustained-release 240 mg, $\frac{1}{2}$ tablet every day (orally).

E. Zantac, 150 mg orally every 12 hours.

F. Lubriderm at bedside, use as needed.

G. Acetaminophen, two tablets orally every 4 hours as needed for headache (or one suppository [strength = 650 mg]).

H. Halcion, 0.25 mg orally every bedtime if needed.

I. Baby aspirin, one tablet orally every day.

J. Lactulose, 15 cc. (tablespoonful) orally every day.

FIGURE D.3

A. Diagnosis: upper gastrointestinal bleeding.

B. Allergy or sensitivity: ibuprofen, diflunisal, penicillin.

C. Diet: clear liquid diet tonight, nothing by mouth after midnight.

D. Maalox, 30 cc. orally every 4 hours.

E. Zantac, 50 mg intravenously every 8 hours.

F. Folic acid, 1 mg orally every day.

G. Potassium chloride, 20 milliequivalents in orange juice every day for 2 days.

H. Call house officer if systolic blood pressure is less than 100 or greater than 180, heart rate less than 60 or greater than 100.

I. Intravenous fluids, $\frac{1}{2}$ normal saline to run at 100 cc. per hour for 3 liters.

J. Vitamin K, 10 mg intramuscularly every day for three days.

FIGURE D.4

A. Intravenous fluids: dextrose 5% in 1/2 normal saline with 20 milliequivalents of potassium chloride to run at 100 milliliters per hour.

B. Ampicillin, 500 mg intravenously every 6 hours.

C. Gentamicin, 80 mg intravenously every 8 hours.

D. Percocet, one or two tablets orally every 4 hours as needed.

E. (or Demerol 50 mg and Vistaril 50 mg intramuscularly every 4 hours as needed).

F. Lasix, 20 mg intravenously now.

G. Captopril, 25 mg orally twice a day.

H. Hydrochlorothiazide, 25 mg orally every morning.

I. Trental, 400 mg orally twice a day.

J. Halcion, 0.25 mg orally every bedtime as needed.

FIGURE D.5

A. Activities: up as desired.

B. Intravenous fluids: dextgrose 5% in 1/2 normal saline with 10 milliequivalents per liter for 3 liters. (*Note:* The order does not specify the drug to be used that will supply 10 mEq. You know the drug must be potassium chloride. However, you *do not* assume the physician wants potassium chloride. Call the physician and be sure to secure a Physician's Order rewritten by the physician for the appropriate drug order.)

C. Cefuroxime 0.75 Gm intravenously every 8 hours. The first dose is to be given immediately.

D. Alupent inhaler, two puffs every 6 hours.

E. Tonight: arterial blood gases.

F. 40 milliequivalents of potassium chloride is to be returned to stock.

G. 10 milliequivalents of potassium chloride (in 100 cc. of normal saline for four runs, each to run for 1 hour).

H. Take temperature rectally. Acetaminophen, two tablets (650 mg total strength) for temperature greater than 101.5 degrees.

I. Halcion, 0.125 mg orally now. Verbal order by phycian.

J. Start gentamicin, 55 mg every 8 hours.

FIGURE D.6

A. Allergy or sensitivity: no known drug allergies.

B. Diagnosis: arteriosclerotic cardiovascular disease.

C. Activities: out of bed with assistance.

D. Oxygen, 2 liters per minute via nasal cannula.

E. Digoxin, 0.25 mg orally every morning.

F. Kondremul, 15 cc. (1 tablespoonful) orally every bedtime on Monday, Wednesday, and Friday.

G. Tylenol, two tablets every 4 hours as needed.

H. Digoxin level in the morning.

I. Xanax, 0.25 mg every bedtime as needed. Orally.

J. Discontinue Xanax. Give flurazepam 15 mg every bedtime as needed. Verbal order by physician.

FIGURE D.7

A. Allergy or sensitivity: aspirin.

B. Diagnosis: chest pain, congestive heart failure.

C. Digoxin, 0.25 mg intravenously every 6 hours for two doses, then digoxin, 0.25 mg orally every morning.

D. Demerol, 25 mg intramuscularly with hydroxyzine, 25 mg intramuscularly every 6 hours as needed.

E. Heparin, 5,000 units subcutaneously every 12 hours.

F. Thiamine, 100 mg intramuscularly tonight and every day for 3 days.

G. Magnesium sulfate, 1 gram intramuscularly into each buttock.

H. Intravenous fluids: dextrose 5% in normal saline (normal saline = 0.9% sodium chloride solution) with 30 milliequivalents of potassium chloride to run at 250 cc. per hour for 2 liters, then decrease rate to 125 cc. per hour.

I. Add 1 ampoule of multivitamin infusion and 1 mg of folic acid to bottle number two (i.e. the second liter bottle).

J. Perform an electrocardiogram every morning for 3 days.

FIGURE D.8

A. Allergy or sensitivity: penicillin.

B. Lasix, 40 mg orally twice a day.

C. Aminophylline, 500 mg in 500 cc. of normal saline to run at 40 cc. per hour.

D. Nitroglycerin patch, 100 square centimeters, apply one every day.

E. Tolazamide, 250 mg orally every day.

F. Slow-K, two tablets every morning.

G. Alupent nebulizers, 0.3 cc. per 3 cc. of normal saline every 4 hours.

H. Ampicillin, 250 mg orally three times a day.

I. Laboratory to do an aminophylline blood level tonight and in the morning.

J. Call the house officer for temperature greater than 100.5 degrees, systolic blood pressure greater than 200, or diastolic blood pressure less than 60.

FIGURE D.9

A. Phenytoin, 100 mg every 8 hours.

B. Potassium chloride, 25 milliequivalents orally now, then every day.

C. Thiamine, 100 mg orally every day.

D. Folic acid, 1 mg every morning.

E. Multiple vitamin, one orally every day. (The oral indication, p.o., indicates that the vitamin is not an infusion.)

F. Intravenous fluids: dextrose 5% in normal saline to run at 75 cc. per hour for 2 liters.

G. Verbal order by physician.

H. 1 gram of magnesium sulfate in each buttock one time.

I. Triazolam, 0.125 mg every bedtime as needed for sleep.

J. Call the house officer if the patient has shortness of breath or seizing.

FIGURE D.10

A. Allergy or sensitivity: none.

B. Vital signs: every 4 hours for two times, then every shift.

C. Dextrose 5% in $\frac{1}{2}$ normal saline with 20 milliequivalents of potassium chloride per liter to run at 100 cc. per hour.

D. Discontinue the intravenous fluids when the patient is able to take drugs, food, and liquids by mouth well.

E. Meperidine, 50 mg intramuscularly every 3 hours as needed for pain.

F. Vistaril, 25 mg intramuscularly every 3 hours as needed for pain.

G. Halcion, 0.25 mg orally every bedtime as needed.

H. Laxative of choice as needed.

I. Cefazolin, 1 gram intravenously in the recovery room

J. Call the house officer if the temperature is greater than 101.5 degrees, the blood pressure is greater than 180/100 or less than 80/60.

Index

A

A-200, 350
Abbreviations, 121
  drugs (table), 14–15
  hospital (table), 15–19
  intravenous admixture programs (table), 140
  medical orders (table), 12–13
Absorption, 184
ACE inhibitors, 214, 221
Acetaminophen, 12, 172, 174, 176, 181, 192, 227, 252–253, 347, 348, 349, 350
Acetaminophen and codeine combination, 157
Acetaminophen with codeine, 253–254
Acetohexamide, 188
Acetylsalicylic acid, 259
Acne, 347
Acronyms for drug profiles, 252
Action, 208
Activan, 316
Acyclovir, 170, 305–306
Adalat, 289–290
Additive (ad), 133
Administration sets, 140
Admixtures, 133
  programs, abbreviations in (table), 140
Adrenal glands, 185
Adrenalin, 186
Adrenocorticosteroids, 236
Adrenocorticotropic hormone (ACTH), 188
Adriamycin, 184
Adsorbents, 229
Advil, 349, 350
Afferent nerve cells, 177
Afrin, 351
Air (as detriment to patient), 149
Albuterol, 114, 254–255
Aleve, 349, 350
Alginic acid, 184
Alka-Mints, 349
Alka-Seltzer Gold, 350
Alkylamine derivatives, 230
Alkylating agents, 232
Alkysulfonates, 232
Allergy, 347
Allopurinol, 172, 255
Alpha- and beta-adrenergic blocker, 239
Alpha-glucosidase inhibitor, 245
Alprazolam, 255–256
Aluminum hydroxide, 184, 225, 349
Alveolar ducts, 181
Alveolar sacs, 181
AMA Drug Evaluations, 40
Ambulatory patients, 3
Ambulatory pharmacy, 206
Americaine, 350
American Drug Index, 152
American Hospital Formulary Service Drug Information, 40, 152
American Medical Association (AMA), 151
American Medical Association (AMA) Drug Evaluations, 152
Amino acids, 133, 134, 148
Aminoglycosides, 184, 230
Aminophylline, 181
Amitriptyline, 306–307
Amlodipine, 256–257
Amoxicillan/clavulanic acid, 258
Amoxicillin, 43, 181, 190, 191, 225, 257–258
Amoxil, 257–258
Amphetamine, 176
Amphetamine agents, 251
Amphotericin B, 170, 176
Ampicillin, 43, 118, 119, 176, 181, 184, 190, 191
Anabolism, 184
Anacin, 349
Analgesics, 9, 117, 172, 174, 176, 181, 184, 192, 211, 219, 224, 227, 248, 347, 348
Anaprox, 288–289
Anatomy, 129
Anbesol, 348
Androgens, 188, 236
Anesthetic drugs, 128, 183, 192, 244
Angina pectoris, 209–210
Angiotensin-Converting Enzyme (ACE), 239
Anhydrous cholestyramine, 157
Antacids, 184, 225
Anti-infective agents, 117, 244, 248–249
Anti-inflammatory drugs (agents), 9, 45, 117, 132, 244, 248, 249
Antiacne agents, 250
Antianemic agents, 246
Antianginals, 234
Antianxiety agents, 219, 221
Antiarrhythmic agents, 179, 234
Antiarthritic agents, 229
Antibacterial, 230, 251
Antibiotic, 57, 81, 117, 127, 128, 170, 172, 176, 179, 181, 190, 191, 213
  reconstituted liquid, 116
Anticholinergic agents, 247
Anticholinergics, 174, 233
Anticoagulants, 117, 179, 212, 223, 246
Anticonvulsants, 174, 176
Antidepressants, 9, 215, 237–238
Antidiabetic agents, 188, 237
Antidiarrheal agents, 183, 217, 219
Antidiuretic hormone (ADH), 189
Antidopaminergic derivatives, 246

Antiemetics, 176, 183, 219, 224
Antiflatulence medications, 183, 349
Antifungals, 117, 170, 176, 184, 192, 231, 249, 250, 349
Antiglaucoma, 244
Antigout drugs, 211
Antihistamine derivatives, 246
Antihistamines, 9, 43, 117, 121, 170, 179, 181, 183, 192, 248, 249, 347, 348
Antihypercalcemic agents, 172
Antihyperlipidemic agents, 212, 222, 223
Antihypertensive agents (hypotensive agents), 179
Antihypertensives, 235
Antilipemics, 235
Antimalarial agents, 211, 243
Antimetabolites, 232
Antimicrobials, 184
Antineoplastic agents, 179, 184, 211
Antineoplastic antibiotics, 233
Antineoplastics, 170
Antiparasitics, 232
AntiParkinson agents, 176
Antiprotozoans, 191, 232
Antipsoriasis agents, 250
Antipyretic drugs, 218, 181, 348
Antiseborrhea agents, 250
Antiseizure agents, 217
Antispasmodic, 183
Antitrichomonal agent, 250
Antitubercular agents, 181, 231
Antitussives, 181
Antiulcer agents, 132, 184
Antiviral/antiherpes agents, 249
Antivirals, 170, 231
Anusol, 350
Anusol-HC, 220
Anxiolytics, 117
Apex, 181
Apnea, 181
Apothecaries' system, 94, 96
  concentration relationships (table), 102
Apothecary conversions (table), 96
Appendicular skeleton, 172
Applied Therapeutics: The Clinical Use of Drugs, 153
Areola, 191, 192
Arterial blood pressure (BP), 178
Arteries, 179
Artherosclerosis, 212
Arthritis, 210–211
Articulations, 172
Ascriptin, 349
Aseptic technique, 125, 136
Aspirin, 45, 172, 174, 176, 181, 192, 227, 259, 349
Asthma, 211–212
Atenolol, 305
Atrophy, 174
Atropine, 174, 219
Atropine sulfate, 183
Atrovent, 314–315
Attapulgite, 349
Attire, IV personnel, 147
Augmentin, 258
Aurothioglucose, 172
Automatic stop order (ASO), 11
Autonomic nervous system (ANS), 175
Auxiliary labeling
  general information labels, 116
  hospital strip labels, 118
  instructional labels, 116–117
  route of administration, 118
  warning labels, 117–118
Aventyl, 320
Avoirdupois measure, 94, 95
Axial skeleton, 172
Axid, 290–291
Axid AR, 350
Axons, 177
Azathioprine, 172, 259–260

B

Baciguent, 349
Bacitracin, 170, 349
Bacitracin-neomycin, 349
Bacitracin-polymyxin, 349
Bacterial derivatives, 229, 231
Bactrim, 325
Barbiturate derivatives, 242
Basal metabolic rate (BMR), 184
Base, 181
Basic Skills in Interpreting Laboratory Data, 153
Bayer, 349
Benadryl, 350
Benoxyl 5, 347
Benzedrex, 351
Benzocaine, 348, 350, 351
Benzodiazepine derivatives, 243
Benzodiazepines, 238
Benzoyl peroxide, 347
Beta-adrenergic blockers, 239
Beta-blockers, 214, 221, 223
Beta-blocking agents, 179, 210
Beta-lactam antibiotics, 45, 230–231
Betamethasone, 157
Bethanechol chloride, 184
Biaxin, 266
Biguanides, 245
Billing parties, 123, 151
Bisacodyl, 183, 348
Bismuth subsalicylate, 225
Bleomycin, 179
Blistex, 348
Blood, 178
Blumgarten, A. S., Dr., 95
Body water content, 131
Bonine, 350
Bottle techs, 127
Brand/trade name, 208
Breathing, 181
Bromocriptine, 186
Brompheniramine, 170, 181
Bronchi, 181
Bronchial tree, 181
Bronchioles, 181
Bronchodilators, 181, 211, 213

C

Calan, 303–304
Calciferol, 188
Calcitonin, 172, 186
Calcium, 172
Calcium carbonate, 186, 225, 348, 349

Calcium channel blockers, 210, 214, 223
Calcium chloride, 186
Calcium gluconate, 186
Calcium lactate, 186
Calcium supplements, 348
Calories, 184
Cancer Chemotherapy Handbook, 153
Cankaid, 348
Canker sores, 348
Caphalexin, 263–264
Capillaries, 179
Capoten, 260–261
Captopril, 260–261
Carbamazepine, 176
Carbamide peroxide, 348
Carbenicillin, 176
Carbidopa, 176
Carbohydrates, 182
Carbon dioxide, 180
Carbonic anhydrase inhibitors, 235–236
Cardiac agents, 179
Cardiology, 177
Cardiovascular/circulatory system
  components, 177
  disorders, associated, 178
  drug classes/drugs, 179
  function/responsibility, 177
  information about, 177–178
  terms and definitions, 179–180
Cardizem, 271–272
Carisoprodol, 307
Cartilage, 172
Casanthranol, 348
Cascara sagrada, 183, 348
Catabolism, 184
Catapres, 309
Catapres-TTS, 309
Catheters, 139
CBC (complete blood count), 179
Ceclor, 261–262
Cefaclor, 43, 261–262
Cefadroxil, 308
Cefprozil, 262
Ceftin, 263
Cefuroxime, 263
Cefzil, 262
Cell membrane, 168
Cell-stimulating agent, 250
Cells, 168
Celsius, 101–102
Centi-, 97
Central nervous system drugs, 118
Central nervous system (CNS), 175
Central processing unit (CPU), 150
Centrally acting agents, 248
Cepacol, 351
Cepastat, 351
Cephalosporins, 172, 230
Cephamycin, 231
Cerumenolytic, 249
Cervix, 192
Cetirizine, 301–302
Cetylpyridinum, 351
Chapped lips, 348
Chapstick, 348
Chelating agents, 172, 211
Chemo dispensing pin, 139
Chemotherapeutic agents, 137, 147, 186
Chemotherapy, 121, 132
  sleeves, 147
Chenodeoxycholic acid, 184
Child-resistant containers, 157
Chlor-trimeton (CT), 41
Chloral hydrate, 6
Chlorambucil, 179, 192
Chloramphenicol, 176
Chloraseptic, 351
Chlordiazepoxide, 217
Chlorpheniramine, 170, 181, 347, 348
Chlorpromazine, 176
Chlorpropamide, 188
Cholinergic agents, 184
Cholinergic drugs, 174
Cholinesterase reactivators, 174
Chronic obstructive pulmonary disease, 212–213
Chronotherapy, 115
Cimetidine, 184, 264–265, 349
Cipro, 265–266
Ciprofloxacin, 117, 170, 265–266
Circulatory system, 130
Circumcision, 190
Citrate of magnesia, 183
Clarithromycin, 225, 266
Claritin, 285
Clean room, 125, 147
Clemastine, 347
Cleocin, 308–309
Clindamycin, 170, 184, 308–309
Clomiphene, 186, 192
Clonazepam, 266–267
Clonidine, 179, 309
Clorazepate, 310
Clordiazepoxide, 170
Clotrimazole, 170, 184, 349
Codeine, 6, 157, 172, 176, 181, 192, 227
Coding and Reimbursement Guide for Pharmacists, 153
Colace, 348
Colchicine, 172, 267–268
Cold, 348
Colestipol, 157
Collagen diseases, 243
Collyrium, 349
Communication, 153–156
Compendium of drug therapy, 40
Components of words, 56
Compounders, 150
Compounding, 125, 137
  general procedures, 126–127
  intravenous, 127–133
    mixing, rules for proper, 136–146
    nutritional support, 135–136
    therapy, selection of, 133–135
Computilization, 149–150
  pharmacy needs, specialized, 150–151
Concentration relationships
  in the apothecary system (table), 102
  in the metric system (table), 101
Concentration (strength), 126
Congestive heart failure, 213–214
Conjugated estrogens, 186, 192, 268–269
Connector nerve cells (interneurons), 177
Connectors, 140

Conn's Current Therapy, 153
Constipation, 214, 348
Container selection, 118–119
Containers, 139
Continuous quality improvement (CQI), 152
Contraceptive preparations, 157
Controlled drug substances, 6, 8, 123, 159
  schedules of, 157
Controlled drugs, 6
Controlled Substances Act (CSA), 156
  Section 290.05, 118
Controlled substances (CDS), 6
Conversions, 99
  apothecary (table), 96
  of measures (table), 99
  pharmacy (table), 95
Corticosteroids, 117, 241
Cortisol, 184
Cortisone, 128, 186, 220
Cotazyme, 184
Cough suppressant, 348
Coumadin, 304
Cowper's glands, 190
Cranium, 172
Crepitation, 172
Critical areas, 149
Cromolyn, 211
Cruex, 349
Crush fractures, 173
Cubic centimeter, 98
Cuprimine, 294
Cutaneous layers (figure), 129
Cuts, 349
Cyanocobalamine, 179
Cyanotic, 170
Cyclizine, 350
Cyclobenzaprine, 310–311
Cyclophosphamide, 172, 174, 179, 192, 269
Cytarabine, 184
Cytochrome P-450 enzyme system, 193
Cytology, 168
Cytoplasm, 168
Cytotoxic chemotherapeutic agents, 192
Cytotoxic drugs, 146
Cytotoxic materials, 147
Cytoxan, 269

D

Darvocet-N, 298–299
Data, 150
Databases, 151
Debridement agents, 250
Deci-, 97
Decimals, 82–85
Decongestant, 249
Defecation, 184
Deltasone, 321–322
Dendrites, 177
Depen, 294
Depigmenting agents, 250
Depo-Provera, 286–287
Depression, 214–215
Dermatology, 169–170
Dermis, 170
Desenex, 349
Desoxycorticosterone, 186
Desquamation, 170
Destroamphetamine, 176
Desyrel, 324–325
Dexamethasone, 176, 179
Dextromethorphan, 181, 348
Dextrose, 98, 133, 134, 135, 136
Dextrose and electrolyte solutions, 134
Diabeta, 278–279
Diabetes mellitus, 215–216
Diagnostic agents, 244–245
Diagnostic suffixes, 56
Diarrhea, 216–217, 349
Diastolic reading, 178
Diazepam, 6, 170, 172, 174, 176, 192, 217, 311–312
Diazide, 302–303
Dibucaine, 192, 220, 350
Diclofenac sodium, 270
Diethylstilbesterol, 186
Differential white count, 179
Diffusion, 169
Diflucan, 275–276
Digestion, 184
Digestive system
  components, 182
  disorders, associated, 183
  drug classes/drugs, 183–184
  function/responsibility, 182
  information about, 182
  terms and definitions, 184–185
Digitalis, 179
Digitoxin, 179
Digoxin (dig), 41, 179, 270–271
Dihydrotachysterol (vitamin D), 188
Dihydroxycholecalciferol, 188
Dilacor, 271–272
Dilantin, 295–296
Diltiazem, 271–272
Dimenhydrinate, 176, 183, 350
Diphenhydramine (DPH), 121, 170, 179, 181, 192, 347, 350
Diphenoxylate, 219
Diphenoxylate/atropine, 217
Diphenoxylate with atropine, 183
Diphenylheptane derivatives, 229
Diphenylhydantoin, 121
Directions, clarity of, 8–9
Disaccharide, 234
Discs (skeletal), 171
Disease states and drug associations, 206
  condition-format explanation, 207–208
  drug-format explanations, examples, 208–225
Disk operating system (DOS), 150
Dispensing, 114, 115
Dispensing systems, 38
Distributive process, 112
  distribution begins, 115
    auxiliary labeling, 116–118
    container selection, 118–119
    final review, 119–120
  drug delivery process
    drug distribution, 114–115
    drug transferal, 113
  handling the unexpected, 122
  information knowledge, importance of, 123
  patient monitoring, 122
    patient profiling, 123
  safe medication practices
    high-risk drugs, 121–122

refills, 120–121
storage of medications, 121
unexpected, handling the, 122
Diuretics, 179, 184, 186, 192, 214, 221
Doctor, 3
Docusate, 214, 220
Docusate sodium, 183, 348
Donnagel, 349
Dopamine, 179
Dopamine-elevating drugs, 248
Dopamine-releasing drug, 248
Dorland, Gould, or Stedman's Medical Dictionary, 153
Dosage form, 11
Dosage limits, 42–43
Dosage range, 208
Doxorubicin, 179, 186, 192
Doxycycline, 312
Doxylamine, 350
Drachm vial, 118
Dramamine, 350
Dristan, 351
Drug abbreviations (table), 14–15
Drug and/or food interactions, 43
Drug class, 42
Drug classes, 208
Drug classes and representative drugs, 227–228
analgesic, 228–229
anti-infective, 230–232
anti-inflammatory, 240
antiarthritic, 243
anticonvulsant, 242–243
antidiarrheal, 229
antigout, 240
antihistamine, 229–230
antinauseant/antiemetic, 245–246
antineoplastic, 232–233
antiobesity, 251
antiParkinson, 247–248
antispasmodic, 247
antitussive, 248
antiulcer, 233–234
blood modifier, 246–247
bronchodilator, 241–242
cardiovascular, 234–235
dermatologic, 249–250
diuretic, 235–236
drug monographs, 305–325
hormone, 236–237
hypoglycemic, 245
hypotensive, 239
laxative, 237
muscle relaxant, 240–241
opthalmic, 244–245
otic, 248–249
pharmacotherapies, common, 251–304
psychotherapeutic, 237–239
supplement, 242
vaginal, 250–251
Drug delivery process
See Distributive process
Drug delivery systems, 38
Drug distribution, 114–115
Drug effect on existing disorders, 43
Drug Enforcement Administration (DEA), 6, 8
Drug/food interactions, 209
Drug formulary, 11
Drug Information Handbook for the Allied Health Profession, 99, 152
Drug Interaction Facts, 153
Drug interference on lab tests, 43–44
Drug monograph
pharmacy practice, status of, 38
pharmacy technicians, 38
changing roles, 39
competencies required, 39–40
confidence builds on competence, 40
patient's responsibilities, 39
patient's rights of expectations, 39
references, 40
reviewing, 40
format (12 points), 41–45
side effects, when significant, 45–48
significant groupings, 46–48
signs, symptoms, and side effects, 45
Drug order, 3, 114
pharmaceutical notations, 12–19
drug abbreviations (table), 14–15
hospital abbreviations, 15–19
medical order abbreviations (table), 12–13
medical order symbols (table), 13
Physician's Order, 10
elements, 11–12
(figure), 5
script
elements, 4, 6–7
prescription label, 9–10
problem areas, 7–9
Drug profiles, acronyms for, 252
Drug review, 119
Drug review format (12 points), 41–45
Drug transferal, 113
Drugs
light-sensitive, 116
multiple uses of (table), 42
popularly prescribed (table), 44
Drugs in Pregnancy and Lactation, 153
Dry skin, 349
Ducts, 185
Dulcolax, 348
Duodenum, 184
Durable medical equipment (DME), 114
Duricef, 308
Dyspnea, 181

E

Edema, 179
Effectors, 175
Efferent nerve cells, 177
Ejaculation, 190
Elavil, 306–307
Electrolyte replacements, 179, 186, 217
Electrolytes (lytes), 130–135, 133, 184, 224, 242
Electronic mail, 151
Electronic technology (electech), 150
Embolus, 179
Enalapril, 272–273
Endocrine glands, 185
Endocrine system
components, 185
disorders, associated, 186
drug classes/drugs, 186, 188
function/responsibility, 185, 187–188
information about, 185–186
terms and definitions, 188–189

Endocrinology, 185
Endometrium, 192
Enteral pumps, 38
Enzymes, 233
Ephedrine, 176, 181
Epidermis, 171
Epilepsy, 217–218
Epinephrine, 128, 179, 181, 186
Equilibrium, 169
Equipment for compounding, 126
Erythromycin, 170, 172, 179, 181
Erythromycin ethylsuccinate, 157
Erythropoiesis, 173, 179
Esidrix, 314
Esophagus, 184
Estrogen, 158, 172
Estrogen-progestin combinations, 192
Estrogens, 236
Ethacrynic acid, 186
Ethambutol, 181
Ethanolamine derivatives, 229
Ethinyl estradio, 192
Ethinyl estradiol/levonorgestrel, 273
Ethinyl estradiol/norethindrone, 273–274
Ethinylestradiol, 186
Ethionamide, 181
Ethylenediamine derivatives, 229
Ethylenimines, 232
Etodolac, 312–313
Etoposide, 170
Excedrin IB, 349
Exocrine glands, 185
Expectorants, 213, 348
Extemporaneous, 125
Exterorecptors, 175
Extracellular, 131–132
Eye irritation, 349

F

Facsimiles (fax), 151
Facts and Comparisons, 152
Fahrenheit, 101–102
Fallopian tubes, 192
Famotidine, 274–275, 349
Fat emulsions, 134, 135, 136
Fats, 133, 182
FDA Pregnancy Category X, 118
Feces, 184
Federal Food, Drug, and Cosmetic Act (FDCA), 156
Feed and breed, 175
Female reproductive system
  components, 190–191
  disorders, associated, 191
  drug classes/drugs, 191–192
  function/responsibility, 191
  information about, 191
  terms and definitions, 192
Fenoprofen, 172, 174
Ferrous gluconate, 179
Ferrous sulfate, 179
Fertility drugs, 186, 192
Fertilization, 192
Festal, 184
Fever, 218
Fibrinogen, 182
Filters, 139, 148
Filtration, 168–169
First Data Book, 152
5-fluorouracil, 184, 192
Flatulence, 349
Flexeril, 310–311
Floor stock, 118
Flora, 182
Fluconazole, 275–276
Fludrocortisone, 186, 236
Fluid/electrolyte therapy, 132
Fluid therapy, 132–135, 134
Fluids, 133
Fluoroquinolones, 231
Fluorouracil, 170
Fluoxetine, 276
Flurazepam, 12
Flush, 170
Folex, 287–288
Folic acid, 179
Folic acid antagonists, 118
Food, 182
Food and Drug Administration (FDA), 151
Fostex 10% Wash, 347
4 Ps, 112
4-Way, 351
Fungus, 349
Furosemide, 179, 184, 186, 277

G

Gallstones, 184
Gantrisn, 190
Gastroenteritis, 218–219
Gastroenterology, 182
Gastrointestinal agents, 225, 247
Gastrointestinal stimulants, 184
Gaviscon, 350
Gemfibrozil, 313
Generic, 208
Generic drug name, 41
Genitalia, 190
Genitourinary, 189
Gentamicin, 176
Gestation, 192
Glands, 189
Glipizide, 188, 277–278
Glitazones, 245
Glucocorticoids, 185, 236
Gluconeogenesis, 189
Glucotrol, 277–278
Gly-Oxide, 348
Glyburide, 188, 278–279
Glycerin, 349
Glycogen, 182
Glycogenolysis, 189
Glynase, 278–279
Goiter, 189
Gold compounds, 172, 211
Gold derivatives, 243
Gold sodium thiomalate, 172, 279–280
Gonadotropins, 236
Grain, 96
Gram, 97, 98
Groupings of side effects, 46–48
Growth hormone (GH), 189

Guaifenesin, 213, 348
Guaifenesin with codeine, 157
Guanethidine, 179
Guide to Parenteral Admixtures, 153
Gustatory, 177
Gynecology, 190

H

H_2-receptor antagonists, 234
Haloperidol, 176
Haloprogin, 170
Handbook of Injectable Drugs, 153
Handbook of Institutional Pharmacy Practice, 152
Handbook of Nonprescription Drugs, 356
Hansten's Drug Interactions, 153
Hardware, 150
Hartmann's solution, 134
Headache, 219, 349
Heart, 177
Heartburn, 349
Heavy-metal antagonists, 243
Helicobactor pylori bacteria, 225
Hematology, 177
Hemoglobin, 179
Hemorrhoids, 219–220, 350
Hemorrheologic agent, 246
Hemostasis, 179
Hemostatic agents, 246
Heparin, 179
Heroin, 157
Hexylresocinols, 351
Hgb, 179
High-efficiency particulate air (HEPA) filter, 148
High-risk drugs, 121–122
Histamine H_2-receptor blockers, 184, 349
Homeopathic Pharmacopoeia of the United States, 156
Homeostasis, 130, 168, 169
Hormones, 172, 185, 186, 189, 192, 233, 245, 251
Hospital abbreviations (table), 15–19
Hospital orders for practice, 457–0
Hospital pharmacy, 206, 357–358
Household measure, 94, 95
Human anatomy and physiology, 167
  anatomical systems
    cardiovascular/circulatory, 177–180
    digestive, 182–185
    endocrine, 185–189
    female reproductive, 190–192
    integumentary system, 169–171
    male reproductive, 189–190
    muscular, 173–174
    nervous, 174–177
    respiratory/pulmonary, 180–181
    skeletal, 171–173
  cells, 168
  physiologic processes, 168–169
Human functioning
  See Human anatomy and physiology
Humulin, 282
Hydantoins, 243
Hydralazine, 179, 214, 221
Hydrochloric acid (HCl), 117, 182
Hydrochlorothiazide (HCTZ), 41, 179, 186, 192, 314
Hydrocodone, 181
Hydrocortisone (HC), 86, 99, 100, 170, 174, 181, 184, 186
Hydrodiuril, 314
Hydromorphone, 176
Hydrophilic drug, 193
Hydroxychloroquine, 280–281
Hydroxyurea, 170
Hydroxyzine, 170
Hymen, 192
Hyperalimentation, 81
Hypertention, 220–221
Hypertonic solution, 133
Hypertrophy, 174
Hypodermic syringes, 149
Hypoglycemic drugs, 117, 216
Hypophysis, 189
Hypotensive agent, 239
Hypoxia, 181

I

Ibuprofen, 43, 172, 174, 192, 281, 347, 349, 350
Ilozyme, 184
Immunosuppresive drugs, 172, 174, 211, 243
Imodium A-D, 349
Imuran, 259–260
Inderal, 322–323
Indications for use, 42, 208
Indolines, 235
Indomethacin, 43, 172, 174
Information knowledge, importance of, 123
Infusion medications, 114
Inotropic drugs, 214, 234
Input, 150
Inscription, 4
Insomnia, 221, 350
Insulin, 116, 127, 184, 186, 189, 216, 282
  syringe, 137
Integumentary system, 56, 129
  components, 169–170
  disorders, associated, 170
  drug classes/drugs, 170
  function/responsibility, 170
  information about, 170
  terms and definitions, 170–171
Interneurons, 177
Interoreceptors, 175
Interstitial, 132
Intestinal lubricants, 237
Intestinal stimulants, 237
Intestines, 182
Intracellular, 131
Intradermal, 171
Intramuscular, 174
Intravenous admixtures, 81, 125, 127, 129
Intravenous antibiotic, 132
Intravenous therapy selection (figure), 132
Inventory review, 119
Iodine, 186
Ipratropium, 114
Ipratroprium, 314–315
Iron preparations, 179
Irrigation solutions, 125
Isoniazid, 181
Isopropyl alcohol, 101, 126
Isoproterenol, 179, 181
Isoptin, 303–304
Isopto-Frin, 349

Isordil, 315
Isosorbide, 214
Isosorbide dinitrate, 116, 157, 315
Isoxsuprine, 179
IV pharmacy environment
  environmental procedures, 149
  IV preparation supplies, 148–149
  laminar airflow hood, 148
  personnel attire, 147
  spill protection, 147–148
IV therapy, anatomy and physiology involved in (table), 131

J

Jargon, 56
Jaundice, 170
Joint Commission on Accreditation of Healthcare, 153
Joint Commission on Accreditation of Healthcare Organizations (JCAHO), 156

K

K-Lyte/CL, 296–297
K-Tab, 296–297
Kanamycin, 176, 191
Kaochlor, 296–297
Kaopectate, 349
Kay Ciel, 296–297
Keflex, 263–264
Keftab, 263–264
Kefurox, 263
Keratin, 171
Keratolytic agent, 250
Ketoconazole, 184
Ketorolac, 282–283
Keyboard, 150
Kidney, 168, 193
Kilo-, 97
Klonopin, 266–267
Knowledge, skills, and abilities (KSAs), 354
Konsyl, 348

L

Labeling, 10, 127
  auxiliary, 116–118
  See also Auxiliary labeling
Lactated Ringer's solution, 134
Lactulose, 183
Laminar airflow hood, 121–122, 125, 126, 136, 148
Lamisil AT, 349
Lanacane, 350
Lanolin, 350
Lanoxin, 270–271
Larotid, 257–258
Larynx, 181
Lasix, 277
Laws, 156–160
Laxatives, 12, 183, 214, 237, 348
Learning, 177
Legend, 156
Legend drug, 156
Lesions, 171
Letter combination sounds and pluralization of medical terms (table), 57
Levarterenol (norepinephrine), 179
Levigating ointments, 126
Levodopa, 176
Levothroid, 283–284
Levothyroxin, 283–284
Levothyroxine, 98, 186
Lice, 350
Lidocaine, 128, 174, 192, 348
Ligament, 173
Light-sensitive drugs, 116
Lincomycin, 172
Liothyronine, 98, 186
Liotrix, 186
Lip Treatment, 348
Lipid disorders, 222
Lipids, 148
Lipophilic drugs, 193
Lisinopril, 284
Liter, 97, 98
Liver, 168, 182, 193, 194
Liver extract, 179
Lodine, 312–313
Loop diuretics, 235
Loperamide, 183, 217, 219, 349
Lopid, 313
Lopressor (tartrate salt), 318
Loratidine, 285
Lorazepam, 170, 316
Lotrimin, 349
Lovastatin, 285–286
Lubricants/artificial tears, 245
Lymphatic system, 130, 178

M

Maalox, 349, 350
Macule, 171
Mag-Ox, 350
Magnesium, 225
Magnesium carbonate, 184, 350
Magnesium citrate, 348
Magnesium hydroxide, 184, 350
Magnesium oxide, 350
Magnesium trisilicate, 184, 350
Male reproductive system
  components, 189
  disorders, associated, 190
  drug classes/drugs, 190
  function/responsibility, 189
  information about, 190
  terms and definitions, 190
Mammary glands, 192
Manual of Medical Therapeutics, 153
Marezine, 350
Marijuana derivatives, 246
Martindale's The Extra Pharmacopoeia, 152
Mastication, 182
Maxzide, 302–303
Measure, systems of, 94–96
  See also Apothecaries' system; Metric system
Mechlorethamine, 179
Meclizine, 176, 350
Medicaid, 123
Medical dictionaries, 40
Medical order abbreviations (table), 12–13
Medical order symbols (table), 13
Medical terms
  components, 56
  letter combinations sounds and pluralization (table), 57

prefixes, 56
prefixes (table), 58
roots, 56
cardiovascular (table), 59
digestive system (table), 59
genito-urinary system (table), 60
integumentary system (table), 60
musculoskeletal system (table), 60
nervous system (table), 61
respiratory system (table), 61
sense organs (table), 61
suffixes, 56
diagnostic (table), 62
operative (table), 62
symptomatic (table), 62
Medicare, 123
Medications, storage of, 121
Medrol, 317
Medroxyprogesterone acetate, 158, 192, 286–287
Meglitinides, 245
Melphalan, 179, 192
Menopause, 191, 192
Menstrual cycle, 191
Menstrual pain, 350
Menstruation, 192
Menthol, 351
Meperidine, 172, 176, 184
Meprobamate, 174, 176
Merck Manual of Diagnosis and Therapy, The, 40
Merck Manual, The, 153
Metabolism, 181, 184
Metaclopramide, 184
Metamucil, 348
Metaproteranol, 114
Metaraminol, 179
Methadone, 176
Methicillin, 172, 179
Methimazole, 186
Methotrexate, 170, 174, 192, 287–288
Methyldopa, 179
Methylphenidate, 176
Methylprednisolone, 157, 317
Methyphenidate, 316–317
Metoclopramide, 183
Metoprolol, 179, 318
Metric system, 94, 95, 97–102
concentration relationships (table), 101
Metrology, 94
Metronidazole, 117, 170, 184, 191, 225
Mevacor, 285–286
Micatin, 349
Miconazole, 170, 349
Microgram, 98, 99
Micronase, 278–279
Midol, 350
Milk of magnesia, 183
Milli-, 97
Milligram, 98
Milliliter, 97, 98
Mineralocorticoids, 185, 236
Minerals, 184, 242
Minim (unit), 96
Minimum Inhibitory Concentration (MIC), 99
Minipress, 297–298
Minocin, 318–319
Minocycline, 318–319
Mitomycin C., 184
Mixing, rules for proper, 136–146
Modane, 348
Monitor (CRT or cathode ray tube), 150
Monoamine oxidase (MAO) inhibitors, 43, 239
Monographs
See Drug monographs
Morphine, 157
Morphogenetic function, 185
Motion sickness, 350
Motrin, 281
Motrin IB, 349, 350
Multiple electrolyte solutions, 134
Murine, 349
Muscle relaxants, 117, 172, 174
Muscle tone, 174
Muscosal strengthening drugs, 225
Muscular system
components, 173
disorders, associated, 173–174
drug classes/drugs, 174
function/responsibility, 173
information about, 173
terms and definitions, 173–174
Mycelex, 349
Mylanta, 349, 350
Mylanta Gas, 349
Myocardial infarction, 222–223
Myochrysine, 279–280
Myology, 173–174

N

Nabumetone, 288
Nadolol, 210, 214, 221, 223
Nafcillin, 172, 179
Naphazoline, 181, 349, 351
Naphcon-A, 349
Naprosyn, 288–289
Naproxen, 172, 174, 192, 288–289
Naproxen sodium, 349, 350
Narcotic analgesics, 176, 228–229
Narcotic medications, 118, 123
Narcotics, 172, 227
Nasal congestion, 351
Nasal decongestant, 348
Nasogastric tube (NGT), 11
National Formulary, 152, 156
National Pharmacy Technician Certification Examination, 435
Natural alkaloids, 247
Natural derivatives, 239, 240
Nausea and vomiting, 223–224
Nebulizer drugs, 114
Needles, 123, 137, 148, 149
Neo-Synephrine, 351
Neomycin, 170
Neosar, 269
Neosporin, 349
Neostigmine, 174
Nerve blocking agents, 172, 174
Nervous system
components, 174
disorders, associated, 176
drug classes/drugs, 176
function/responsibility, 175
information about, 175–176
terms and definitions, 177
Networks, 151

Neurology, 174–177
Neurons, 177
Neurotransmitters, 177
New drug application (NDA), 41
Nifedipine, 289–290
Nitro-Bid, 319–320
Nitro-Dur, 319–320
Nitrogen mustards, 232
Nitroglycerin (TNG or NTG), 41, 82, 97, 118–119, 157, 179, 210, 319–320
Nitroprusside sodium, 119
Nitrostat, 319–320
Nix, 350
Nizatidine, 290–291, 350
Nodule, 171
Nolvadex, 323
Non-narcotic derivatives, 248
Non-sterile formulations, 125
Nonamphetamine agents, 251
Nonpharmaceutical products, 356
Nonsalicylates, 172, 243
Nonsteroidal anti-inflammatory agents (NSAIA), 117, 172, 174, 192, 227, 240
Nonsteroidal anti-inflammatory drugs (NSAID), 211, 227, 229, 243, 347, 350
Nonsteroidal estrogen antagonist, 192
Nonsympathomimetics (xanthines), 241
Noradrenalin, 186
Nordette, 273
Norepinephrine, 179, 186
Norethindrone acetate, 158
Nortriptyline, 320
Norvasc, 256–257
Notable comments, 209
Noteworthy facts, 44
Novolin, 282
Nucleus, 168
Nupercainal, 350
Nuprin, 349, 350
Nutrients, 133
Nutritional agents, 172
Nutritional supplements, 174
Nutritional support, 132, 135–136
Nylidrin, 179
Nystatin, 170, 184, 192
Nytol, 350

O

Occult blood, 185
Ocu Clear, 349
Olfactory, 177
Omeprazole, 116, 225, 291
Omnibus Budget Reconciliation Act of 1990 (OBRA 90), 156, 158
ONCOlink, 151
Ondansetron, 291–292
Opcon-A, 349
Operative suffixes, 56
Ophthalmic, 177
Ophthalmologic preparations, 125
Opiate derivative, 229
Optic, 177
Orabase gel, 348
Orphenadrine, 174
Ortho-Novum 7/7/7 28, 273–274
Oscal, 348
Osmosis, 169
Osmotic diuretics, 235
Ossification, 173, 189
Osteoarthritis, 173
Osteology, 171–173
Osteomalacia, 56
Otic, 177
Otrivin, 351
Output, 150
Ovals, 118
Over-the-counter drugs (list), 347–351
Ovulation, 191, 192
Oxacillin, 172
Oxandrolone, 172
Oxy 10 Wash, 347
Oxymetazoline, 349, 351
Oxytocin, 189

P

Paclitaxel, 292–293
Pain, 224
Pallor, 170
Pamabron, 350
Pamelor, 320
Pamprin, 350
Pancreas, 186
Pancreatic supplements, 184
Pancrelipase preparations, 157
Papaverine, 179
Papule, 171
Para-aminophenol, 227, 228
Parasympathetic nervous system, 175
Parchment papers, 126
Paregoric, 183
Parenteral drug routes (table), 131
Parenteral feeding, 135
Parenteral hyperalimentation, 135
Parenteral nutrition, 132, 148
  total, elements (figure), 136
Parenteral nutrition formulas, 114
Parenteral pumps, 38
Parenteral therapy, 127–136
  (figure), 128
Paroxetine, 293
Partial parenteral nutrition (PPN), 135
Patent holders, 41–42
Pathogenic bacteria, 57, 117, 125
Patient monitoring, 122–123
Patient profiling, 123
Patient review, 119
Paxil, 293
Pazo, 350
Pediculicide agents, 250
Pen Vee K, 41, 294–295
Penicillamine, 172, 294
Penicillin, 43, 45, 117, 121, 170, 172, 179, 181, 190, 191
  injectable intramuscular suspensions, 128
Penicillin G, 176
Penicillin VK, 294–295
Penis, 190
Pentazocine, 184, 192
Pentids, 41
Pentoxifylline, 321
Pepcid, 274–275
Pepcid AC, 349

Percentage, 86–88, 137
Peripheral nervous system (PNS), 175
Peripherally acting agents, 248
Peristalsis, 185
Permeability of a cell, 168
Permethrin, 350
Perphenazine, 176
Petrolatum, 349, 350
Pharmaceutical Calculations, 153
Pharmaceutical notations, 12–19
  drug abbreviations (table), 14–15
  hospital abbreviations (table), 15–19
  medical order abbreviations (table), 12–13
  medical order symbols (table), 13
Pharmaceutical products, 355–356
Pharmaceutically elegant, 38, 119
Pharmacodynamics, 192
Pharmacokinetics, 167, 192–194
Pharmacologic Basics of Therapeutics, The, 152
Pharmacologic treatment (drug-format explanation examples), 208–225
Pharmacology, 192
Pharmacy calculations, 81
  apothecaries' system, 96
  decimals, 82–85
  metric system, 97–102
  percentage, 86–88
  ratio and proportion, 92–93
  systems of measure, 94–96
Pharmacy conversions (table), 95
Pharmacy environments
  hospital pharmacy, 357–358
  overview, 354–355
  retail pharmacy, 355–357
Pharmacy equivalents (table), 96
Pharmacy manufacturing log, 126
Pharmacy practice, status of, 38
Pharmacy rules, 156
Pharmacy skills (special)
  communication, 153–156
  compounding, 125
  "computilization", 149–150
    pharmacy needs, specialized, 150–151
  general compounding procedures, 126
    following the preparation, 127
  intravenous compounding, 127–133
    mixing, rules for proper, 136–146
    nutritional support, 135–136
    therapy, selection of, 133–135
  IV pharmacy environment
    environmental procedures, 149
    IV preparation supplies, 148–149
    laminar airflow hood, 148
    personnel attire, 147
    spill protection, 147–148
  law, 156–160
  reference sources, 151–153
Pharmacy symbols (table), 96
Pharmacy Technician COACH—real pharmacy orders examples, 360–411
Pharmacy technicians
  changing roles, 39
  competencies required, 39–40
  confidence builds on competence, 40
  patient's responsibilities, 39
  patient's rights of expectations, 39
  professional appearance and demeanor, 436
  references, 40
  role of, 38
Pharynx, 181, 185
Phazyme, 349
Phenanthrene derivatives, 228
Phenazopyridine, 116
Phenobarbital, 82, 157, 176, 183, 192
Phenol, 351
Phenolphthalein, 183, 348
Phenothaizine derivative, 248
Phenothiazine derivatives, 230
Phenothiazines, 238
Phenylbutazone, 172, 174
Phenylephrine, 86, 181, 349, 351
Phenylpiperidine derivatives, 228
Phenytoin, 174, 176, 295–296
Phillips' Milk of Magnesia, 350
Physician, 3
Physician's Desk Reference for Nonprescription Drugs, 356
Physicians' Desk Reference (PDR), 40, 99, 152
Physician's Order, 3, 10
  elements, 11–12
  (figure), 5
Physiology
  See Human anatomy and physiology
Phytonadione, 179
Piloerection, 189
Piperazine derivatives, 230
Piperidine derivatives, 229
Piperonyl butoxide, 350
Pituitary, 236
Place values, 85
Placenta, 192
Plaquenil, 280–281
Plasma, 132, 178
Platelets, 178, 179
Podophyllotoxin derivative, 232
Poison Prevention Packaging Act (PPPA), 156, 157–158
Poisons, 123
Polymox, 257–258
Polysporin, 349
Portals, 148
Posology, 94
Postganglionic adrenergic blockers, 239
Potassium chloride (KCl), 134, 179, 296–297
Potassium iodide (KI), 86
Potassium (K), 98, 174, 179
Potassium-sparing diuretic, 235
Potassium supplements, 157
Practice Standards of the American Society of Health-Systems Pharmacists, 153
Pralidoxime, 174
Pramoxine, 350
Pravachol, 297
Pravastatin, 297
Prazosin, 297–298
Predisone, 157, 170, 174, 176, 179, 181, 184, 186, 192, 211, 321–322
Prefixes of medical terms, 56
  metric system, 97
Prefixes of medical terms (table), 58
Prefrin, 349
Premarin, 268–269
Premsyn PMS, 350

Preparation, following the, 127
Preparation H, 350
Prescription, 114
  examples for practice, 437–456
Prescription label, 9–10
Prilosec, 291
Primidone, 176
Prinvil, 284
PRN (*Pro Re Nata*), 11–12
Probenecid, 172
Procainamide, 179
Procaine, 172, 174
Procarbazine, 179
Procardia, 289–290
Prochlorperazine (phenothiazine), 183, 219, 224
Product selection, 115
Product waste, 137
Progestins, 236
Promethazine rectal suppositories, 116
Proportion and ratio, 92–93, 137
Propoxyphene, 12, 172, 176
Propoxyphene napsylate/acetaminophen, 298–299
Propranolol, 179, 210, 214, 221, 223, 322–323
Propriorecptors, 175
Propylthiouracil (PTU), 186
Proteins, 182
Prothrombin, 182
Proton pump inhibitors, 234
Proventil, 254–255
Provera, 286–287
Prozac, 276
Pseudoephedrine, 92, 181, 348
Psyllium hydrophilic fiber, 348
Psyllium hydrophilic mucilloid, 183
Pulmonary, 180
Pulmonary circuit, 177–178
Pump infusions, 139
Purchasing, 151
Purine antagonists, 232
Pustule, 171
Pyrazinamide, 181
Pyridostigmine, 174
Pyridoxine, 179
Pyrimidine antagonists, 232

Q

Quinidine, 179
Quinine, 174

R

Ranitidine, 184, 299–300, 350
Ranitidine bismuth citrate, 225
Ratio and proportion, 92–93, 137
RBC (red blood cell), 179
Receptors, 175
Record review, 119–120
Red Book, 152
Reference sources, 151–153
Refills, handling, 120–121
Regulating action, 132
Relafen, 288
Remington's Pharmaceutical Sciences, 152
Repigmenting agents, 250
Representative drug trade name(s), 41–42
Reserpine, 179
Respiration, 181
Respiratory inhalation products, 211
Respiratory/pulmonary system
  components, 180
  disorders, associated, 180–181
  drug classes/drugs, 181
  function/responsibility, 180
  information about, 180
  terms and definitions, 181
Restoril, 323–324
Retail pharmacy, 355–357
Review of distribution process, 119–120
Rheumatrex, 287–288
RID, 350
Rifampin, 181
Rigor mortis, 174
Ringer's solution, 134
Ritalin, 316–317
Robotics, 150
Root portion of medical terms, 56
  cardiovascular (table), 59
  digestive system (table), 59
  genito-urinary system (table), 60
  integumentary system (table), 60
  musculoskeletal system (table), 60
  nervous system (table), 61
  respiratory system (table), 61
  sense organs (table), 61
Rounding off, 84
Rules of similarity for drug classes, 45
Rx, 4

S

Safe medication practices
  See Distributive process
Salicylates, 172, 227, 228
Satient agents, 251
Scabicide agents, 249
Scanners, 150
Schedule, 209
Script, 3
  elements, 4, 6–7
  (figure), 6
  prescription label, 9–10
  problem areas, 7–9
Scrotum, 190
Sebaceous, 171
Secundum artem, 38
Sedatives, 176, 183, 192
Sedatives/hypnotics/anxiolytics, 238
Selective serotonin reuptake inhibitors, 239
Semen, 190
Semisynthetic derivatives, 247
Senna compound, 214, 220
Septra, 325
Sertraline, 300
Serum, 180
Sex hormones, 186, 236
Side effects, 209, 251
  groupings as significant, 46–48
  "how long", 45
  "how much", 45
  "how unbearable", 45
  when significant, 45–48
Signature, 6
Signs, symptoms, and side effects, 45
Simethicone, 183, 349

Simvastatin, 301
Skeletal system
  components, 171
  disorders, associated, 172
  drug classes/drugs, 172
  function/responsibility, 171
  information about, 171–172
  terms and definitions, 172–173
Skin portion of integumentary system, 129
Sleepinal, 350
Sleeping aids, 221
Sodium bicarbonate, 350
Sodium chloride, 133, 135, 169
Sodium chloride (NaCl), 99, 100
Sodium fluoride, 157
Sodium nitroprusside, 116
Solu-Medrol, 317
Solute, 100
Solvent, 100
Soma, 307
Somatic nervous system (SNS), 175
Somatic receptors, 175
Sominex, 350
Sore throat, 351
Spermatic cord, 190
Spermatogenesis, 190
Spermatozoa, 190
Sphygmomanometer, 178
Spill protection, 147–148
Spironolactone, 179, 184
Spleen, 178
Starches, 182
STAT, 118
Stedman's Specialty Word Books, 153
Sterile compounding, 125
Sternum, 173
Steroids, 170, 174, 176, 179, 181, 184, 185, 186, 192, 211, 240, 243
Stimulants, 176, 238
Stomach acid, 182
Stool softeners, 220, 237
Storage of medications, 121
Strength (concentration), 127
Streptomycin, 179, 190, 191
Strip labels, 10, 116
Subcutaneous, 56, 171, 129
  layers (figure), 130
Subscription, 6
Succinate salt, 318
Sucralfate, 184, 225
Sucrets, 351
Suffixes of medical terms, 56
  diagnostic (table), 62
  operative (table), 62
  symptomatic (table), 62
Sugars, 182
Sulfamethoxazole/trimethoprim, 117
Sulfasalazine, 184
Sulfinpyrazone, 172
Sulfonamide derivatives, 240
Sulfonamide diuretics, 236
Sulfonamides, 117, 190, 231
Sulfones, 231
Sulfonylureas, 245
Sulindac, 172, 174
Sunscreen, 250
Suppositories, 116
Suspensions, 116
Symbols
  medical orders (table), 13
Sympathetic nervous system, 175
Sympathomimetic drugs (adrenergics), 241
Sympathomimetics, 179
Symptomatic suffixes, 56
Synapses, 176, 177
Synthetic compounds, 247
Synthetic drugs, 247
Synthroid, 283–284
Syringes, 123, 125, 137, 148
System, 168
Systolic reading, 178

T

Tachycardia, 56
Tacky mats, 147
Tactile, 177
Tagamet, 264–265
Tagamet HB, 349
Tamoxifen, 192, 323
Tartrate salt, 318
Tavist, 347
Taxol, 292–293
Technicians
  See Pharmacy technicians
Telangiectasia, 171
Temazepam, 12, 323–324
Temperature conversions, 101–102
Tendons, 173, 174
Tenets of pharmacy, 112, 120, 122
Tenormin, 305
Terazosin, 221
Terfenidine, 170
Terminology, 56–62
  skeletal system, 172–173
Terms and definitions
  cardiovascular/circulatory system, 179–180
  digestive system, 184–185
  endocrine system, 188–189
  female reproductive system, 192
  integumentary system, 170–171
  male reproductive system, 190
  muscular system, 173–174
  nervous system, 177
  respiratory/pulmonary system, 181
  skeletal system, 172–173
Testosterone, 172, 186, 192
Tetany, 174
Tetracyclic compounds, 238
Tetracycline (TCN), 41, 170, 176, 179, 181, 184, 190, 191, 225, 231
Tetracyclines, 117
Tetrahydrolozine, 349
Textbook of Adverse Drug Reactions, 153
Textbook of Materia Medica and Therapeutics, 95
Theophylline, 181
Therapeutic drug levels, 81
Thiamine, 179
Thiazid diuretics, 235
Thiazide derivative, 239
3-in-1 solution, 148
Thrombolytic agents, 247
Thrombus, 180
Thyroid agents, 98, 186, 236–237
Thyroid extract, 82, 186
Thyroid hormone (thyroxin), 185

Tinactin, 349
Ting, 349
Tissues, 168
Titralac, 349
Tolazamide, 186, 188
Tolazoline, 179
Tolbutamide, 186, 188
Tolfanate, 170, 349
Tolmetin, 172, 174
Topical analgesic/anesthetic agents, 250
Topical anesthetic, 348
Toprol XL (succinate salt), 318
Toradol, 282–283
Total parenteral nutrition (TPN), 135
(figure), 136
Toxic levels, of drugs, 81
Trace elements, 133
Trachea, 181
Tranquilizers, 9, 170, 176, 183, 192, 217
Transfer sets, 148
Transfer spikes, 139
Traxene, 310
Trazodone, 324–325
Trental, 321
Triamcinolone, 170
Triameterne, 179
Triamterene/hydrochlorothiazid, 302–303
Triazolam, 221
Tricyclic compounds, 238
Trimethobenzamide, 219, 224
Trimethoprim/sulfa (co-trimoxazole), 325
Trimethoprim-sulfamethoxazole, 184
Trimox, 257–258
Tripelennamine, 192
Triphasil 28, 273
Tritin, 349
Troy weight, 94
Tuberculin syringe, 137, 149
Tucks, 350
Tums, 348, 349
Turbinafine, 349
Tyenol, 252–253
Tylenol, 349
Tylenol PM, 350
Tylenol with codeine, 253–254

U

Ulcer, 224–225
Undecylanate, 349
Unexpected occurrences, 122
Unisom, 350
United States Pharmacopeia (USP) (1890), 97
United States Pharmacopoeia Dispensing Information (USPDI), 152
United States Pharmacopoeia, 152, 156
Unwanted drug effects, 43
Urea, 349
Urea derivative, 232
Uricosuric agents, 172
Urinary anesthetics, 116
Urinary antiseptics, 231
Urinary drugs, 247

V

V-Cillin K, 41, 294–295
Vagina, 191
Valium, 311–312
Vancomycin, 170
Vaso Clear, 349
Vasoconstrictors, 181, 349
Vasodilators, 179, 214, 221, 235
Vasopressin, 186
Vasopressors, 179
Vasotec, 272–273
Veetids, 41, 294–295
Veins, 180
Venous route, 135–136
Ventolin, 254–255
Verapamil, 303–304
Verelan, 303–304
Vesicle, 171
Vibramycin, 312
Vicks, 351
Vinca alkaloids, 232
Vincristine, 179, 192
Viokase, 184
Visceral receptors, 175
Viscous lidocaine, 183
Visine, 349
Visine L.R., 349
Vitamin B-12 preparations, 179
Vitamin K preparations, 179
Vitamin preparations, 179
Vitamin therapy, 188
Vitamins, 133, 185, 242
Voice mail, 151
Voltaren, 270

W

Warfarin, 304
WBC (white blood cell), 180
Weight to weight (w/w) measurement, 99–100
Wheal, 171
White petrolatum, 348
Windows (Microsoft), 150
Wintergreen oil, 101
Witch hazel, 350
Wycillin, 41

X

Xanax, 255–256
Xanthines, 240
Xylometazoline, 351

Z

Zantac, 299–300
Zantac 75, 350
Zestril, 284
Zilactin-L liquid, 348
Zinacef, 263
Zinc oxide, 350
Zinc undecylanate, 170
Zocor, 301
Zofran, 291–292
Zoloft, 300
Zolpidem, 221
Zovirax, 305–306
Zyloprim, 255
Zyrtec, 301–302